To Bobbi
Here's to
22 years more.

CALIFORNIA
ART THERAPY
TRENDS

CALIFORNIA ART THERAPY TRENDS

Edited by

Evelyn Virshup, Ph.D., ATR

Magnolia Street Publishers — Chicago

© 1993
Published by
MAGNOLIA STREET PUBLISHERS
1250 W. Victoria
Chicago, Illinois 60660

ISBN: 0-9613309-3-7
Library of Congress Catalog Card No. pending
Cover Design: Evelyn Virsup
Printed in the USA

Contents

Art Therapy with families and the Abused

Art Therapy in Hospitals

Art Therapy and —

Old Concepts /New Ways

Introduction

When I first entered the field of art therapy in Los Angeles, there were only a handful of art therapists in California, and not a lot of jobs, either. It seemed amazing to me that so few people knew about or valued this incredibly effective therapeutic modality!

Now, twenty years later, there are almost six hundred members of the American Art Therapy Association in California, practicing up and down our state. Stories about some person, residential treatment center, school or clinic being helped by art appear regularly in the newspapers.

Even more remarkable has been the development of the ways in which art therapy is being used. Initially, being the product of a public school education, I thought there was one way to do art therapy, the way I was taught in school. I soon learned the contrary to my amazement, when one of my supervisors asked me to create an original exercise for a particular problem. For me, in the early 1970's, a time when women in general, and I in particular, did not question authority, it was a powerful revelation. I finally gave myself permission to use my inner resources!

Now I fully understand and teach that among the many joys of practicing art therapy is the ability, not only to understand the various psychological theories, but to be inventive and innovative, and give new ideas space to grow. With that spirit, you and your clients can deal creatively with the plethora of problems we all face. One of the outstanding attributes of the process of art therapy is that the risks you take on paper can generalize into your life. We and our clients can draw out the past, sketch in the present, and graphically plan for the future.

In your hands is a collection of essays by thirty art therapists in California who bring awareness and the experience of expressing themselves both visually and verbally to a multitude of people with a multitude of dilemmas. As we continue to share our graphic tools with our clients through and beyond their stressful times, we offer them ongoing ways of exploring and helping themselves to better health and to new ways of expressing themselves through the arts, which we know are basic to the human condition.

The contributing art therapists responded enthusiastically to my request that they tell us what they are doing, and how they are doing it. The book is hands-on, clinically oriented, how thirty art therapists who live in California practice—a day in their life, as it were. We cannot claim they are typical—there are almost 600 others, each with their own individual style, but it is how *these* California art therapists practice. You will find a wide range of topics here, with different attitudes and orientations, from treating abused children, and helping bereaved children grieve, to exploring women's roles as therapists and planning art therapy in-service programs, from using movement and art in unique combination, to inner exploration using one's own art. Teenagers under fire, teenagers incarcerated, multiple personalities, the aging, the trauma of adoptees, a sexually abused homosexual with AIDs, a left hemisphere stroke victim: you will read about how art therapists have helped these people help themselves through the power of graphic language.

You will read about how to write grants to create your own job, how to set up an art and play program in a medical hospital, as well as in a state psychiatric hospital, how to bring art therapy to art schools, how to do sand tray work. If you are a complete novice, you will learn about how art therapists have entered the field by volunteering to do art weekly with abused children. Mask-making in a meditative manner with adolescents with short attention spans, helping the depressed elderly express their unresolved sadness, learning how to work with children of different ethnicities, working with families, battered women and children, even working with many families simultaneously, all are described here in detail to give you the range and flavor of the experience.

The writers have shared their expertise and their suggestions for exercises freely. However, not only are there many different schools of art therapy, but there are at least two different schools of thought about using other people's exercise, possibly in a rote manner. Some readers, especially those new to the field, may find such exercises useful because it relieves anxiety and insecurity about using art materials creatively and innovatively for therapy.

For them, suggestions for techniques for dealing with different populations can be invaluable. However, when anxiety has subsided for you, and you feel comfortable, your creative juices will flow and you will know how best to communicate with your clients and structure the hour in your own style. As Jung recommended, after you've studied the various theories, just be your authentic self and intuitively you'll know what to do. Art therapy validates intuition.

California has the reputation of being innovative. I hope you will find here, as I have, a rich collection of different approaches and concepts to stimulate you to read further and, if you haven't already, to incorporate art and/or art therapy into your life.

In closing, I wish to thank Dorothy Royer, Tobe Reisel and Virginia Rothman, three of the Los Angeles avant-garde, for introducing me to the process of art therapy. I am also deeply obliged to the many contributors from all over our state, without whom there would be no *California Art Therapy Trends*.

I wish to thank my publishers, Kathryn Stern and Sarah Reinken, for responding to my suggestion to create this book. And finally, most thanks to my husband, Bernie, who has also integrated the art therapy process into his own professional work. Without his active encouragement, this book would have remained a fantasy.

Evelyn Virshup
Woodland Hills,
California
October, 1993

Rethinking Outpatient Adolescent Art Therapy Treatment
by Shirley Riley, MA, A.T.R., M.F.C.C.

Shirley Riley received her M.A. in Art Therapy in 1975 from Immaculate Heart College in Los Angeles, became a registered art therapy in 1976, and a licensed Marriage and Family Therapist in 1979. She has practiced family art psychotherapy at a community mental health center and been a faculty member of the Loyola Marymount University Master's program in Marriage and Family Therapy (Clinical Art Therapy) since 1979.

Having taught family art therapy in university programs nationally and internationally, presented papers at conventions and published articles in art therapy journals, Ms. Riley received the 1990 American Art Therapy Award for outstanding clinical services to families. She has been a board member involved in many committees of the American Art Therapy Association.

> *Problems facing America cluster around the values and culture of the society...a deepening race and poverty problem, widespread crime and violence, the spread of a massive drug culture, the inbreeding of social hopelessness, the profusion of sexual license, the massive propagation of moral corruption by the visual media, a decline in civic consciousness, [and] the emergence of potentially divisive multiculturalism...*
> Zbigniew Brzezinski

Introduction

Clinical art therapy has been a preferred method for adolescent treatment, both individual and group, in many mental health clinics during the past several decades. However, external accelerated stimuli have resulted in accelerated developmental pressure on young people without giving them adequate time to integrate their adolescent developmental tasks.

After a decade and a half of specializing in adolescent treatment, I have noticed a dramatic shift in their responses. This change stimulated my curiosity about the continued validity of traditional therapy with adolescents.

Some of the questions I ask are:

- Has the escalating pressure of the socio/economic environment and violence in the home caused a dramatic change in the developmental tasks of the youth?

- Has early exposure to sexualized experiences been so pervasively stimulating that it is no longer an issue to be explored?

- Have family values buckled under the loss of structure and tradition?

- How can we continue in judgment and in the security of our knowledge if, for example, a boy's understanding of male behavior is that it is "correct" to invite danger, and fight his helplessness by breaking laws and accept jail as the inevitable ending?

- What about the girl whose oppositional and aggressive behaviors are her only defense against repeated sexually abusive attacks in her home?

- How can a therapist leap the generation gap when each decade (or less) our children pass through experiences that previously took a life-time of change?

- Is it my inadequacy or the adolescents' changes that are deciding factors in their lack of participation in therapy?

- Are these stressors only the irritants we are willing to recognize? Is it easier to turn away from the real problems, rather than face the greater issues of ethnic and shifting demographic pressures?

Can we still say with conviction that art therapy is the therapy of choice with this age group? Or has the pace of life and the reduced attention to aesthetics of living and learning reduced the efficiency of a therapy that encourages and celebrates the creative approach to learning? My reflections and explorations of these and other issues comprise the body of this paper.

The adolescent boys and girls we see in treatment do not represent their entire age group. Our clients are the unfortunate fraction of teenagers that have been so damaged that their behaviors have called attention to their plight. These children who come to us are in the greatest need, the sorriest state and with the least resources.

These youths have experienced the entire gamut of adolescent challenges by the time they first add "teen" to their chronological age. Their exposure to sex, violence, drugs, and temptations of every sort, as well as to domineering and aggressive peer groups pressures, are all compressed in a time warp that allows for little if any integration or resolution of adolescent tasks.

Middle class and lower income families alike are beset with overwhelming insecurities, often functioning in economic chaos. Sons and daughters of families more fortunate financially are also at risk—attempting to deal with divorce, two parent incomes that keeps both mother and father fully engaged outside the home, and conflicting ethical values in a troubled world. An extraordinary number of these youths have single parents, often who are not psychologically much older than themselves. Killings, jail and divorce have removed the man from the home in a high percentage of cases. When present, mother is too exhausted from working two jobs to do much mothering and father is overworked and rarely at home.

Mysterious questions around sexuality and romance, commitment and loyalty are de-mystified in elementary school, if not before. The teacher/parent who shows the child how to love or live a good life often comes over the TV screen—an electronic relationship limited to half-an-hour or an hour with time-out for commercials. Role models are disposable and interchangeable and on the whole manufactured and unauthentic (Goldner, Penn, Sheinberg, Walker, 1990, p. 343).

It is hard if not impossible to rebel against family values when the family itself is fractured. The children cannot test the rules of the home if the only sensible rule is "survive at any price." They cannot examine their gender-defined roles by measuring their values against the beliefs of their same sex parent if the parent is not available.

It still comes as a shock to find a 15-year-old in the recovery phase of substance abuse, already an old hand at this destructive game. The histories of our young clients are often so brutally sad that we wonder how anything can help! Therapy may seem like an exercise in futility.

There is little comfort in the belated focus on family values in the governmental politics which cause both distress at the distortions, and only a glimmer of hope for many of us who have seen the changing circumstances that pressure our young people today (Hersch, 1993, p. 41).

3

Foundations of Clinical Art Therapy Treatment with Adolescents

In spite of changing times and variations in the speed of maturation of our children, there are many fundamentals of clinical art therapy that remain valid and effective when working with this population. The developmental stages, tasks and needs of youth can be explored successfully with art expressions in a therapeutic environment.

The grand task of adolescence is to individuate and complete the process of separation from the family of origin (Blos 1962). The modality of art therapy is uniquely responsive to these needs since

- It reflects the youths' desires by offering a form of therapy that gives them control over their expressions—the young clients reveal only what they wish to reveal in the art or in the explanation of the art
- They find using media stimulates their creativity
- It provides a pleasure component
- It utilizes personal and age/group metaphors and symbols.

The adolescent believes that his/her control effectively keeps the adult (therapist) from making intrusive interpretations. By rejecting "talk" therapy and the concomitant request to expose "feelings" the adolescents experience autonomy (control) and this comfortably feeds into their narcissistic stance (Riley 1988). Since the experienced art therapist is not concerned with establishing control, he/she rarely needs to probe. However, the clinician continues to provide the young client with opportunities to create products that address issues of ambivalence and immediate concern in their world. Thus, in their own art, they may find new views and solutions to their dilemmas.

Group treatment is often the preferred choice, since it reflects the adolescents' desire to utilize a peer group as a replacement for parental influence and structure (Linesch, 1990). Today, this preference has escalated to a point where the parents' influence is so diminished that the dominant attachment is to a gang, crew or clique. This type of attachment has increasingly become the focal point of adult concern and fears concerning adolescent development and behaviors.

In group or individual treatment, the general stance of the art therapist is one of interest, positive curiosity (Checchin, 1993), and an attitude of extreme caution about any form of interpretation—either of the art product or the meaning of the verbal expressions. The therapist can rely on the art to do the communicating and trust that the message will be shared at a pace that fits this population. The boys and girls are encouraged to set their own group rules and decide on procedure. The results may be more rigid than normally set by the adult, but as long as they feel in control, that they are "beating the system," then they will be more compliant.

Past and Present

These general considerations and guidelines worked very well for me and my colleagues until recently. Now my observation is that adolescent group is rarely successful in an outpatient setting. Let us look at the issues that must be considered to reconstruct a theoretical approach for today's society (Gergen, 1991).

Case Vignette. The social/sexual confusion of the adolescent.

A client (a 13 year old girl) chose to use adolescent art therapy group to help her make the decision,"When should I lose my virginity?" Since, to this group, the state of virginity was not a particularly desired or precious status to preserve, the matter really became a mechanical discussion around social acceptance and gender roles. The person with whom she would have her first sexual encounter was less important than weighing the succeeding change of social status and the peer approved advantages or disadvantages that would accompany this passage.

My struggle to introduce questions of vulnerability, risk, and opportunity for physical harm or disease was my own issue. I wrongly worked too hard to encourage the group to discuss the emotional component of sexual coupling, but, as one might expect, I was not successful. The information on "how to" and "where to" was so clearly explicated on TV and in teenage gossip, that my attempts to help her explore her decision was impotent. I recall one of my questions, "Is it important for the woman to have orgasm as well as the man?" was met by blank looks and disbelief that women did, or indeed could, have orgasm. Babies yes, pleasure no.

This example demonstrates how social opinion affects many of the issues that the therapist for adolescents ordinarily anticipates to be part of treatment. The "therapy" resided only in the fact thatthe adolescent chose the group to be her audience and her sounding board.

Basic Attitudes

The following are some attitudes that therapists must integrate into their skills and belief systems in their attempts to find a way into the world of the adolescent.

The stance of "not knowing" (Goolishian and Anderson) is basic to learning about the many experiences our youths of today have lived and which we can only imagine. Making assumptions, coming forth with interpretations, finding your meaning in their art is presumptuous.

Deciding that you "know" an adolescent's feeling or belief system is unrealistic since they have little idea of how or what they feel or believe. When your client is in a state of flux you must join them in their uncertainties. Swimming together upstream and rescuing each other from drowning is the way adolescent treatment should be conducted. To push this metaphor a little more, it may be that your client only knows how to dogpaddle, you know the Australian crawl, back stroke and how to float. What you don't know is which of these swimming techniques are going to be acceptable to your adolescent, or even if you had better learn to dogpaddle because it works better in these muddy waters! Teaching a young person more ways to swim gives him a sense of survival and new skills to navigate his own personal rapids. When an adolescent recognizes that he has some options on how he will direct his life, when he sees that he is not irrevocably bound to act out his delegated role (Stierlin, 1985) in the family script, he has made a major move toward autonomy.

We have to examine carefully the notions that it is best to get past defenses, get in touch with feelings, stay attached to the family; depending on circumstances, perhaps none of these changes would benefit our clients.

We must develop our ability to let the adolescent teach us, through his/her art expression together with the related description, where they are in their lives and, more importantly, where they want to go.

Unless treatment allows for long term involvement with a teenager, a crisis intervention mode of problem-solving is perhaps our best choice of therapy most of the time (Belnick, in Linesch, 1993). Fortunately, although the goals may be pragmatic, the modality of art therapy introduces the notion of creativity. Not creativity in the art product (although that is a precious possibility) but creativity in gaining coping skills. Creatively finding a new solution allows the pattern of behaviors to take a new direction. Imaginative crisis intervention allows the therapist to embrace untried and unique solutions that are formed to fit and support each client in a personal manner. In this form of art therapy the therapist approaches the session in a manner not unlike forming an aesthetic art expression—knowing, for example, that you desire to have a painting as an end product, understanding that all the elements of making that painting, the canvas, the media, the tools, the environment, the audience, and your thoughts as the painting develops, all have unpredictable but dominant influences on how the end results will be accomplished. That process is not unlike good art therapy. The difference is that the painting has no deadline; the crisis must be resolved within a six or eight week period.

Social Challenges to Trust

Teen-age treatment has always had as a first concern the establishment of safety and trust. Today this is a major issue. Consider, the adolescent may have had to cross over gang lines just to visit the clinic. Is death or a beating worth chancing just to get to therapy? When he/she does find a way to get to the clinic, and if it is group treatment, why would he/she risk saying anything that may evoke dire consequences from other group members who may be in an opposing gang? Why say anything that might be "leaked" to the enemy, resulting in physical violence? The group is no longer a safe place.

Also, since a high percentage of cases now seen are those resulting from sexual abuse or other acts of violence on their person, we must realize that the threat of exposing the perpetrator is another basic retardant to a young client's communication. They know only too well how the system intervenes and breaks up homes, sends children into foster care and punishes everyone in the family. Their lack of naiveté keeps the silence. They are wise beyond their years; not with the wisdom we would desire for our children, but the wisdom of the streets that has rules and beliefs not necessarily in synchrony with the law or the values we hold as mental health professionals.

Once a core group of adolescents begins to attend therapy regularly, it is very difficult to introduce a new member without setting the group back to the first phase of testing trust. To refuse treatment presents an administrative difficulty for the clinic, but having a new child thrust into an established group is a serious frustration for the art therapist leader. Often, in today's mental health world, expediency takes precedence over therapeutic concerns. Pragmatic concerns conflict with the aesthetics of treatment.

As a result the therapist experiences uncertain attendance and, when they do appear, the members are not willing to be verbal and often refuse to make an art object.

Modified Goals for Adolescent Treatment

We can see how the acceleration of external stimuli and the diminished parental role as interpreters of value force the therapist to abandon tradition and search for a realistic approach to adolescent treatment.

Preparatory Phase of Treatment

Today's treatment has to start so slowly that it may seem to be in reverse rather than proceeding. A useful time frame may be to project the first six months solely as preparation for group. Just the experience of being with a safe adult and fellow adolescents over a period of time is of such great value to the young client that it may comprise one of the main goals of therapy.

First attempts to chance an art task will be more likely to succeed if they arise from dialogue or special interests of the adolescent. To mark down anything is perceived as risky so the therapist must take the attitude that s/he is willing to be helpful but will not decide what can be safely discussed. The early art experience is presented as an opportunity to learn a skill, a product—a function similar to the one an arts and craft teacher performs. When discussion touches on stress points it is wise to be prepared to quickly move away before the group becomes silent, again. However, the seeds of future discussion are being sowed.

There are exception to this rule of slowness. There have been times when the teenager is so desperate to move out of the situation that he or she opens up quickly and promptly describes every detail of the difficulties. This rapid disclosure is more likely to happen in individual treatment, sometimes in groups, and rarely in family work. The therapist has to respond in a variety of ways, such as preserving confidentiality and being protective, while convincing the youth that not keeping secrets and involving the family is essential to relieving the problem.

Sharing art work may be the first step in breaking through old power struggles since it provides a new avenue on which to base a dialogue. The emotional visual impact of disclosure makes the picture more powerful than words! Often the art products that lay out the trauma become objects that can engage the family in a problem-solving dialogue that they have avoided. It is hard to deny concrete evidence of problematic situations. There is less misunderstanding of the truth (as the adolescent presents it), when all concerned look at the product instead of relying solely on words.

Some Techniques for Early Treatment

At this phase the therapist's creativity is taxed through the quest for activities that fit the interests and sophistication of the group. Art therapy tasks are required that do not threaten their safety with rapid exposure and have the flexibility to be a long or short term project, depending on the ability of the adolescents to stay involved.

The art task might reflect the adolescents' uncertainties by creating games "of finding a way out of a maze," drawing their neighborhood and making changes they would like, telling stories, illustrating their tales, and "doing graffiti." These are the type of tasks that introduce some graphic expression but stay clearly and safely within the range of metaphor and the familiar.

I find this time of treatment the most challenging to my skill and my impatience to be "helpful." Realistically, the art tasks should be created to last over some period of time. Since members have poor attendance, they find some reassurance if they can fit back into the "game" and, upon returning, recognize the same project. It may also be a reality that the therapy does not go much beyond this stage as far as the drawing tasks are concerned. Under most circumstances, adolescent art has a tendency to stay within safe stereotypes and familiar symbology. However, in due time, the therapist may begin to speculate on values and problems that are of meaning to the group. The basic stance of "not knowing" (Anderson and Goolishian, 1988) is of the greatest value to the therapist. If the youth will "teach" you, then you have made it over the barrier of adolescent suspicion and therapy may follow.

Treatment Issues

When trust has finally been established, the therapist has to redirect her/his thoughts toward projecting treatment goals.

The complexity of difficulties the adolescent brings to therapy is truly extraordinary. This generalization is perhaps colored by the fact that mental health treatment today is continuously narrowed down to those clients in the "greatest risk" category. In community mental health and hospital treatment, preventive therapy is a lonely memory of the past. State funding and insurance-sponsored therapy clearly demand a severe, dysfunctional diagnosis to qualify for therapy and payment. In addition, they fund only short term or projected outcome treatment.

This framework is in conflict with the issues of timing we have discussed in the previous section of this paper. It is not easy to be forced to have a treatment plan that contradicts the basic needs of the client. However, we do continue to treat and we do find some success.

One of the strengths of art therapy treatment, particularly under the above constraints, lies in the ability of an art expression to contain a multiplicity of meanings. Although a limited amount of this material may be explored in the session, the youth has brought these problems forward into visual awareness and may examine them on his/her own. A therapy session is only a stimulus to the problem-solving or changes that go on after the therapy hour is over, particularly since art therapy allows the client to take away (either in memory, or in hand) a product that enriches the field of contemplation and invites the embedded meanings to emerge and deepen the client's understanding.

Looking at the Historical and Primary Socialization of the Young Client

One of the helpful tasks that give the adolescent and the therapist "a way to go" is to do a picture story of the family without attempting to impose the formal family genogram or family map format on the client. This traditional tool should never be offered to the adolescent in the traditional way (McGoldrick and Gerson, 1985). Each history of the family should be a trip of discovery which is individually created. As the art expression comes into being, the opportunities to look at the difficulties of adolescence are externalized in a natural manner. Through the concrete expression of generational patterns of the family, the stories that were told, the family's myths and traditions (or lack of), the gender-defined roles, the redundant patterns of, for example, violence, incarceration or the strength to rise above adversities—many vital issues arise that help an adolescent on his primary search to establish an identity.

It is important to bear in mind that the client chooses the combination of media, personal color coding, and personal symbols to represent his/her own family. Through this process, the therapist can understand more clearly the world view of the client, the family, and the social environment from which the youth developed.

Considering the financial constrictions of treatment in these times, as well as the natural desire of the adolescent to "get on with it" and finish therapy, often this major task and the sessions that evolve from the family history may comprise the treatment.

A Scroll-type Genogram: Case Example

One of the most remarkable life stories I have observed, produced by an adolescent, was a twelve foot scroll depicting his sixteen years. This drawing described his life from birth to present time, including all the family members that had impacted his world, as well as the numerous abandonments and abuse situations he experienced. The scroll started as a four-foot length of white butcher paper upon which he first drew himself in utero and then drew outstanding memories year by year. When the four feet of paper became filled, we attached another four feet, and again another piece, until his life was drawn up to the present. The purpose of the life-scroll was to enable him to stand back and review his life, to place before himself his remarkable ability to survive and to make difficult decisions for his own welfare. At first, he constantly depreciated himself. For example, when he was seven he was sent to an ashram in India. Instead of empathizing with this little seven year old boy who had been sent to India without any knowledge or understanding of the situation, he was critical that he had not adjusted more quickly to his trauma. He maintained the same critical attitude when he saw how early he used drugs and alcohol to deaden his grief, and did not admire his fortitude to have joined AA and DA at age fourteen and remain sober for two years.

The observant stance allowed him to evaluate himself as though he was another person, and over time, begin to appreciate his difficulties and success in a new way. He understood the roots of his depression. As his life unfolded on the paper, he relived the pain of abandonment, he "remembered" the sexual assault when he was hospitalized in India, he grieved over the rejection he experienced from his father, and he allowed some anger at his dependent and chronically depressed mother. I believe that very few of these crucial clinical issues would have emerged so powerfully had they not been externalized and re-experienced in the context of his own re-creation of the flow of his life in his art therapy expression.

The choice of the visual narrative form was his invention. My role was to encourage him to join me in an observing position and help him realize his strengths. He displayed in the drawing many situations where he survived and which would have defeated most of us, myself included. The art task provided such a broad field of knowledge about the primary and secondary socialization of this client that the direction leading to further art therapy opportunities were rich.

Ethics and Ambivalence

The following clinical vignette is an example of a dilemma presented by a youth of our society which challenged the values (ethics) of therapy.

A fourteen year old Hispanic male client was forced into art therapy by his parents who were extremely anxious because Hector had threatened to join a gang and thus disgrace their family. He would not utter a word in his family sessions with another therapist, who subsequently referred him to art therapy.

His school performance had dropped to total failure and, although he did not cause a behavior problem in class, neither did he show the slightest interest in academics. He was a competent artist for his age. In art therapy, he willingly produced an art product, discussed his family and talked about his ambitions, but never seemed to move beyond social communication. He once said he hoped that his family would move to another neighborhood so that he would not have to deal with gang pressure.

Narcissistically, he believed he would be a television star and was taking professional lessons to accomplish this goal. His narcissistic stance was dramatically revealed through a clay sculpture, where his self-representation stood in the crossed beams of two spotlights that shone on him alone as a camera recorded his acting. Visually it was a delightfully executed sculpture and Hector felt proud of himself both as artist and as the "star" of the television show he created.

Some weeks later we were working with graffiti as an art therapy tool. He felt graffiti was able to express more than just "marking" gang territory. As we worked in this format the boy talked about spray paint as a medium and I moved the discussion to airbrushing and the similarities between commercial spray paint and airbrushing as an art form. Hector was enthusiastic and interested. He opened up in a more affective manner than I had so far experienced. We spoke of his future as an artist and I felt gratified that I had found an entré into his interests. The following session Hector proudly came in with a complete professional airbrush kit—compressor, spray tool, special nozzles and various inks and other paraphernalia for spray painting. He showed me how he intended to use this equipment to work as the artist for the school yearbook and how pleased he was that I had introduced him to this medium. He felt that he had found a new niche for himself in his peer group at school.

Of course, I was pleased for him and encouraged his involvement and development of an anti-gang persona. However, I knew what this equipment cost and I was painfully aware that we were looking at several hundred dollars worth of very fine tools. If I suggested that he had stolen this air brush, I might very well lose this client. If I ignored the issue, I was colluding with a thief. If I reported him to his family, who consistently excused his behaviors, Hector would have felt betrayed by yet another adult. What was I to do?

I decided to question him directly, but he declared he had purchased the airbrush with his savings. The issue was never resolved. We continued seeing one another for several more sessions but no further change occurred. He left therapy because he said "he had been helped a lot." Adolescent sanction of stealing had triumphed over adult ability to problem-solve.

Where to Establish Adolescent Treatment

Adolescent treatment, particularly in group, can be more successful if it is offered at a site that does not place the child at risk to attend. The risk is not only physical, such as crossing through gang territory, but also can be emotional, if by coming to a clinic they feel labeled as "crazy" or "nerd" which connotes "different."

At hospital, day treatment and residential settings the adolescent, forced into attendance, is often non-compliant, but the threats which he perceives to his person are usually internal rather than external. In these settings the challenges to the art therapist are ones that fall in the realm of treatment difficulties for which we are trained. Another choice which has become increasingly more practical and popular is to take the therapist to the children. School groups or after school meeting places are logical sites and provide a better understanding of the immediate crisis or social stressors in the adolescent environment. In this school/rap setting, the therapist needs administrative support to design the group therapy as a privilege for many, rather than a punishment for a few. By following the plan suggested above—of starting slow and letting the adolescent shape the direction, the experience can become acceptable and even desired by the larger youth community.

The Los Angeles Riots And Art Therapy

The aftermath of the upheaval in south-central Los Angeles in 1992 presented a massive crisis wherein therapeutic ethics, values, confidentiality and empathy were all stretched to a new dimension. In the immediate aftermath of the riots, when the adolescents drew in a school-based art therapy group, their memories of the days of the rebellion, they often drew themselves inside their homes looking out.* They preferred to take an uninvolved position in the crisis and in the therapy. They were very guarded about the information they shared. Some of us were equally protective of our feelings and possibly conflicted about how to evaluate the issues of repression versus retribution, disadvantage versus opportunistic greed, and in particular how to be the "therapist in charge" when all values were problematic. The crisis presented clinicians with serious questions on how much to share. Some remained inside their own protective walls of theory, looking out at the world, just as our adolescent clients stayed in their homes rather than face questions with no answers. Perhaps we both closed our eyes rather than face the painful reality of destruction, injustice, and subsequent hurtful outcomes of the L.A. uprising.

The nonjudgmental quality of the art therapy made a difference by providing distance and concretizing the issues. The youth could draw what she/he saw, externalize the behaviors of society, both good and bad, and make some comments about the art expressions. This was less threatening than making the same remarks about real people or real neighborhood situations. The city flamed again on the paper and the ruins were resurrected by the young people in the art. In art therapy the values and judgments of the members were respected and their pain and loss accepted.

Through their art expressions the fires, the looting, the tragedies and the unnoticed deeds of bravery became alive again. The therapist and the adolescents had the opportunity to co-create a view of the events which lead to a shared speculations about avoiding the same situation in the future. Only when we each came out from behind our walls could we meet on grounds that might lead to some positive change (Riley, Walter, Newborn, 1992).

The Post-Modern Art Therapist—Summary

In no other age group do we, as art therapists for adolescents, need to be less knowing and more wise. Our clients, caught between traumatic childhood experiences and adult stressors, at the mercy of societal uncertainties and escalating violence in the world and on the streets, have their own internal tumultuous world which is all too syntonic with the tumultuous external world. There are few places for them to seek out structure and ongoing values that stay in place long enough to serve the needs of an adolescent seeking to form an identity and find a satisfactory world view of her/his own (Gergen, 1991). Therefore, adolescent art therapy treatment can still provide a therapeutic service to our young people of today's world.

To continue to offer treatment in a traditional way while our children and society are fluctuating in a composite of untraditional amalgams of the old and the new, is to offer therapy that lacks substance.

As many of us try to be useful to this age group, let's make a pact to experiment and follow these children in ways that meet them in the world in which they live. Who can tell—the city-wide visual markings, known to us as graffiti, may successfully make its mark on all of us. We may be able to channel it into a new form of art therapy, where each youth's "tag" no longer needs to destroy, but can constructively reflect their own worth.

14

References

Allen, J. (1988). *Serial drawing: A junior approach with children.* In C. C. Schaefer (ed.) Innovative Interventions in Child and Adolescent Therapy. NY: John Wiley & Sons.

Anderson, H. and Goolishian, H. (1988). *Human systems as linguistic systems.* Family Process 27(4), 371.

Belnick, J. (1993). *Crisis intervention model for family therapy.* In D. Linesch (ed.) NY: Brunner/Mazel.

Blos, P. (1962). *On adolescence.* NY: The Free Press.

Brzezinski, Z. (1993) *Out of control: global turmoil on the eve of the twenty-first century.* NY: Chas. Scribner.

Cecchin, G. (1987). *Hypothesizing circularity and neutrality revisited.* Family Process, 26(4), 405.

Cox, K. (1990). *Breaking through: Incident drawings with adolescent substance abusers.* Arts in Psychotherapy 17(4), 333-337.

Dickerson, V. and Zimmerman, J. (1992). *Families with adolescents: escaping problem lifestyles.* Family Process. 31, 341.

Emunah, R. (1990). *Expression and expansion in adolescence. The significance of creative arts therapy.* Arts in Psychotherapy 17(2), 101-107.

Finkelhor, D., Gelles, R., Hotaling, G., and Straus, M., eds. (1983). *The dark side of families.* Beverly Hills: Sage Publication.

Gergen, K. (1991). *The saturated self.* NY: Basic Books.

Hull, J. (1993).*A boy and his gun.* Time Magazine. NY: Time Inc.142(4), 20.

Johnson, D. (1987). *The role of the creative arts therapies in the diagnosis and treatment of psychological trauma.* Arts in Psychotherapy 14, 7-13.

Landgarten, H. (1981) *Clinical art therapy: a comprehensive guide.* NY: Brunner/Mazel.

Linesch, D. (1988) *Adolescent art therapy.* NY: Brunner/Mazel.

Pynoos, R. and Eth, S. (1986). *Witness to violence: the child interview.* Journal of the American Academy of Child Psychiatry, 25(3), 306-319.

Riley, S. *Art therapy with families who have experienced domestic violence.* In E. Virshup, (ed.) California Art Therapy Trends. Chicago: Magnolia Street Publishers, in press.

Riley, S. (1988). *Adolescents and family art therapy.* Journal of American Art Therapy Association. 5, 2 43.

Riley, S., Newborn, M., Takasumi, Y. and Walter, J. (1992). *Art captures the impact of the Los Angeles crisis.* Journal of the American Art Therapy Association. 9(3), 139-144.

Rinsley, D. (1980). *Treatment of the severely disturbed adolescent.* NY: Jason Aronson.

Sgroi, S., Ed. (1988). *Handbook of clinical intervention in child sexual abuse.* Lexington, MA: Lexington Books.

Smolowe, J. (1993). *Choose your poison.* Time Magazine. NY: Time Inc. 142, 4-56.

Stierlin, H. (1981). *Separating parents and adolescents.* NY: Jason Aronson.

* This situation was reported by a colleague, N. Hass-Cohen, M.A., in the El Nido Outreach program.

Clinical Art Therapy with Adolescents of Color
by Anna Hiscox, M.F.T., A.T.R.

Anna Hiscox, M.F.T, A.T.R., a native of New York City, received her Master's degree from the College of Notre Dame in Belmont, California. She works with adolescents at a mental health hospital in San Francisco, where she also supervises art therapy interns. Ms. Hiscox is on the Mosaic Committee, a multicultural subcommittee of the American Art Therapy Association, founded in 1990, working toward increasing the sensitivity and insight of art therapists as well as other professionals working with clients of different cultural and racial backgrounds.

Introduction

Intercultural diversity is a fact of social life, and one which the culturally competent worker must be able to handle (Green, 1982, p. 87). The cultural polarity and ethnic diversity of the Bay Area mandates that art therapists and others in the mental health profession have a responsibility to become familiar with cross-cultural and inner-cultural systems and ideology. Implicit in the education and training of people in cross-cultural issues is the development of cultural sensitivity, empathy and genuineness.

San Francisco and the Bay Area have encountered dramatic changes within the past 10 years which have affected children and adolescents economically, socially, and psychologically.

This geographic area has become a mecca for new immigrants wishing to fulfill the American dream. As cited in the 1990 U.S. Census, the San Francisco Bay Area population breakdown by race and ethnicity is as follows: White 57%, Blacks 9%, Asian and Pacific Islander 15%, Hispanics 12%, and other 6%. Figures for San Francisco itself shows: Whites 47%, Blacks

11%, Asian and Pacific Islander 29%, Hispanic 14%, Native-American .04%, and other .02%.

The socio-economic spectrum of inner cities includes the economically disadvantaged, drug addicts and alcoholics, one-parent families, step-families/blended families and gangs. The past two decades have witnessed a marked increase of children and adolescents of color admissions to inpatient and residential treatment facilities. In the San Francisco Bay Area, 60% of the adolescent population on hospital units are a mixture of cultures, creating new challenges for the mental health field.

This chapter discusses the role of art therapy in the assessment and treatment of adolescents of color in brief inpatient hospitalization.

Art Therapy in Short Term Hospitalization

The goal of brief inpatient hospitalization is to minimize and/or reduce the crisis and return the teen to his or her baseline functioning. Hospitalization can effectively accomplish this goal by providing a safe and caring environment. Due to the rising cost of coverage for hospitalization and mental health care, the average length of stay for adolescents in many psychiatric facilities has decreased significantly. Pharmacological treatment is used when applicable. In order to effect change quickly and efficiently, an integrated team approach to crisis intervention, treatment, and diagnosis which includes both verbal and creative expressive components has been found useful.

Art therapy is an integral part of the care plan. The job of the art therapist in a brief inpatient facility is to work with other disciplines and professionals to assess, evaluate and provide structure through which the adolescent can record his or her difficulties.

Art therapy is an important modality in providing care and treatment to the kaleidoscope of ethnic and cultural diversity seen in mental health facilities today. Drawing and painting are frequently the most effective way to motivate non-English-speaking children to express themselves. Symbols drawn by children of color are not different from other adolescents with similar cognitive and developmental skills. However, minority children's differences are observed in their manner of relating to art itself, and in the therapist's understanding of what he or she is seeing. The non-verbal aspect of art psychotherapy gives the clients an opportunity to listen with their eyes (Landgarten 1981). Clinicians from various disciplines have all cited the universality of art-making. Arnheim (1969), Kellogg (1969), Piaget (1968), DiLeo (1973) and Landgarten (1981/1987) agree that the use of symbols and images bypass the cultural and language differences which occur in verbal therapies. Kramer posited that art adapts itself readily in service to the important issues in the cultural life of a people (Kramer, 1977).

The Therapist's Use of Self

McGoldrick (1982) perceptively noted, "We are always a part of the systems we are trying to observe, and our participation affects our observations." This perspective sensitively describes the framework for intervention with minority adolescents. Boyd-Franklin (1989), supporting McGoldrick, asserts, "In working with any ethnic group, the ability of the clinician to effect change is greatly increased by the exploration of what aspects of his or her own culture, ethnic group, and family of origin she or he likes and which ones she or he does not."

Because of the non-threatening process of art making, the art therapist is frequently the first to provide information to the treatment team. Obtaining assessment information is contingent upon the therapist's use of self. Kwiatkowska (1978), Riley (1988), and Arrington (1991) are researchers and pioneers who have successfully combined family therapy and art therapy to create change within the individual and/or family. In order to effect the changes described by these authors, it is imperative that we first get in touch with our own transference issues, which may be significant when interacting with culturally diverse adolescents.

A Systemic Framework

When working with patients in general, but especially when working with minority adolescents, it is very important that the therapist's attitude and approach be compatible with changing social, individual and family attitudes and customs, all of which form a system within which therapy and art therapy must function. With these children, to be useful, art therapy must be integrated with their culture.

Intercultural diversity is a fact of social life, and it is one which the culturally competent worker must be able to handle (Green, 1982). The cultural polarities and ethnic diversity of the Bay Area mandate that art therapists and others in the mental health profession become familiar with cross-cultural and inner-cultural systems and ideology. We must educate and make both clients and therapists aware of cross-cultural issues to develop cultural sensitivity, empathy and genuineness.

The structural approach to art psychotherapy provides useful boundaries for the art activity and group. However, the therapist must be willing to let the client lead and teach in order for cultural nuances to be addressed.

Adolescents in groups are frequently the best co-therapists, providing the key to unresolved conflicts. Systemic learning depends on whether the worker-as-help-provider is willing to adopt the role of worker-as-learner (Green, 1982). This dual relationship is important in a culturally diverse environment where the therapist must adapt the art process and product to the culture of the minority adolescent, by-passing language and cultural differences.

When working with teens, it is important for the therapist to be aware of the teen's music; terminology in verbal expressions (cultural language in adolescent subsystems); and the color of clothing, which may represent the alliance to subgroups within the community. Language, music, and clothing continuously change within the adolescent cohort. Conflicting adolescent terms used to describe drugs, hair styles, and dress challenge clinicians to remain abreast of the ever changing terminology.

Music

Music is very important to these adolescents. It is a means of communication, and often tells a story. The range of music may vary from Rock, Hip-Hop, Reggae, and Rap, to Rhythm and Blues. The social messages of songs come through regardless of the type of music used as a vehicle of expression.

In the 60's, the songs of the day documented a cultural revolution of immense proportions. Today, Rap music documents a similar struggle. Rap music has become a universal language for teenagers, crossing all ethnic barriers. Current musical lyrics are sometimes graphic and violent. Not all teenagers are attracted to Rap music, but Rap appears to be intrinsic to the adolescent subculture.

Today's young people are proclaiming things are different than they were in the 60's and 70's. There is a new surge of self-esteem in children of color. There is also a renewed awareness and pride in ethnicity. Stories of this new revolution are being told lyrically. The heroes of the revolution are Rap artists. On April 29th, 1992, Los Angeles exploded in anarchy and chaos in response to the Rodney King verdict. In this writer's opinion, Rap music predicted the events of the times, mirroring deep changes in American society today, just as it did in the Watts Riots of 1965.

As clinicians, we can use music not only to hear, but also to validate the pain, anger, and confusion which is so concretely conveyed through lyrics and music. Our interventions can provide boundaries as well as provide a safe environment for our clients/patients to create, enlarge, and document their stories. Music and art are very effective means of communication.

Subgroups and the Color of Clothing

Young people have found intriguing ways of compensating for the decay of family and community support systems. Two of the most publicized adolescent and young adult families today are the Bloods and the Crips. These two groups function as surrogate families for many teens, especially minority adolescents. By joining groups such as these, many teens receive familial bonding and a sense of belonging which is frequently missing in their own families of origin. These subgroups are recognized in their community by adorning themselves with specific colors of clothing.

One of the major components of building rapport and effective intervention with teens may be our observational skills. Being aware that a patient or client's clothing may represent an allegiance to a particular subgroup may reduce resistance, increase communication, and assist with therapeutic goals.

Methodology

It is within the context of cultural awareness and personal vulnerability that a systemic approach to treatment and intervention is most successful. Listening and hearing with one's eyes when teens are acting out and being resistant is important in staying attuned to the therapeutic process. The therapeutic intervention and resolution of conflict is often depicted in the first drawing: resistance is also reduced and acting-out is transferred into a concrete form of representation.

Adolescent art in brief hospitalization necessitates a structured, direct, process-oriented group or task-oriented individual session. In group and/or one-on-one sessions, patients have the opportunity to draw out their problems and have their feelings validated.

The clinical model emphasizes working with the family as well as the individual. However, this ideal situation is not always possible. Therefore projective drawings provide an opportunity for the art therapist to work with the patient's family of origin, extended-family and microsystems without all the members present.

In order to elicit information, provide structure, reduce resistance and increase motivation, art activities are at first directive. Group themes are generalized and adapted to problems affecting teenagers in the 90's, such as drugs and alcohol, family conflict, and abuse. Teenagers frequently indicate who they are, both as individuals and in the context of family and community, within the first two sessions.

The directive approach to art psychotherapy that involves structured art tasks is limiting because it minimizes primitive spontaneous expression. However, it provides the structure necessary for teens in crisis. It also provides boundaries within the scope of creativity. Within this kind of art-making, patients are offered choices in media which greatly increase their creative expression.

Exercises:

The Metaphor of a Bridge—Historical information, assessment and evaluation of adolescents in treatment may be obtained by having the teenager draw a bridge. According to Hays and Lyon (1981), the metaphor of a bridge represents a symbolic link between humans, society and the individual. C. G. Jung speaks of crossing a river as a symbolic image for a fundamental change of attitude. Drawing a bridge may make visible our feelings about our control or lack of control over the environment. Assessment and evaluation can be determined by the response to several variables in the drawing, including directionality of the bridge, placement of self in relation to the bridge, actual bridge construction and attachment. This projective drawing has proven to be a valuable tool in pre/post evaluation and in accurately identifying the stage of crisis upon admission, as well as a springboard for further communication.

Abstract Family Drawing—Kwiatkowska (1978) worked with entire families, helping them to identify family conflict by the use of pictorial expression to increase communication. One of her techniques within her family assessment continuum is the "Abstract Family Drawing." Kwiatkowska emphasizes the use of color, motion, lines and shapes to represent the personality of each family member. This procedure vividly conveys the intense feelings about family interactions.

Draw Your Place of Birth—Draw Your Place of Birth (or homeland) provides implicit and explicit information about the patient and his or her family, providing invaluable metaphorical data.

Draw Your Family — Burns and Kaufman (1972) found that *Kinetic-Family-Drawings (K-F-D)* helped to identify the client's perception of the quality of feelings and interactions among family members. The Abstract Family Portrait and the K-F-D have been useful in the assessment of family issues.

Projective Figure Drawing — Hammer (1980) and others have written about the value of *Projective Figure Drawing*. This technique helps in depicting the metaphorical schemata of the individual and his or her self-concept. Again, given short hospitalizations, this method of assessment provides much information quickly.

Accuracy in Evaluation and Assessment

In providing services to children and adolescents of color, one must be cautious about misinterpreting symbols. Accuracy in evaluation and assessment must include the patient's own interpretation. Levy (1980) asserts that the interpretation of projective figure drawings is without sufficient experimental validation, rarely yields unequivocal information and frequently misleads the unwary, the naive, the reckless and the impulsive. It is imperative that the methodology of administering instruments of assessment is consistent with Levy's philosophy. Most assessment tools are not designed with ethnically and culturally diverse people in mind.

Many of the teens seen in hospitals and mental health facilities do not come from intact families. Abstract family drawings and the K-F-D alleviate the stress of teens having to project their family realistically. These two exercises counteract the tendency to invent or fantasize when the patient may not be able or ready to discuss family issues and circumvent resistance.

Self "Objectification" — The adolescent finds it much easier to relate to the picture than to the self. Wadeson (1980) entitles the process of viewing the art from a distance prior to integrating the images as part of the self "objectification." Wadeson says "I call this process objectification because feelings or ideas are at first externalized in an object (picture or sculpture). The art object allows the individual, while separating from his or her feeling, to recognize their existence."

Discussion

A systemic approach and methodology was conceptualized as a means of developing and implementing art therapy groups and individual sessions with children of color. Art therapy assessment tools have not been developed that are applicable to any one particular ethnic group. A culturally sensitive approach, a systemic understanding of the individual within his societal culture, and the dynamic use of art are basic to the current trend in art therapy in a multicultural society.

Periodically, historical events happen in communities that affect not only that community but the nation and the world. Last April, this nation witnessed the out-cry of many communities in response to the Rodney King verdict and subsequent Los Angeles riots. Citizens of underdeveloped neighborhoods and cities have been beset by drugs, apathy and the insensitivity of government. Economic disparity and racism continues to divide one of the world's greatest countries. When a predominantly white jury vindicated four police officers for the beating of an unarmed African-American male, the underlying message heard in minority cultures was that as a country, we are not ready for change. The King verdict was only the spark that set fire to the underlying anger and pain of people living in separate and unequal conditions.

Many of the clients/patients seen in mental health facilities today come from these poor neighborhoods. Outpatient clinics and hospitals are challenged to meet the ever-growing demands of administering services to a diversity of ethnic groups. The multiplicity of languages, cultures, spiritual beliefs, racism, as well as depleted funds have made this an extremely difficult task. However, we as art therapists can make a difference using a universal language, intertwined with effective interventions and with awareness of differences in customs and beliefs.

Assisting our clients/patients to resolve issues through art psychotherapy also helps the art therapist deal with his/her own unresolved stereotypical views of a particular client or ethnic group. As art therapists, we are in a unique position. We are in a pro-active position as we work with clients/patients using art, frequently helping our clients make important observations and changes in their behavior.

Conclusion

This text was written with the hope that it will provide some insight in engaging culturally-diverse adolescents in therapy through the use of art therapy techniques as well as the therapist's use of self. There are many techniques, activities and ideologies for implementing art therapy groups as well as individual sessions. The correct therapeutic intervention is the one that successfully engages patients, assists them in objectification, and provides a means of discovery and recovery.

References

Arnheim, R. (1969). *Visual thinking.* Berkeley, CA: U. of Cal. Press.

Arrington, D. (1991). *Thinking systems-seeing systems: an integrative model for systemically-oriented art therapy..* The Arts in Psychotherapy, 18(3), 201-211.

Boyd-Franklin (1989). *Black families in therapy.* NY: Guilford Press.

Brady, T. J. (1992). *Cultures in conflict: psychiatric care of ethnic minority children.* Unpublished paper presented at the 2nd (1992) Child Psychiatry Conference. McAuley Neuropsychiatric Institute, St. Mary's Hospital, San Francisco, CA.

Campanelli, M. (1991). *.Art therapy and ethno-cultural issues.* The American Journal of Art Therapy, 30, 34-35.

Constantine, L.L. (1986). *Family paradigms: The practice of theory in family therapy.* NY: Guilford Press.

Di Leo, J. H. (1973). *Children's drawings as diagnostic aids.* NY: Brunner/Mazel.

24

Erickson, E. H. (1982). *The life cycle completed*. NY: W.W. Norton.

Gibbs, J. T., Huang, L.N. (1989). *Children of color*. San Francisco: Jossey-Bass Publishers.

Green, J. W. (1982). *Cultural awareness in the human services*. Englewood Cliffs, N.J.: Prentice-Hall.

Hammer, E.F. (1980). *The clinical application of projective drawings*. Springfield, Ill.: C. C. Thomas.

Hays, R.E., and Lyons, S.J. (1981). *The bridge drawing: A projective technique for assessment in art therapy*. The Arts in Psychotherapy. 8, 207-217.

Kramer, E. (1977). *Art therapy in a children's community*. NY: Schocken.

Kwiatkowska, H.Y. (1978). *Family therapy and evaluation through art*. Springfield, Ill.: C.C. Thomas.

Landgarten, H.B. (1987). *Family art psychotherapy: a clinical guide and casebook*. NY: Brunner/Mazel.

Levy, S. (1980). *The clinical application of projective drawings*. Projective Figure Drawing, Hammer (ed), Springfield, Ill.: C.C. Thomas.

McGoldrick, M. (1982). *Ethnicity and family therapy: An overview*. M. McGoldrick, J. K. Pearce and J. Giordano (eds). NY: Guilford Press.

Mirkin, M. P., Ricci, R. J. and Cohen, M .D. (1985). *A family and community systems approach to the brief psychiatric hospitalizations of adolescents*. Handbook of Adolescent and Family Therapy. Mirkin, S. and Koman, S. eds. NY: Gardner Press.

Nichols, W. C. & Everett, C. A. (1986). *Systemic family therapy*. NY: Guilford Press.

Oster, G. D. & Gould, P. (1987). *Using drawings in assessment and therapy*. NY: Brunner/Mazel.

Riley, S. (1985). *Draw me a paradox. Family art psychotherapy utilizing a systemic approach to change*. Art Therapy, 2(3), 116-123.

Riley, S. (1988). *Adolescence and family art therapy: Treating the "Adolescent Family" with family art therapy*. Art Therapy, 5(2), 43-51.

Wadeson, H. (1980). *Art psychotherapy*. NY: John Wiley & Sons.

Mask-Making: A Creative Approach with Adolescents in Distress
by Judy Leventhal, L.C.S.W.

Judy Leventhal, M.S.W, a licensed clinical social worker and marriage and family therapist, is an artist and therapist in private practice in Santa Monica who teaches and offers groups and private consultation. Currently she serves as creative arts therapy consultant for Angel's Flight, a Catholic Charities of Los Angeles shelter and Erikson Center for Adolescent Advancement. She exhibits her paintings and sculptures in and around Los Angeles and has exhibited her and her students' masks at the International Festival of Masks since 1984.

As a contemporary art form, mask-making is a powerful and therapeutic tool for working with adolescents in distress. In making their masks, they learn to explore their creativity, their problems and themselves.

Mask-making is the central feature of the creative arts program I offer runaway, homeless, and emotionally-distressed youth, which evolved out of a course initially designed for adults.

Mask-Making As A Therapeutic Tool

In 1982, I developed a mask course to guide adults into their own creative process as part of their personal and professional growth. Initially offered at a women's conference, I brought it to both UCLA Extension and Otis Art Institute/Parsons School of Design. The course is based on mask-making traditions as well as the psychology of creativity, conceptualized by psychoanalyst, Rollo May, in his book, *The Courage to Create.* May gave his support and permission to entitle the class after his book.

During mask-making, participants explore and renew their courage and sense of purpose, and apply their creativity toward addressing important junctures, central issues and transitions in their lives through a series of art activities. These activities include music, movement, mixed media and nature collage, mask making with clay and papier maché, and journal keeping. As part of the course, participants are invited to exhibit their masks and journal notes at the International Festival of Masks in Los Angeles, sponsored by The Craft and Folk Art Museum.

The Festival is an outdoor, grass roots event and includes a Parade of Masks, exhibits and performances. Artist Edith Wyle, founder of both the Museum and the Festival, realized in 1976 that the city had become an historic social experiment, with more than ninety-two various cultures living and working in Los Angeles. The Festival was envisioned to bring together cultural groups from around the city and the region, to celebrate their distinct roots, and to build bonds, networks, and common ground for a larger city-wide culture. Mask making became the unifying theme, since masks exist in every culture and historically are an integral part of traditions marking rites of passage throughout the life cycle. The masks that I display, created by course participants, mirror a moment in time, a blend of past experience, current events and future dreams in the life of their creator. Frequently the masks embody a complex mix of thoughts, feelings, and memories that a participant has not been able to convey adequately through words alone. Through journal notes, the mask makers share more about their own life transitions.

In 1991, I began creative arts programs for adolescents at Angel's Flight, a Catholic Charities of Los Angeles shelter for runaway and homeless youth. Shortly thereafter, I developed a similar program at The Erik and Joan Erikson Center for Adolescent Advancement, a program of the San Fernando Community Mental Health Center, a long-term residential treatment facility in Tarzana, California.

The creative arts offer the adolescents tools for self-empowerment, to reclaim their inner voice and vision for their future. Through mask-making, runaway, homeless and abused youth have learned to cope with their troubled lives. Among the profound issues and concerns they face are:

• Withdrawing from drugs

• Separating from an abusive parent

• Uncovering memories of childhood sexual, physical and mental abuse

• Exploring and reconciling suicidal thoughts and impulses

• Learning how to take responsibility and work through angry feelings

- Expressing and establishing identity through creative ability in art
- Articulating feelings and beliefs of powerlessness and despair.
- Moving away from gang activities and gang-related violence
- Developing relationships built on trust and collaboration
- Building a foundation of competence and accomplishment

These young people possess untapped, unrecognized inner resources for creativity. With the help of a safe, structured environment and artistic support, they are able to build a bridge between the creative life of the spirit and imagination and the realities of the responsibilities of the adult world.

While engaging adolescents in the creative arts, I have heard more about their deepest concerns. Some retreat back into wariness, hostility and despair; others begin to accept the complex and challenging circumstances of their lives. I feel a sense of gratitude for the opportunity of participating with them, as a guide, in their efforts to create meaning in their lives and prepare to enter the world of adult world responsibility.

Working With Adolescents In Distress

The young people with whom I work come from family backgrounds where there are histories of abuse and abandonment, early betrayals of their trust and innocence, drug and alcohol abuse, and physical and emotional abuse and neglect. They come from all parts of Los Angeles, from throughout the United States, and from Mexico, war-torn Central American countries, the Caribbean, Puerto Rico, and the Pacific islands. Often their families have experienced economic and cultural dislocation, the impact of racism, and poverty. They lack the educational and personal resources and the social networks necessary to manage effectively in highly complex and often turbulent urban areas.

The youth have developed survival skills. They are often hyper-alert, fearful of being hurt or left out; quick to react to or challenge authority. They have high internal standards for themselves and others. They have grown up with little structure, safety or support to practice small steps toward solid accomplishment. Often, they vacillate between an exaggerated sense of their own powers and abilities, and a sense of futility and feelings of inferiority. They have been hurt, and frequently are caught up in cycles of vengeance, engaging in hurtful expressions of anger, with temporary feelings of control and mastery, followed by periods of remorse, confusion and helplessness.

In their families, rules are unclear, rigid, inconsistent, or nonexistent; the atmosphere is tense; there is much anger and disappointment. Youth are often fearful and reluctant to explore their inner life. (Claudia Black, Double Duty, 1990.)

Frequently they share histories of sexual abuse, intense feelings of loneliness and isolation, and vague experiences of shame and loss. The complex truths and realities in their families are rarely acknowledged or openly addressed.

At a time when life would normally hold great promise, these young people are dealing with developmental issues beyond the usual challenges of adolescence. Many experiment with alcohol or drugs to numb their pain, to tolerate the companionship of others, or to allow for the expression of aggressive impulses. Others turn to gangs for a sense of structure, family and community.

In designing and facilitating creative arts programs, as an artist, a teacher, and a therapist, I assist my clients in bringing out their creative abilities and applying themselves toward dealing with the limits, challenges and circumstances of their lives. I guide them to tap internal resources they may not have been aware of, or had not had the opportunity to develop.

The immediate focus is to encourage each youngster to sift through events in their daily lives—and to look at their aspirations; how they want their world to be. This process supports both their immediate adaptation to shelter or residential life, and then the transition to a community placement or return to family. The group is designed to offer youth a safe place to deal with central issues in their lives.

Within the context of the art studio environment, youth are encouraged to experiment with a wide range of art supplies and natural materials that stimulate their imagination. They are guided to relax and focus their attention, to actively see with all their senses and, through the language of art, to record their experiences in their very own way. Every thread of initiative is supported as I respond to their requests for a particular color, brush, scissors, collage papers and other materials. I reflect back to them their natural sense of curiosity and wonder, and their enthusiasm for expressing themselves through art. When that enthusiasm and initiative is encouraged, the youth are better able to participate in the process of self-exploration and problem solving and to deal with their emotional pain.

Youth learn that creative work involves relationships based on mutual trust and collaboration. There is a balance between planned, well-organized art activities and opportunities for spontaneous improvisation. The adolescents are involved in learning to work within a system. There are guidelines, limits and ground rules. Agreements are made about the use and purpose of materials, tools and the physical space; they are expected to assist with setup and cleanup, and they need permission to leave the room. Although no explicit sexual or gang-related imagery is permitted, these elements do find symbolic expression in their work.

Throughout the sessions, they choose the level of their participation. There are times when they need to sit in solitude or say "no" to a particular activity. They find that creative work includes moments of frustration and that part of their job is to learn to manage themselves in ways that are safe and constructive.

Step by step they engage in the art activities and in the disciplines of the creative process. Awareness and insights emerge as they interact with the materials offered, work with their hands and give tangible shape and form to the content of their lives. They experience a growing sense of competence as they strengthen their identities as creators, actively participating in the process of shaping their own lives.

Angel's Flight

At the 1991 International Festival of Masks, I met Angel's Flight staff, who suggested that mask-making might be a useful activity for the young people at the shelter. They wanted an art therapy program that offered their young people an opportunity to complete an art project within their two or three week residence; a project that would instill a sense of self confidence in youth through the discipline and emotional commitment necessary to complete the work. They also wanted to offer them recognition and affirmation for their creative efforts and looked forward to exhibits to increase public awareness about the difficulties, challenges as well as the talents and potentials of runaway and homeless youth.

Angel's Flight was organized through Catholic Charities of Los Angeles to respond to the growing population of runaway and homeless youth in the city and the county. The agency provides a 16-bed, 21-day emergency shelter and a community outreach program for youth ages 10 through 17. Using a crisis intervention team approach, youth are assisted to strengthen their abilities to deal the immediate and difficult circumstances in their lives and develop a new perspective on the many challenges they face. From the time they enter the shelter, they are involved in learning social and group living skills, and in learning to exercise their capacities for constructive choice. Whenever possible, agency efforts are focused on strengthening family bonds and community networks of support. Youth are involved in learning to deal with complex issues and emotionally difficult choices and decisions, whether they return to their families or separate and move into short- or long-term placement or independent living programs.

To get a sense of my initial program at Angel's Flight, following are excerpts from my journal notes, centering on one very special young man:

Javier: Separating From An Abusive Parent

I bring a van load of art supplies—poster paints, chalks, bowls, brushes, oil pastels, poster board, magazines, scissors, glitter, fabric swatches, straw, and paste—and am greeted by seven youths sitting at a large table in the main room of the shelter. I introduce myself as an artist, and tell them that for next two and one half weeks, we will meet on Tuesday and Thursday afternoons, and that I will guide them in the art of mask-making. A staff person translates for those who understand only Spanish.

I ask them to tell a story about themselves, through their art: "Where are you in your life today? How do you want your world to be?" Javier, 14, draws a black oval shape and, inside, puts a red brown spot. He shares, "I'm depressed, I got here at one a.m., I'm bored." I gently encourage him to continue; he draws a shelter, "This is where I am now." He shares that he is very angry. "I shouldn't have done that," expressing remorse for an unspecified act. Although curious, I refrain from verbal exploration; I want him to stay focused on his art. He quickly makes a little doll out of fabric and straw and wants to stick pins in it, adding "Just kidding." He talks about returning to school and his swim team.

In the next session I introduce lots of natural materials: desert and beach sand, pebbles, small red rocks, dried flowers, grasses, leaves, small twigs, sea shells, seed pods, assorted fabrics, paints, chalks and blotter paper to revitalize their senses, their connection with the world of nature that surrounds us, and their creative spirit.

With fabric, paint and blotter paper, Javier builds a body form. He adds desert sand, red rock, and dried flowers; the arms are outstretched, the legs firmly planted—a red brown rock man appears. Javier shares, "This is my spirit!"

At the third session, Javier and the other adolescents are eager to start their masks. I tell them that in many cultures, masks are made to call upon creative forces for health, protection, guidance, abundance and knowledge. I show how to prepare an armature by covering a plastic bowl with tin foil and placing it upside down on an 18 by 24 inch masonite board, also covered with foil. (For detailed mask-making instructions, see appendix.) I place three

32

twenty-five pound bags of clay and a bowl of water next to Javier. I tell the group to "Think about what you want to release from your life, who you are angry at, scared of, what hurts inside. Call upon your inner guide and imagine your hopes and dreams, and how you want to shape your life."

Javier declares, "I want this to be big, I have trouble with anger!" I encourage him to give shape and form to the depths of his feelings. Clay is a flexible and forgiving medium. It can be pushed, pulled and pounded and allows for the release of intense feelings of frustration in an immediate way.

As he piles the clay over the armature, Javier quietly reveals more about a family history of violence and his father's drinking and abuse. Javier has been in many placements. He works steadily, using seventy-five pounds of clay. He is proud of the results and tired. He covers his mask with saran wrap to keep it moist.

His clay image serves as a mold, and will be transformed into a papier maché mask. We shred long narrow strips of newsprint, soaking them in a paste solution. Building sturdy, durable masks requires five layers of papier maché. Javier works in steady spurts and arrangements are made for him to continue over the weekend, with staff support.

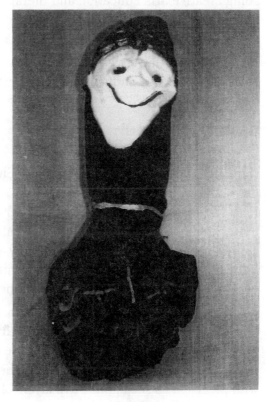

In the last session, Javier applies white gesso as an undercoat to the dry papier maché mask that he has carefully lifted off the clay mold. He paints the lower face dark grey with bits of copper; the mouth, red; the large eyes, dull turquoise. He is preparing to move on to a group home the next morning. At the end of the class, I ask the students in the group to lend their masks to the shelter for exhibits. Javier likes that and agrees to work late into the evening to complete his piece and write a journal note.

Fig. 1 Disturbed

He paints the elongated upper face white, lips, red, deep set eyes, dark blue with a light blue and bronze cap on top (Fig. 1). My immediate impression is that he has depicted himself, with a tentative smile, slowly rising above his father. His powerful mask is accompanied by his equally powerful journal:

> Disturbed
> *This piece took me a week and a half to make. I was inspired by my emotions…I have been feeling very depressed and…you can see the depressed features and you can tell that his face expresses a sign of confusion. My piece was also influenced by my emotional frustration…At times I've felt very disturbed; and through art I can express myself instead of keeping it to myself.*
> Javier

Javier has given tangible shape and form to a complex mix of thoughts and feelings in his mask. He has experienced moments of joy and a glimpse of his strengths and capacities to sort through and release his anger, constructively, rather than on impulse.

Based on the success of the initial class, I continued to develop an ongoing creative arts education and therapy program, now part of a federally funded program for substance abuse prevention with homeless and runaway youth.

The following are vignettes of youth who, in the process of creating their masks, experienced shifts in their perspectives on the many challenges they face.

Celeste: Her Divided Self

Celeste, 15, has been crying. She shares that she and her mother go through cycles. "We don't get along!" She says she has run away several times. "There are two parts to me; a very sad part and a happy part," she says. I suggest that she draw these parts of herself; she quickly draws a self portrait with a line down the center of the image. She adds, with urgency, "I am a deep person, I want to understand myself better!" I suggest that in very difficult situations, people often have conflicting thoughts and feelings and I encourage Celeste to carry the theme from her drawing into a mask.

She selects a round bowl for an armature, and begins to work with clay. She sculpts a deep groove between the left and right sides of her thick round clay mask; she shapes a sun and a smile on the left side; and on the right, she sculpts tears and struggles to get the mouth just right. Celeste works with precision as she applies five layers of papier maché over the clay mold. After her mask is dry, I help her remove it from the clay. Celeste paints her mask white, the deep groove, black; the left side has a bright yellow sun and a red smile; the right side has dark blue tears and a down turned red mouth (Fig. 2). Showing pride in what she has accomplished, she writes:

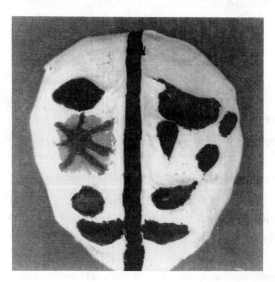

Fig. 2 Celeste's conflicted mask

Smile Now, Cry Later

The side with the sun is for happiness, for example when I'm at the beach or with friends. The other side is for sadness. The tears are for pain and hurt, from the death of a close friend and membe of my family. Celeste

In making her mask showing her inner split, a deep groove down the center of the image, Celeste brings parts of herself into direct relationship with one another. The groove bears information and acts as a bridge between her separate parts. She volunteers that she feels clearer and stronger inside. She is more fully aware of what she wants and needs; less apt to split off her thoughts from her feelings and actions. She is able to talk more openly with her mother about her need for affection and her need to grow and be on her own. As she becomes clearer inside, she is better prepared to deal with her own hurt and anger, and more willing to make conscious decisions about her future.

Carmen: Dealing with Death, Embracing Life

In the art studio today, the youngsters are wary, tense, sullen and subdued. I have brought lots of collage materials including textures of sandpapers, wire mesh, charcoal, and swatches of velvet and other silky, soft fabrics. I direct them to explore the rough and smooth areas of their lives with these materials. The group works quietly and intently, putting some graffiti markings into their collages, in a layered effect with sand and origami papers. Carmen, 17, approaches me and whispers, "I want to make a mask; I see a mask of death in my mind!" Carmen has seen a lot of death in her homeland, Nicaragua. Since coming to this country, she has made a number of suicide attempts, has been hospitalized twice, and has worked closely with her therapist on her self-destructive patterns.

35

In the next session, I start with music, a tape of contemporary ballads from Central America, and add reggae from Jamaica and ask everyone to draw from their imagination, to the rhythms and melody. There is intense focus. The group enjoys drawing and the youth are now ready to work with clay. Carmen sculpts an image of death, with deep-set eyes, teeth that jut out, indented cross bones on the chin, and a cross on the forehead, with a deep curved shape that frames the facial features.

Carmen requests clay and papier maché to work with over the weekend, "to deal with what is on my mind." When I see her the following Monday, her mask is complete; the image is compelling and her papier maché construction is sturdy. She is pleased, then wavers, comparing herself to others, "I don't like what I did." I tell her she showed a great deal of courage to explore the issue of death and form such a clear and forceful image.

The art studio is a place that offers safety and support for youth to explore their deepest thoughts and feelings about central issues in their lives, without requests for analysis. My focus is to offer constructive ways to deal with suicidal thoughts and impulses through the non-verbal language of art. Carmen decides to paint her mask on her own. At our next art session, she shows me her work (Fig. 3). The deep-set eyes are painted black with dots of green at the centers. The face is bright white and there are bold accents of red all around. I encourage her to write a journal note to go with her mask. Carmen writes:

Death

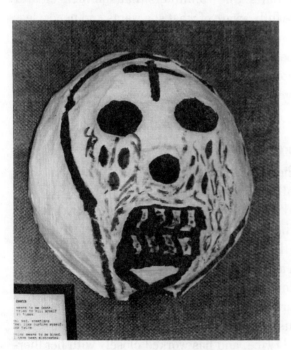

This mask means to me death, because I tried to kill myself more than 20 times. When I feel sad, sometimes I still feel like hurting myself, but I think twice. The red color means to me blood, because I have been mistreated. The black color means to me darkness and emptiness inside my body. White means to me the color of the mask. White is the color that can reflect other color.

Carmen

Fig. 3 Carmen portrays her image of death

This art activity has given Carmen a constructive way to shape and form her raw pain, communicating her sense of despair. In the process of creating her mask, her energy shifts. She takes pride in her work, a sign that she has hopes for her future. Carmen will remain at the shelter for the next three months until she turns eighteen. Although at times she talks of suicide, she does not make an attempt. The care and commitment of the Angel's Flight staff has helped her believe in her future. She is now focused on finding work, a place to live and a dream of completing her high school education.

Francisco: Strengthening His Commitment To Stay Off Drugs

Francisco, 15, in his first art session, focuses on making a flag of Mexico. He slowly cuts wide strips of red, white, and green tissue paper, carefully gluing each strip to poster board. He is pleased with his efforts; I help him hang his flag above a doorway in the main room.

At the next session, Francisco is having a difficult day. He is restless, irritable, disruptive; picking fights and asking for lots of attention and reassurance. Our challenge is to help him redirect his energy, explore his deeper issues and to learn to manage himself.

Today, I am teaching the adolescents how to work on clay masks and invite Francisco to participate. Staff assist in translation. Francisco immediately responds in Spanish, "Drugs are the demon; I want to make a mask of the Drug Demon!" Francisco has lots of energy. He quickly sculpts a clay mask, wrapping the clay in saran wrap to keep it moist, before he starts the papier maché. It's just about time to end the class. Francisco rushes to apply his first layer of papier maché.

Over the weekend, he helps others clean the multi-purpose room and places his mask outside in the sun, where it dries and cracks. At our next session, I tell him it is unworkable and he will need to start over. Willingly, he quickly sculpts another clay mask, wraps it in saran wrap and slaps large, wide strips of papier maché over the clay. This time I'm firm with him about the requirements of the materials, telling him how important it is to work slowly and carefully. I appeal to his sense of pride and desire for quality and remove the papier maché layers he has just applied. Francisco pours out his frustration to a staff person who listens patiently. I join them and ask staff to let Francisco know that frustration is a necessary part of the creative process. They know that Francisco is experiencing another frustration—withdrawing from marijuana and glue, which he used daily on the streets. Francisco regroups, returns to his work, and slowly applies three layers of papier maché, molding the wet narrow strips of paper into the contours of the wet clay mask.

37

At our next session, he is eager to paint. He selects black, bronze, red and ultra- marine blue. With a flourish, he quickly paints his mask and adds a red feather. He writes a journal note about his work, struggling in Spanish. He asks another staff person to help him. While he writes, she translates his words into English.

Francisco is pleased. He has demonstrated the power of choice and self-responsibility, both to himself and to staff, in the process of creating his mask. He has exercised his will, sustained his sense of purpose and shown his competence. From a developmental perspective, these are important steps in early intervention with adolescents who have issues with substance abuse. The staff has stood by him

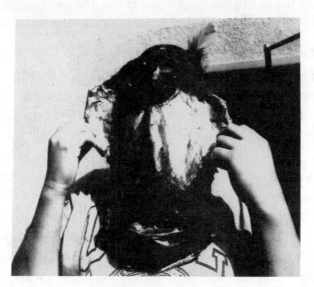

Fig. 4 Francisco's image of drug withdrawal

without attempting to rescue, with the expectation that he could work through his frustrations, and he has begun to blossom. He writes:

Drug Withdrawal

This mask is my crazy imagination...this is the reason...this mask shows a nervous reaction for the need for drugs; and wanting to use drugs. Each color shows how I was feeling.   Francisco

Jason: Exploring His Sense Of Powerlessness

Jason, 17, is invited to make a mask; to address what hurts, what he is angry, sad or scared about, and to bring into focus his aspirations for his future. He responds with enthusiasm and devotes an entire session to sculpting, continually smoothing over the surface of the clay until an image emerges. He sculpts a tear drop on the corner of the left eye and struggles about whether or not to sculpt a mouth. After encouragement to trust his instincts, he decides the mask will have no mouth.

In the next session, he carefully applies five layers of papier maché. He is eager to paint his mask, but he is leaving to complete a sentence on assault charges at a youth detention center. Another shelter resident agrees to paint the mask, provided he gives her explicit directions. Jason does a paint sketch of what he wants, and adds written directions (Fig. 5). I encourage him to write a journal note.

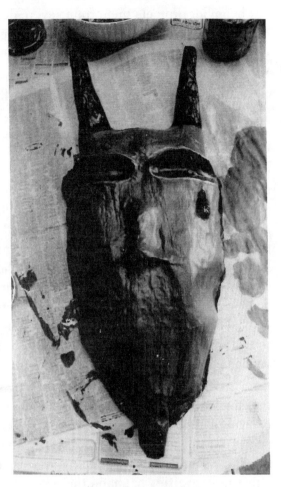

Fig. 5 Jason's mask of powerlessness

The meaning of this mask is about how I feel when I am being viewed from the outside, what/how other people see me. The tear represents my true feelings and no mouth represents that I have nothing to say in what people think of me.
Jason

In his brief shelter stay, Jason has brought into focus his view of himself and the world. As he identifies and accepts his sense of power- lessness, he exercises new choices and explores new pos- sibilities.

The Erikson Center

The Erikson Center, a program of the San Fernando Valley Community Mental Health Center, is a long-term, residential treatment facility for seriously disturbed adoles- cents. This 66-bed facility specializes in working with adolescents from ages 14 to 17 with backgrounds of severe emotional and physical abuse and neglect, who have gotten into trouble in their communities and in other placements. An open setting, the Center offers youngsters an alternative to a corrections facility, juvenile hall or mental hospital. Placements are court-ordered. Agency efforts are focused on education and habilitation, and on assisting youth to develop previously unrecognized potential.

From a developmental perspective, the goal is to help youth relearn the first steps in trusting themselves and their capacities to form mutually caring relationships, and to help them strengthen their sense of will and learn to exercise capacities for choice and self control throughout each day's activities.

Erikson Center clients have experienced profound loss. Their acting out behavior protects them from severe depression. Initially, they tend to express wariness and hostility to protect themselves from further hurt. They test the limits and parameters of each new relationship. The work has been very challenging.

The program philosophy is based on the pioneering work of psychoanalyst Erik Erikson and artist Joan Erikson. Their theory of human development examines what central strengths emerge in each period of life, when things go well. The theory, drawing from the fields of biology, cultural anthropology, and psychology, is based on the premise that eight basic strengths emerge as we go through life, each "the outgrowth of a time of specific developmental confrontation. Where a strength is not adequately developed according to the given sequence for its scheduled period of critical resolution, the supports of the environment may bring it into appropriate balance at a later period," (Joan Erikson, Wisdom and the Senses, 1988, p.74). The Eriksons collaborated in establishing treatment programs for young adults and adolescents at Austen Riggs, a private hospital in Stockbridge, Massachusetts, where they worked from 1951 through 1971. In their approach, the role of the arts and of psychotherapy were given equal weight in assisting young people in their recovery and growth.

In *Identity, Youth, and Crises,* Erik Erikson describes adolescence as a time to consolidate earlier stages of development; to incorporate new physical energies and sexual powers; to learn what is involved in being male or female and to develop a unified sense of self. The overall strength that emerges is fidelity, a sense of loyalty to one's own values, and confidence and competence in capacities to shape the present and commit to future roles and responsibilities.

Adolescence is a time of turbulence, exploration and struggle. The contrary pull is toward identity diffusion, with a sense of inner fragmentation, an interruption in capacities to concentrate and complete tasks—commitments are avoided. Erikson observes that the community often underestimates how long and intricate childhood history has restricted youth in their choices of identity. Youth engage in delinquent patterns of behavior or become mental patients when they sense no hope for a positive future or to gain a moratorium from responsibilities to which they are not yet ready to commit.

Their loss of a sense of self is often expressed in disdain for roles offered as constructive or desirable by family or community, in partial identification with those who have been most harmful and influential, and in identities based on their beliefs in their own badness.

Joan Erikson, throughout her career, has focused on developing ways to expose emotionally disturbed youth to creative activities, to encourage their recovery and growth. At Austen Riggs and more recently at Mount Zion Hospital in San Francisco and in San Francisco City Schools, she has observed that psychiatry has taken a long time to acknowledge the role of communality and activity in the recovery and growth of individuals; that participation in the arts restores one's sense of active and creative participation in life as a whole.

Erikson's model Art Activities Program was conceptualized on the premise that everything done in the Basic Workshop is therapeutic; the word "therapy" is left out. In the workshop, youth are trusted with tools and know that they are trusted. Rules and regulations for the management of the shop involve a patients' activities committee, which also participates in planning the activities. Teaching and learning involve a contract; all parties come to an agreement as to what is to be accomplished and how all will benefit from fulfilling the contract. Consistent with her perception that agencies need to be prepared to give special recognition and support to client's developmental potential, at the Erikson Center, the variety of planned activities, guided by artist consultants who are uninterested in diagnostic classifications, can offer remarkable insights.

Following are journal notes that highlight the participation of youth at the Erikson Center, who worked through moments of inevitable frustration in completing their mask work. These adolescents present a host of different challenges—they are not able to manage themselves, they are frequently hostile and many have backgrounds of assaultive behavior. While the pace is more gradual than Angel's Flight, the work is as intense. They initially express enthusiasm for an art activity, then moments later experience frustration which they express as either disdain for further involvement or despair, with a decision to stop. I am alert to these trends and assist them in regrouping and refocusing. They appreciate the support in standing by them in their frustration and assisting them, gently yet firmly, to persist and work through their anxiety and frustration.

Dionne: Celebrating Her Cultural Roots

Dionne, the first to arrive, helps me unload the van and arrange assorted drawing, collage, and origami papers, magazines, oil pastels, glitter, bowls of small sea shells, beads, poster paints, brushes and paste, all around the art studio. Nine more adolescents file in quietly and are warmly greeted by the staff of two. All take seats at counter space or at the round center table. I introduce myself as an artist; the mood is cautious, tense, reserved. I tell them that we will be on a journey together during the next four weeks; that we will explore the art materials, the life of the imagination, and learn about one another. Next week, we will start making masks.

With sheets of newsprint fastened to the counter and table tops, we begin. I ask each person to choose two oil pastel colors, one for each hand, and to draw to the rhythm of the music—reggae tapes. With dark brown oil pastels, Dionne draws a sturdy tree trunk and exclaims, "That's ugly!" She switches to lettering the name of a friend from stencils, then splatters paint over the stencil and paper. Now she is having fun.

At the second session I add the more natural materials: dry leaves and grasses, textures of earth, small branches, fresh spring flowers, and large sheets of blotter paper, asking them to create collages out of these materials. Dionne draws a series of snow-capped mountain forms and arranges beach sand, shells, flowers, and desert sage on blotter paper, adding a perimeter of blue paint. She studies masks I've brought, made by adult students from my private practice.

Next time, Dionne carefully builds a large, thick clay mask, over a square bowl armature. She sculpts the eyes, large and round; the nose, flat and wide; the mouth, thick and broad. She genuinely smiles as she works in silence and wraps her clay mask in saran wrap to keep the surface moist. Next session, she applies a layer of papier maché over her entire mask and announces that she is done. I validate her effort thus far and suggest that to be strong and durable, the mask will need four more layers of papier maché. She lets me know she is finished for the day and leaves.

At our next session, I wanted to offer the young people a constructive way to focus their energies. Many grew up in South Central Los Angeles, where civil unrest began this week, following the Rodney King verdict in Simi Valley. I want to somehow convey to them the importance of having a positive and meaningful say in their own futures. On impulse, I bring them flowers. Dionne quickly puts the flowers into a vase and asks to take them with her after class. She adds that she loves to garden and knows how to grow tomatoes. I share with the class that the day after the verdict, I worked downtown, near the civil unrest. I ask what they think and feel about what is going on in the city right now. I ask them to put their thoughts and feelings into their art.

42

Everyone works. Dionne designs an African-American flag, skillfully applying strips of red, black and green paint onto a large piece of blotter paper. She playfully dips her hands into the paint bowls and covers another sheet of paper with her hand prints. She also adds more layers of papier maché to her mask and returns to her unit, carrying the vase of flowers.

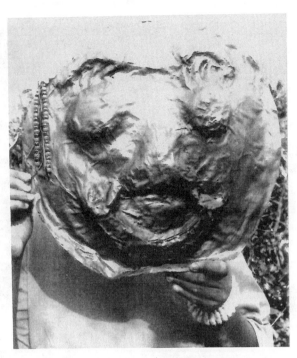

Fig. 6 Dionne chooses not to write a journal note.

Step by step, Dionne works to finish her mask; she applies a coat of black acrylic over black gesso and asks for beads for the hair. At the closing session, she greets me in the parking lot and admires the black and red-brown beads I've brought. She decides to repaint, working burnt umber over the black satiny color. The mouth becomes dark red; the eyes remain black. A white lace bow and beads are added to the hair (Fig. 6). She has softened the mood of her mask considerably. She is shy and, with coaxing, agrees to pose for a photograph with her mask. She likes the color print that I give her to acknowledge her and her work.

Julie: Sharing A Dilemma About Her Special Friend

Julie focuses quietly throughout the art sessions. She begins carefully, and in her initial collage, works with small white sea shells, beach sand and paint, forming the words, "I love you." She volunteers that she is enjoying herself.

In the second session, she arranges small twigs into the shape of the words, "Be Happy," surrounding these letters with blue chalk. She adds the words, "Don't Worry," and paints a colorful heart shape. She selects a round bowl as an armature, and builds a thick, clay mask with small, round eyes, tiny nostrils; the mouth is slightly heart-shaped and wide open. As she begins to work with papier maché, I observe that she is rushing and I encourage her

43

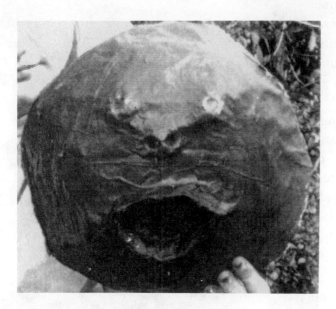

Fig. 7 Julie's friend, Fred

to slow down for the best results. Julie paints the surface of her mask bright lemon yellow; the round eyes, blue; the mouth, crimson red (Fig. 7). She writes a journal note:

Fred is the name of my special (mask) friend. I can talk to him whenever I want, and he will listen to me and not laugh at me. My friend has a big mouth, but never talks to me. That's what pisses me off. I want him to talk to me.
Julie

Mark: Revealing and Containing His Wild Side

At first, Mark is tense and hesitant, sharing that he does not know how to draw. He quickly switches to stencils, tracing a snow flake. During the next session, he continues to struggle and asks for a ruler, "I can't draw a straight line!" I encourage him to scribble with oil pastels, using both hands, as he listens to reggae music. He asks for paint and wants me to select the colors— "any colors." I suggest orange and red; he adds black and purple and paints a series of angles and lines on blotter paper, working tentatively, carefully and slowly. He is moving through his uncertainty.

Mark likes working with clay and builds his mask over an oblong shaped bowl. Absorbed in his work, he repeatedly smooths over the surface of the clay as he shapes the facial features. There is a delicate quality to his work. He carefully applies layers of papier maché. As he prepares to paint his mask, he slowly applies an undercoat of black gesso, then adds white and alizarin crimson. We mix an orange-red-violet color for the mouth.

The mask is cohesive and the image is strong; he is pleased (Fig. 8). Only when I ask him to write a journal note, do I learn that he reverses most of his letters. He asks Julie to type what he writes:

(This) face is a wild, and crazy face, that I somehow formed out of a ball of clay. I say it's wild and crazy, because I'm wild; I don't know

44

about crazy, but I'm very wild. Me and my face have a lot in common; We share everything, including secrets. Mark

Exhibits As Therapeutic Tools

Exhibits are part of the creative and therapeutic process. Adolescents' self-confidence and self-respect are strengthened as they receive recognition and appreciation of their creative efforts.

At the Erikson Center, the students and I carefully arranged the masks in the main reception area, where they are seen by staff and visitors. The tone of the reception area has been tangibly changed—the potential of the youth is made visual, as is their pain. The youth experience their ability to have a positive impact on their environment.

At Angel's Flight, the work of the adolescents attracts the

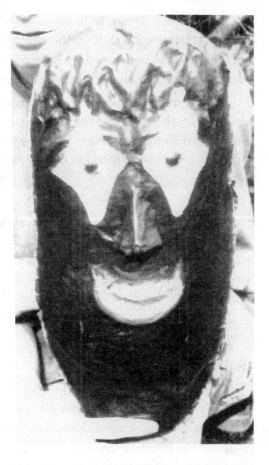

Fig. 8 Mark's wild and crazy face

attention of the Craft and Folk Art Museum and is featured at the 1992 International Festival of Masks. Both former and current shelter residents volunteer their time in the Angel's Flight exhibit booth and share more about their masks with Festival attendees. The exhibit at the Festival and the adolescents participation in the on-going art classes are featured in the Los Angeles Times.

From my journal notes, it is clear that for these young people, a bridge to the adult world of responsibility has been formed:

Jason: Jason was allowed to attend the festival from the honor camp where he was completing his sentence. He watches closely as others view his work; he has softened. He tells me he is working as a cook for other boys at the camp and that he has received good feedback on his cooking skills.

45

Today, he is receiving validation for his efforts to reveal his views about himself and his world.

Carmen: Carmen tells me she is working as a cashier for a fast food chain on the evening shift so she can complete her high school studies during the day. She is dressed up in honor of her participation in the festival. She is mindful that she will need to return to work by mid-afternoon.

Festival-goers: Festival-goers are moved by the exhibit; some feel overwhelmed by the raw emotion contained in the masks and share more about their own difficult histories. Inspired, energized and deeply moved by the intensity, color and directness of the youths' work, some look on in silence.

In the spring of 1993, by invitation from the City of Santa Monica's Ken Edwards Center for Community Services, Angel's Flight exhibits the adolescents' masks for six weeks. The mask work and personal notes of thirty former and current residents are displayed. A reception is held to honor the mask makers and provide a forum for runaway and homeless youth to share their life experiences with the community. Their work is featured in *another* article in the Los Angeles Times. As part of the exhibit, several youth demonstrate how to make a mask. The adolescents respond positively to the recognition they receive.

Conclusion

Mask-making is a powerful and therapeutic tool for working with runaway, homeless and emotionally distressed adolescents. Step by step, as they engage in mask making with clay and papier maché, they explore the disciplines of the creative process. They learn that creative work involves relationships based on mutual trust and collaboration and they learn to apply themselves to the many challenges in their lives. Through their participation youth strengthen their sense of trust and hope, and exercise their capacities to explore their inner thoughts and feelings. Awareness and insights emerge as they interact with the variety of materials offered and work with their hands.

As they begin to work with clay, images emerge from inside that are surprising and at times startling. They are encouraged to explore these powerful images and experience their courage as these image are developed. Through the process of building sturdy masks with layers of papier maché over the clay molds, they continue to sort through a complex mix of inner thoughts and feelings.

Each mask tells a story—a blend of past experience, current events and future dreams. Through mask-making, youth give tangible shape and form to their deepest concerns and this is what is at the heart of the artistic creative process.

Exhibits are an important part of the therapeutic mask-making process. Exhibiting their work is a way to honor and acknowledge the youth for their creative efforts. The concerns they share through their masks are concerns that touch us all. The mask is a bridge to what matters deeply.

Appendix

How to Make a Mask

Step 1: To prepare the armature, cover an 18" x 24" masonite board with aluminum foil. Cover the outside of an 8" round or 12" oblong bowl with aluminum foil and place the bowl, upside down, on top of the masonite board.

Step 2: Have on hand two or three 25-pound bags of soft moist clay. Using your hands, apply a layer of clay over the armature and build up the clay until you've used at least 12 1/2 pounds of clay. This forms the clay mold. I recommend using a full 25-pound of clay for the mold.

Step 3: The features of the mask can now either be carved into the clay or more clay can be added on to build up the features. This process takes time—allow at least one hour. As you interact with the clay, images will spontaneously emerge. The clay can be pushed, pulled or pounded and worked and reworked until the image is satisfying to you, emotionally and aesthetically.

Step 4: Carefully cover the clay mask with saran wrap to keep the clay soft and moist. Apply saran wrap to the detailed contours of the clay mask so the saran wrap is molded to the features. Leave an ample amount of saran wrap at the edges of the clay mask.

Step 5: To prepare the papier maché, hand-tear long, narrow strips of newspaper and leave the edges rough. For glue, I recommend methycellulose paste (brand name "Archivart") which is archival and non-toxic and widely used for book-binding. It is available at fine art stores. The paste comes in powder form. To mix, work with a clean, clear plastic bowl with an airtight lid. Fill the bowl with ice cold purified water. Mix paste according to the directions on the package—adding the powder 1 tablespoon at a time, for a total of 3 tablespoons to 4 cups ice cold water. Stir intermittently until thick—about 10 minutes. Spoon a little paste into a clean bowl and add purified water to thin it down to the consistency of thick cream. Soak newspaper strips in this mixture.

Note: A one-pound jar of paste powder will yield 6 to 7 gallons of paste. A mask of average size uses about 1 quart of paste.

Step 6: Apply one layer of paste-soaked strips over the saran-wrapped clay mask. Work carefully and slowly, molding the papier maché to the contours of the mask. The mask takes on a different form as the features are amplified through sculpting with papier maché. I recommend 5 layers of papier maché to create a strong mask. This process can take 3-5 hours, depending on the size of the mask.

Step 7: Let the clay and papier maché mask dry for about 5 days. Store in an airy, dry place. Do not place the mask to dry in direct sunlight or in a car trunk. The drying process can be aided by using a hand-held hair dryer.

Step 8: Once the mask is dry, the papier maché can be removed from the clay mold. The papier maché will be bonded to the saran wrap, preventing it from sticking to the clay. Carefully lift the papier maché off the clay, starting with the outside edges of the saran wrap.

Step 9: Apply a coat of white or black gesso to the papier maché mask and let the gesso dry thoroughly.

Step 10: The mask is now ready to be painted. I recommend an assortment of high-grade acrylic paint or high-grade poster paints. A well-rounded palette will include ivory black, titatium white, alizarin crimson, cadmium red light, cadmium yellow light, pthalo blue, ultramarine blue, raw and burnt sienna, raw and burnt umber, bronze, and silver.

The resulting mask is museum quality—a point I emphasize to the adolescents. I use archival paste for several reasons: the mask will have a long life, withstand variations in temperature and humidity, and can be reshaped.

Critical to the development and success of these creative arts therapy programs has been the support and enthusiasm of key individuals associated with each facility. The author wishes to express her appreciation especially to Heidi Amundson, L.C.S.W., Director of Angel's Flight, and to Gary Crouppen,Ph.D., Clinical Services Director of the San Fernando Valley Community Mental health Center, Inc., for their enthusiasm and support.

References

Alkema, C. (1971). *Masks*. NY: Sterling.

Arnheim, R. (1969). *Visual thinking*.Berkeley: University of California Press
————(1966). *Towards a psychology of art*. Los Angeles:University of California Press.

Baranski, M. (1954). *Mask-making*. Massachusetts: Davis Press.

Black, C. (1990). *Double duty*. NY: Ballantine.

Blakley, R. (1978). *African masks.* NY: St. Martin Press.

Chastang, C. (1992). *Unmasking the hurt.* Los Angeles Times View section, Oct. 7th.

Cordry, D. (1980). *Mexican masks.* Austin: University of Texas Press.

Edwards, B. (1979). *Drawing On the right side of the brain.* Los Angeles: Tarcher.

Erikson, E. (1968). *Identity, youth, and crises.* NY: W W. Norton.
————(1986). *Childhood and society.* NY: W.W. Norton.

Erikson, J. (1976). *Activity, recovery, growth: the communal role of planned activities.* NY: W. W. Norton.
————(1988) *Wisdom and the senses: the way of creativity.* NY: W. W. Norton.

Goulding, M. (1979) *Changing lives through redecision therapy.* NY: Grove Press.

Hirabayashi, B. (1993). *Unmasking emotions.* Los Angeles Times Westside Section, May 20th.

Jung, C. G. (1959). *Four archetypes.* NJ: Princeton University Press.
————(1966). *Man and his symbols.* NY: Dell.

Kiebert, C. (1982). *All of a sudden.* Santa Cruz: Sentient Systems.

Kandinsky, W. (1977). *Concerning the spiritual in art.* NY: Donner.

Kramer, E. (1971). *Art as therapy with children.* NY: Schocken.

Levin, P. (1988). *Cycles of power.* Florida: Health Communications.

Lippard, L. R. (1983). *Overlay: contemporary art and the art of prehistory.* NY: Pantheon.
————(1990). *Mixed blessings: new art in a multicultural world.* NY: Pantheon.

Lommel, A. (1970). *Masks: their meaning and function.* NY: Excalibur.

May, R. (1976). *The courage to create.* NY: Bantam.
————(1972). *Power and innocence.* NY: Delta.
————(1968). *The meaning of anxiety.* NY: Bantam.

Miller, A. (1984). *Thou shalt not be aware: society's betrayal of the child.* NY: Farrar-Straus-Giroux.

Oaklander, V. (1978). *Windows to our children.* Utah: Real People Press.

Rank, O. (1932). *Art and the artist.* NY: Alfred A. Knopf.

Rogers, C. (1961). *On becoming a person.* Boston: Houghton Mifflin.

Segy, L. (1976). *Masks of black Africa.* NY: Donner.

Sivin, C. (1986). *Mask making.* MA: Davis.

Wherry, J. (1969). *Indian masks and myths of the west.* NY: Funk & Wagnalls.

Art Making at a Probation Camp
by Anne Nathan-Wlodarski, M.A., A.T.R.

Anne Nathan-Wlodarski is the founder and executive director of HEARTWORLD, a non-profit arts center for abused and underprivileged children. She holds master's degrees in behavioral psychology and art therapy and is a professional artist, exhibiting her work in the Los Angeles area. Ms. Nathan-Wlodarski is an educational outreach coordinator for the Los Angeles Cultural Affairs department and curatorial assistant at their ARTSPACE Gallery.

Introduction

In spring of 1992 the nation was forced to listen to the voices of the inner city. Through the smoke and broken glass of riot-torn America, we were forced to react to the obvious and unmistakable reminder that many Americans lead lives not of their own choosing. For a moment, we ceased comparing the less fortunate with the fortunate, and were acutely aware that a major problem could no longer be ignored.

Today, we lie at the crossroads of great change. The choice lies in how to heal ourselves and how to stop the escalating violence. At the core of the issue are those who perpetrate the crimes which threaten the functioning of our society. Are they victims of the society they punish? Violence can no longer be treated solely as a law enforcement issue, but rather must be addressed as an epidemic which affects each and every one of us.

In a world filled with pain, abuse, and neglect, many children live in fear, denied the right to imagine, create and express feelings that have been locked inside. Unable to grow with hope for a better future, and be nourished by understanding and love, they have become prisoners without the necessary means to escape. They are victims who oftentimes victimize. They are already behind veritable bars by the time they enter society, bars created by dysfunction and hopelessness.

Communities must begin to address violence at its core, by targeting the beginnings of societal turmoil and by developing specific ways and means of breaking the cycles of violence into which certain populations are born. Many of society's ills—gang violence, drug abuse, teen pregnancy, suicide and AIDS can be attributed to child abuse and neglect.

Nationwide statistics tell a grim tale of the effects of child abuse. The National Center for Child Abuse and Neglect estimates that ninety-seven percent of the individuals incarcerated for violent crimes were victims of child abuse. Further, those who abuse others were most likely abused at one time in their lives. Incidents of child abuse have increased over 250 percent in the past ten years, with reports of child sexual abuse in the state of California increasing at the alarming rate of over 1,000 percent during the same period.

Due to the growing numbers of reported cases of abuse and neglect, facilities face increasing difficulties in providing these young victims with anything more than basic needs. They have little time or money to expose these children to the necessary healing processes. This vicious cycle will not be broken until the level of concern, evidenced by both community support and involvement as well as financial assistance, is met.

Those behind bars, particularly the growing number of incarcerated adolescents, must be given the opportunity to break out of the cycle of abuse and become healthy, functioning members of society. Art therapy provides a positive way to address the causes of violence by providing a creative outlet for anger and frustration, and by increasing self-awareness.

Literature Review

An article by Day and Onorato (1989) states, "The world of art therapy has scarcely penetrated the walls of correctional facilities." I was unable to find any other material which specifically dealt with art therapy in a jail setting or a probation facility. However, I found one book (Brandreth, 1972) related to the subject. *Created in Captivity* discusses art-making (rather than art therapy) with prison inmates. Brandreth suggests that because prison inmates have time on their hands, they turn to the creative arts. He feels that art can be the antidote for boredom. Since prisoners are cut off from commercial entertainment and the everyday distractions of domestic life, it is natural that they should take advantage of the opportunities and materials provided inside, even though they might not choose to do so on the outside.

52

Brandreth states, "Even those who protest their contempt for anything vaguely artistic, can be persuaded to take an active interest, simply by example. They see their colleagues getting pleasure out of something unexpected, and they decide, because they've got nothing to lose, that it might be worth their while to investigate. The desire to create exists in all; the ability to create is dormant in many; the opportunity to create is denied to the majority in the present structure of society. Incarceration does not engender creativity of itself; it simply provides the time, the materials and the guidance in the form of instructors and craftsmen."

Oaklander (1969) suggests that the troubled adolescent has introjected many faulty messages. He has feelings of loneliness, fear, and anxiety which he finds difficult to share. He needs help in learning how to express these feelings.

Setting

This Los Angeles county probation facility was formed in the 1950s as a forestry camp, nestled in a woody setting of the Santa Monica mountains. It was later converted into a probation facility for juvenile boys. There are twenty camps in all which house some 2,000 wards from the ages of twelve through eighteen. The ethnic makeup of the camps is seventy percent Hispanic, twenty percent African-American, and ten percent Caucasian.

The wards are all felons, having committed burglary, armed robbery or murder. The camp is geared for control and treatment of the most seriously delinquent offenders at the county level. They stay at the camp an average of six months to one year. If the wards reach their nineteenth birthday at the camp, they are automatically transferred to the California Youth Authority (CYA), or tried for their crimes as adults.

Vocational training at the camp is accomplished primarily through assignment to work crews. In order to be considered for the privilege of a work crew, the ward must meet requirements of the academic program. Work crews perform culinary duties, dormitory and camp maintenance, and school-sponsored work.

Sixty percent of the wards at the camp participate in a full-time school program. The other forty percent are engaged in a work experience program in which they earn school credit for work. These wards attend school every other day.

53

Counseling Program

Deputy probation officers integrate counseling with behavior modification, scholastic potential, and vocational planning. Treatment modalities include both individual and group counseling. All wards are seen individually, a minimum of once a week, by their counselor. Areas discussed include camp behavior, personal responsibility, communication skills, achieving academic potential, vocational planning, complying with court orders, and emancipation.

Group counseling is held among the eight living-groups at the camp with an advisor, and occurs at least once a week. In-house matters are discussed; the purpose is seen as problem-solving rather than therapeutic. Great attention is devoted to increasing group living skills through cooperation and respect for others (Los Angeles Probation Department 1992).

In a recent study known as The Eight Percent Problem (Orange County Probation Department, 1992), it was reported that seventy-one percent of the wards do not return to the the camps; fifteen percent returned once more, and six percent returned two more times. Eight percent returned three to thirteen more times. This group was booked or referred to the camps again a total of 1,068 times after their initial contact. Each re-referral increased the workload of probation and the courts. The Eight Percent Group was responsible for fifty-five percent of that added workload.

This group is at high risk for repeated offenses. Typically, they are referred to the camps again within six months of the first referral. Most of these offenders can be identified early in the referral process. The majority of this group:

- are fifteen years old or younger
- lack effective parental supervision and control
- have substance abuse problems
- have academic, behavioral, and/or attendance problems at school
- have had one or two prior police contacts before camp referral

The conclusion of this report states that "intensive individual attention and support are a requisite for helping high-risk youth improve performance and succeed. We invite the help and participation of all youth-serving professionals, organizations, and concerned citizen groups." I felt that as an art therapist volunteering time, I was indeed lending support as a "youth-serving professional."

While some probation camps are open, or unlocked facilities, this camp remains closed, or locked. Although there are no cells, the wards have rooms with restricted access. There are three dormitories (A, B and C), with "A-dorm" being the holding cell, used for punishment. Here, a ward remains in isolation from his peers and activities until a designated time of release.

The outer doors and gates of the camp are permanently locked. Parental visitations, including siblings, wives and/or girlfriends are allowed on Sunday afternoons between 1:00 and 4:00 p.m. During the time I worked at the camp, I was told that twenty of the wards were parents of one or more children.

Format

I served as an art therapy intern at this facility on a weekly basis for approximately nine months. I worked with a different group of five wards each week. Sessions lasted approximately one-and-one-half hours. The supervisor sent a different group of wards each week, but on occasion, I worked with one or two of the same wards in different groups over the nine-month period.

Initially, most of the obstacles I encountered were staff-related. While most of the personnel were congenial and helpful, my presence there was sometimes an inconvenience. It was rumored that the camps would be forced to close due to financial necessity, and because of this, there had been a hiring freeze. The staff was "overworked and underpaid," as it were. As far as they were concerned, I was an added responsibility that they didn't need. This "problem" corrected itself as time went by, however, as the staff became accustomed to my presence and the "routine."

In the beginning, finding a suitable location for the group was an issue. Classroom space was at a premium, so it was decided that the group meet out-of-doors at a picnic table. This was quite pleasant most of the time, but occasionally caused distractions when other wards walked over and made teasing remarks and unwelcome comments about the artwork. At this point, I either encouraged the "intruders" to sit down and participate in the artwork, or, if they refused, politely asked them to leave. During inclement weather, we moved to an indoor classroom. On several occasions, group time was cut to one hour because the "head count" was not completed, i.e., all wards were not accounted for by the time the group was to begin.

Other obstacles centered around the wards' behavior toward a female: they were constantly testing their boundaries, to discover what they could "get away with." Once they knew what was expected of them, however, there were no major difficulties. Frequently, the situation was taken care of by well-behaved wards who "protected" the group and put a stop to the misbehavior before I had to intervene.

There was no immediate supervisor present during the group sessions, except on occasions when scissors or glue were used. However, someone was always close at hand. Over the course of the year, there was never a serious problem with the wards. Essentially, they were well-behaved. In fact, they looked forward to their "creative time" with me, and always asked when I would be returning. I found that being consistent, that is, showing up every week and on time, was extremely important to them. They were so accustomed to being disappointed, that being with an adult who kept her word, made an impact; if I knew I would be unable to return the following week, I made a point to inform them. Additionally, the fact that I was a "volunteer" seemed to make a positive impression. Many times the wards made comments indicating that they thought highly of the fact that I did this work without pay.

Because I was unable to work on a regular basis with the same wards each week, a sense of trust and group cohesiveness that normally occurs in group therapy sessions never developed. This in turn prevented establishing more in-depth relationships. Since their files were inaccessible to me, there was no way of knowing the level of their family dysfunction. Only by limited verbal communication and using art therapy directives, was I able to get a glimpse at their backgrounds.

Another minor obstacle within the groups was occasional boredom whenever they were working on an "art therapy directive" (as opposed to an "art project"). When this occurred, I realized that it was not in fact boredom, but rather fear, or being uncomfortable with feelings the artwork brought forth. At this point, I tried to talk with the wards and gently encourage them to continue. At times this did not work, however, and often time and circumstances did not permit further discussion. Because the wards needed to trust and be able to simply express creatively, I allowed them to begin an "art project."

Art projects were varied, and sometimes continued over a period of several weeks. Many of the wards were quite artistic and thoroughly enjoyed these projects. Often, I was asked to take snapshots of their work, which I did on various occasions.

During the sessions, I tried to engage the wards in conversations about their feelings regarding their incarceration, as well as their lifestyles before and afterward (there were always a number of repeat offenders in a group). The same pattern emerged in virtually every group: Wards were often reared by a single parent (usually the mother) and were frequently neglected; there was a history of alcohol or drug abuse within the family; almost every ward had been, or still was, a member of a gang, and the gang became his "family." Additionally, there was frightening apathy, both toward killing, i.e. drive-by shootings, and being killed. Many of the wards seemed to feel they had nothing to live for, and therefore death was not as feared as it might be for the average adolescent. Over and over I heard, "So what; if we die, we die." In fact, on two occasions over the nine-month period, a ward I had worked with was killed in a gang-related shooting.

Confidentiality

Information and artwork were considered confidential. However, on occasion, I did share artwork and certain information with the immediate supervisor on hand. At the beginning of each session, I advised the wards that this would be a possibility, and they understood. I also told them that the artwork and content of the sessions would be documented. Occasionally, a ward would ask to keep his artwork. This was allowed after being approved by the supervisor.

Art Material

Due to security factors, art materials were limited, and painting (water based) and drawing media comprised the primary supplies. Felt-tip markers and pencils were available at every session. Scissors, glue and clay were considered contraband, and used only on specially structured sessions.

Art Projects

Art projects included drawing, painting, collage, woodwork, and photography. The project which proved most enjoyable and educational was "Pictures into Paintings." For this venture, I obtained permission from the camp and brought in another volunteer who was a photographer. She came in one afternoon with several 35mm cameras, and taught the wards the basic skills necessary to operate them. They were very eager students and learned quickly. We walked around the camp, and the wards photographed landscapes, animals (the camp had adopted two dogs), the photographer volunteer and me, as well as each other.

By the following week, the photographer had developed the photographs and mounted them on colorful matte boards. I brought them to the session (this was the only time I was able to have the same wards two weeks in a row) and instructed the wards to make paintings from their photographs. I encouraged them to take a more "abstract" approach, not worrying about trying to make the painting look exactly like the corresponding photo. This served to alleviate the usual "I can't draw" fear associated with drawing and painting, and allowed the wards to be less inhibited in their work (Fig. 1).

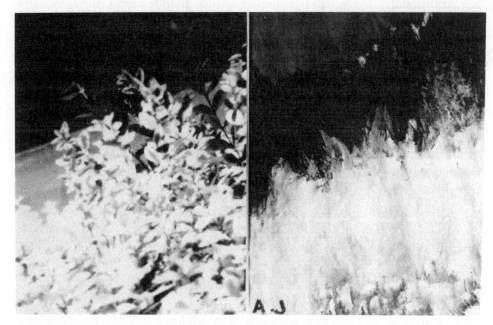

Fig. 1 Abstract art from life

The project was a great success. The wards were proud of their work, and decided to display it the following Sunday during family visitation. Additionally, the wards had learned the basic skills necessary to operate a camera. Several of them stated that they "would like to be photographers someday." This project had served to not only allow them to express themselves creatively, but to realize that there might be something artistic *and* feasible to which they could aspire in the future.

Another art project lasted for six weeks and involved the use of scrap wood pieces, which had accumulated from the wood shop classes. I collected these and had the wards paint them to make into a wood mosaic. I was careful not to allow any gang signs; however there were a number of African and Mexican flag designs used. After painting all the pieces, the wards glued them onto a large (six foot by nine foot) piece of plywood. After the wards were dismissed, I applied varnish to the entire piece to protect it from the elements and took snapshots of the wards standing near the piece, which was displayed on a wall inside the facility (Fig. 2).

The art projects served to create a sense of group cohesiveness and trust, which had been lacking. Additionally, they increased self-esteem, in that the wards were pleased with the way the projects looked. They also received special attention from the staff, their peers, and others who viewed the works.

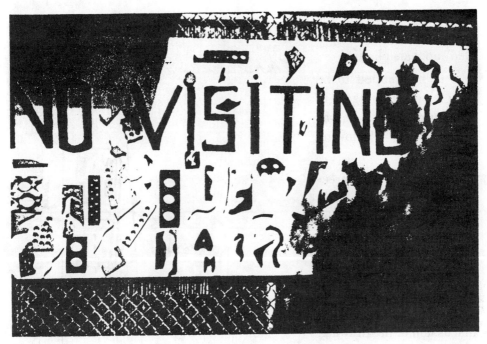

Fig. 2   A group art project

Art Therapy Directives

Art therapy directives were used in an attempt to bring the wards more in touch with their feelings. I found this to be extremely difficult because they were very guarded, and exhibited great resistance to expressing or discussing emotions.

Examples of Directives:

In the directive, "Draw a symbol of yourself or your life," wards were encouraged to think about their identity and how they viewed themselves. In Fig. 3, Juan, sixteen, drew himself sitting against a brick wall with his head between his knees, under which he wrote, "When I'm lonely." To the right of the figure is a car with a gunman inside shooting a figure on the street. Juan wrote, "About a drive-by shooting which happens every day." He stated that this was a symbol for his life and "probably always will be." The drawing reflects the sense of hopelessness shared by so many of these wards.

In Fig. 4, Mike, thirteen, draws "his greatest fear" as being "Devil-Dad," and writes he is "scared at night. Mom says he's real and he is mean." Mike was very resistant to discussing this drawing. I asked about his father. He told me his father had left the home three years earlier when Mike was ten. Mike also said his father had indeed been "mean to him." From the drawing, it could be inferred that Mike's father may have molested him; Mike wrote that he was "scared at night," and the end of the tail on "Devil-Dad" appears phallic.

I had hoped to be able to see Mike again in another group, but he was released the following week.

In Fig. 5, the directive "Where will you be in one year?" is depicted by Kevin, sixteen, as "Me, getting shot." Kevin drew a figure shooting him with a gun. The gunman wears a smile on his face. In our discussion of the drawing, Kevin stated that "There are people in my neighborhood who like to shoot people," and he was sure this will happen to him. I asked Kevin if he thought

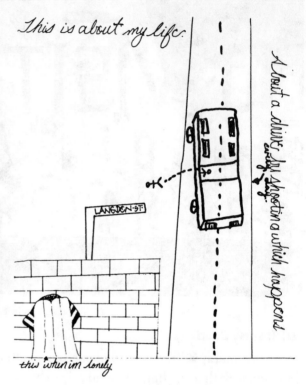

Fig. 3 "When I'm lonely."

there was a way of preventing this from occurring. He replied that the only thing he could do was to move away. He added, however, that this was not very likely, and that he just had to "accept life as it was." Again, here was the sense of resignation which I so often encountered.

A marked contrast in attitude about the future was exhibited by José, thirteen, in Fig. 6. In response to the same directive, José made a drawing of himself "At home in my backyard with my girlfriend and my friends." He revealed that he is not in a gang, and had no fear of getting shot. It is of interest to note the three-year difference in the two wards' ages; additionally, while Kevin had been returned to the camp twice, this was Jose's first visit. Both drawings in Fig. 5 and Fig. 6 appear as crude stick-figures, and lack in basic drawing skills the average adolescent would have acquired. More than simply a lack of talent or ability, this could be attributed to the fact that many of the wards never had the opportunity to draw or paint before.

Marco, a withdrawn thirteen-year-old, draws himself as a dog, in the directive, "Draw yourself as an animal" (Fig. 7). Marco was very shy and with-

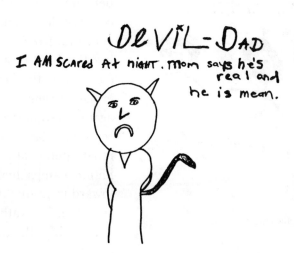

Fig. 4 Mike's "greatest fear."

drawn. He would repeat that he was "happy" over and over again. He expressed great displeasure at having to draw anything, because he "could not draw." However, with some coaxing, I managed to persuade him to make one drawing. On the drawing, he writes that he is "a happy dog." When I asked Marco to tell me about the dog, he replied that the dog was "sad and scared." I told him that I thought the dog was a happy dog. He responded by saying that the dog "used to be happy." I asked Marco what made the dog scared and sad. "Lots of things," he replied. At that point, he became very fidgety, saying that he was "tired" and refused to do any more artwork.

This was the common pattern in my work with this population. They were not ready to deal with any emotions that surfaced, which threatened to expose any vulnerability.

Conclusions

If I were to work in this setting again, I would conduct individual sessions with the wards. They obviously required more attention than I was able to give in the groups.

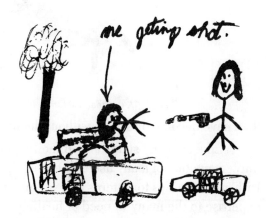

Fig. 5 Where Kevin imagines he will be in one year.

Individual and group counseling the wards received at the camp was behavioral, and geared toward the ward's ability to "fit in" at the facility, toward assimilating into the group. It was not geared toward exploring the

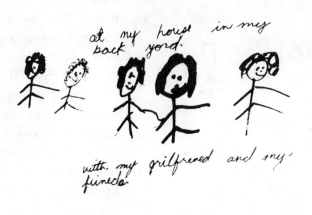

at my house in my back yard.

with my grilfriend and my friends.

Fig. 6 Where José imagines he will be in one year.

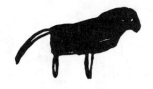

I AM A HAPPY dog that IF I WAS a dog.

Fig.7 "A dog that used to be happy."

cause of his wayward behavior, or what could be done to prevent him from leaving the facility and committing the same crime (or worse) over again. Like other correctional facilities, rehabilitation at probation camps leans toward treating "the symptoms" rather than curing "the disease."

In their world, often filled with pain, abuse, and neglect, many adolescents are denied the right to imagine, create and express feelings that have been locked inside. Unable to grow with hope for a better future and be nourished by understanding and love, they have become prisoners without the means to escape.

Like so many state-funded facilities, financial burdens prevent the the implementation of many useful therapeutic programs. These facilities are ripe with opportunities for interns and volunteers, who could donate their time and expertise to the many in need of healing.

References

Azima, F., Cramer, J, and Richmond, L. H. (1989). *Adolescent group psychotherapy.* Monograph 4, American Group Psychotherapy Association. Wisconsin: International Universities Press.

Bender, D., and Leone, B. (series editors)(1985). *America's prisons: opposing viewpoints.* Minnesota: Greenhaven Press.

Brandreth, G. (1972). *Created in captivity*. London: Hopper and Stroughten.

Kramer, E. (1971). *Art as therapy with children*. NY: Schocken Books.

Landgarten, H. B. (1981). *Clinical art therapy: a comprehensive guide*. NY: Brunner/Mazel.

Los Angeles County Probation Department (1992). *Camp David Gonzales*. Downey, CA: Community Affairs Office.

Strait. E. and Onorato G. T. (1989). *Making art in a jail setting*. Advances in Art Psychotherapy. Edited by Harriet Wadeson and Jean Durkin. NY: Wiley Interscience.

Oaklander, V. (1979). *Windows to our children*. Highland, NY: The Center for Gestalt Development.

Orange County Probation Department (1992). *The eight percent problem*. Santa Ana, CA: Research & Program Planning Division.

Wadeson, H. and Durkin, J. (1989). *Advances in art psychotherapy*. NY: Wiley Interscience.

Weiss, A. E. (1988). *Prisons: a system in trouble*. NJ: Enslow.

Art Therapy, Psychodrama & Sand Tray Work with a Sexually Abused Homosexual AIDs Patient
by Julia Whitney, Ph.D., A.T.R.

Julia Whitney, a registered art therapist, has a doctorate in clinical psychology and is licensed as a marriage and family therapist. She is a certified trainer, educator and practitioner in psychodrama, the president-elect of the American Society for Group Psychotherapy and Psychodrama and a consulting editor of the Journal of Group Psychotherapy, Psychodrama, and Sociometry. She maintains a private practice in San Francisco.

Art therapy and psychodrama are two powerful action techniques that can be used to augment each other in many ways—especially, I have found, in psychotherapy with individuals. This was particularly evident in my work with Michael, a young adult victim of child abuse who turned to therapy when altruism, denial and alcohol were no longer working effectively to help him cope with the stress in his life.

When he first came to see me, Michael's affable, easygoing manner and apparent casualness seemed incongruent with the tremor in his hands. A tall, handsome 30 year old homosexual, he had been doing field work for three years while working toward a Master's degree in counseling. This training had provided him with enough insight to help others understand their psychological processes, and to be aware of his limitations in being able to understand his own.

He acknowledged that he was consuming more alcohol than was good for him, that he found it difficult to feel anger, that fear of his feelings kept him stuck in depression, and that drinking kept him from feeling anything at all. Assigned to write a paper for a class in Family Therapy, using his own

65

life experience to describe a family crisis and prescribe its treatment, he found himself handicapped by depression, unable to write and preoccupied by confused memories of his father. He dropped the class and asked my help in sorting out his life.

Within two weeks of our first session, Michael joined AA and quit drinking. His extensive experience in participating in and leading groups had well prepared him to benefit from the recovery program group work and to use the support he felt from his professional and social networks. Therefore, individual therapy was my treatment of choice to deal with his sense of estrangement from his family and his difficulty with self disclosure in intimate relationships.

Because he was so articulate we agreed that an art therapy approach might provide a new way for him to express and experience himself, gain insight, and attempt to reconcile his emotional conflicts.

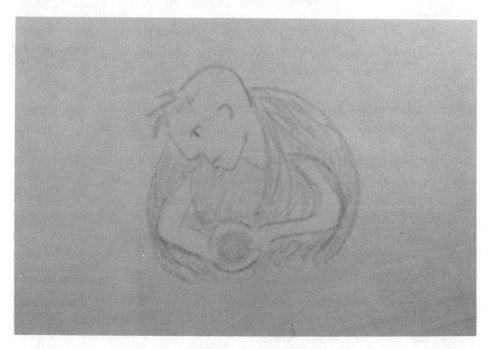

Figure 1   How Michael felt about his life.

Art Therapy Begins

Because he was apt to focus more on everyone else's opinions, needs and desires, I began a series of art exercises that would encourage him to focus on his own. His first drawing (Fig. 1) was in response to the question, "How do you feel about yourself in your life at this time?" (See appendix for detailed descriptions of directives.) The picture shows a male figure from the waist up, shrouded in a purple cloak, hunching over and clutching a gold ball in both hands. Aspects of the self? Yes. But what aspects and why?

Psychodrama Intermingled with Art Therapy

To find out exactly how the purple cloak and gold ball represented him at this time, I used the psychodrama technique of *role reversal*. In role reversal, one assumes the identity and expresses the point of view of a person, an animal, an inanimate object, an abstract concept, or an aspect of oneself. To enable Michael to physically experience the graphic representations of his self image, I asked him to assume their positions physically, as he had shown them in the drawing, and speak as the male figure and as each object.

Choosing to reverse roles with the purple cloak first, he stood behind his chair, and, hovering over the imagined figure seated in it, said, "I will protect you, but not forever."

Then, in the chair, drawing his feet up under himself, clasping his knees and bowing his head, he said as the gold ball: "I am your integrity. Hold onto me. Guard me." As the figure bent over under this protective mantle, he responded to it, "I hope I won't always need you!" and he assured the gold orb, "I will protect you."

Reflecting on this drawing and his responses to it, Michael acknowledged the oppressiveness of the protective shield he'd created around himself. At the end of the session he delightedly recognized his identification with a woman he'd been counseling that morning. He had been irritated by her complaints. Now he was aware of how strictly he prohibited himself from asking anyone for help, which he saw as complaining; and he could appreciate his client's "learning to express herself in a new way" or "showing a formerly unexpressed part of herself." just as he saw himself doing.

A Major Theme

That exercise provided material for the next six weekly sessions during which Michael established the goal of feeling less obligated to defer to others. As he expressed his longing for a strong protective father who would accept and respect him, he saw how his sense of obligation to others was connected to that longing. This began the grief work over his father, a military officer-turned-clergyman who had died the year before. Their mutual anger and disappointment as a result of their idealization and depreciation of each other was a major theme throughout the course of the treatment.

On the seventh week, Michael interpreted something I said as an indication that I cared about him and could be trusted not to disintegrate, disappear or retaliate if he stopped being so careful to protect me by censoring himself. Now we were aware of dealing with the results of his relationship with his mother as well.

Childhood Memories

I introduced the second art exercise (Fig. 2) to elicit childhood memories and emotions emphasizing experiences of pleasure and internalized sources of support. Asked to draw an object important to him when he was a small boy, he drew two figures on the same page: a toy giraffe and a bride doll. In role reversals with these objects he revealed his perceived need to be either ten feet tall and "above it all" or a beautiful woman, "an exquisite treasure worthy of protection." Both were a long way from a frightened, needy little boy.

He remembered this time of his life, around four, as confusing and sad

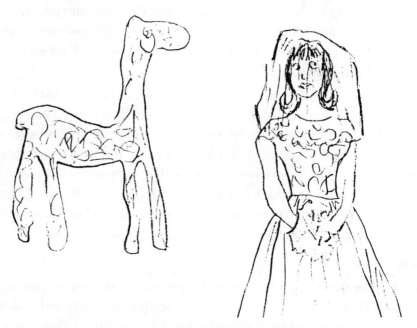

Fig. 2   Objects important to him as a child.

because he felt that his parents considered him disgusting and wrong and had "wrenched" these beloved toys away from him. He said he was sad when I also "made him" give them away in fantasy. Not thinking to choose to give them to himself, he imagined giving the doll to his closest female friend and the giraffe to a male friend who was dying of AIDS.

By the end of that week this sadness had turned into fullblown anger at me. However, because he claimed the anger felt unjustified, he first wept over a TV show he'd seen in which an abused boy feels he should be better so his parents wouldn't have to mistreat him. Then he expressed anger at the government over his tax bill and at his employer for lack of appreciation. I encouraged him to stand and use the physical gestures his parents had squelched in him as he verbalized these grievances. We both noticed at the end of the hour that his hand tremor had ceased.

In the next few sessions Michael became aware that he was not so much afraid of expressing his anger as of appearing less than perfect. To get to the source of this view of perfection and the expectation that he should be able to attain it, I asked Michael to diagram his social atom.

The Social Atom

J. L. Moreno, who originated the concepts of psychodrama and sociometry in the early decades of this century, used this term to designate the group of significant others who make up the reality of a person's life. Moreno described this nucleus of important relationships as a constant that one maintains throughout life, tending to replace absences as they occur with others who fulfill that role.

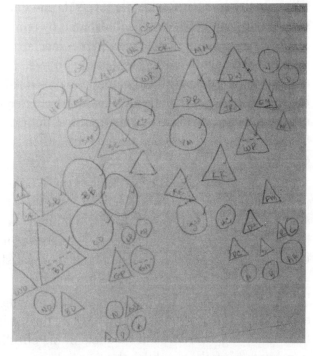

I instructed Michael to include in the diagram all the people, living or dead, whom he would consider essential to a description of his life, depicting males as triangles and females as circles. I asked him to designate their importance to him by the size of the figures, and their emotional closeness to him by their placement in relation to the triangle representing himself. I expected this diagram to provide clues to

Fig. 3 A diagram of all the people in Michael's life.

the basis of his expectations of perfection and a rich source of productive role reversals.

Its most compelling feature was that it involved 58 people (Fig. 3).

The results of Jane Taylor's research project entitled "Diagnostic Use of the Social Atom," published in 1984, indicate clear support for her first hypothesis that over 90% of protagonists would include between 5 and 25 people in their social atoms. She says that "logic would lead one to wonder at a person's ability to maintain relationships of any depth with over 25 persons." Not only did Michael indicate far more than the average number of significant relationships, but at least 23 appear larger than he, and all of them are drawn closer to each other than any of them are to him.

He himself was startled to recognize the accuracy of this graphic depiction of his sense of being overwhelmed by the oppressive awareness of the needs of so many others, and his need to distance himself as the only way he knew to protect himself from the self-imposed mandate to accommodate or, at least, respond to them. Through role reversals he saw how many of them had become internalized, to "live in his head," so to speak. It seemed to him he was carrying the whole cast of characters around with him and feeling accountable to them all.

In the next few weeks role reversals and dialogues with several of these significant people, whom we represented by empty chairs in my office, gave Michael an opportunity to experience a reoccurrence of his parents' expectations for him. He felt they wanted him to live up to their ideas of perfection and fulfill their demands without meeting his needs to be heard or encouraging him to set his own personal standards. He perceived his mother as being unable to bear hearing about his troubles, but expecting him to listen attentively to hers, while he experienced his father's requirements as physically exploitive.

He saw how he had internalized these parental attitudes and was now perpetuating them through projections onto others and by self-deprivation. He also began to see that this attention to others' needs was serving to distract him from his own. As he heard himself express and clarify his own position in these sessions he began to experience more satisfying interpersonal as well as intrapsychic relationships in his current life.

During this period he accomplished moving, finding a new roommate and finding an AA sponsor. In therapy we dealt with the anxiety aroused by the increasing awareness of the facts of his childhood, especially his relationship to his father, and the changes in his current living situation.

70

My Space

I introduced the art exercise called "My Space" to help him focus on and prioritize his own preferences. In response to a guided fantasy through which I led him to envision a spot uniquely his, he drew a realistic picture of the hotel room he stayed in when he first left home to be on his own. A brightly colored room, it was comfortably furnished for one, with an overstuffed chair and a book, a lamp, a picture on the wall of trees and a brook, a fringed and patterned rug, a large window and a door with a huge lock. What a striking contrast to the *other*-focused quality of his social atom diagram!

Drawing a Dream

Soon after this he expressed concern that his newly acquired AA sponsor might not be strong enough, that Michael might be able to manipulate him. He realized that if he let himself show weakness his sponsor might be better able to show strength. This frightening realization preceded a dream of his father, brother and himself in which the father sexually molested the two small boys. I asked him to re-experience the dream in his mind's eye and then represent it graphically with whatever image or images stood out for him.

His drawing shows a bleak scene with one boy literally on the carpet and the other hiding under a desk out of father's reach (Fig. 4). I asked him

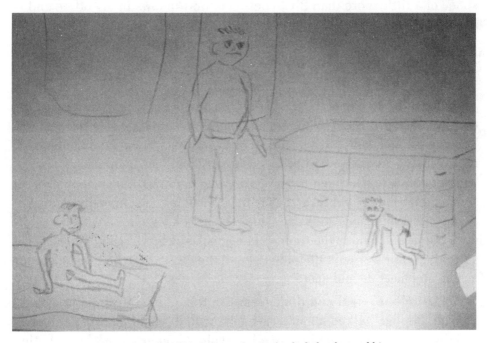

Fig. 4 A dream of his father molesting his little brother and him.

71

to assume the roles of all the figures in the drawing, following self presentations of each one with statements to each of the others. Then he addressed
himself to the little boy under the desk. After he berated him for all the
shameful qualities he'd always attributed to him, he finally expressed his
compassion and understanding, and offered to support him so that he would
no longer have to hide.

Coming to the next few sessions was difficult for Michael. He felt he
was coming to meet his father. However as he focused on confronting himself and his own experience of the past, he became less anxious about remembering the details of what actually happened. In role reversal with the image
of his father, he became aware of his father's dilemmas and conflicts and
how they had affected him. At one moment he'd tell Michael he was a special person, destined for greatness; the next he'd berate him for being con-
ceited and egotistical. As Michael spoke to the image of himself as a child
he heard how he himself alternated between wanting to protect himself from
harm and taking masochistic pleasure in tormenting himself. He realized he
needed to stop trying to annihilate the polarized voices but listen and perhaps
integrate them.

The Sand Tray

At this point Michael showed an interest in the sand tray. It occupies a
space of a little more than 2'x 3' between the windows in my office and is
filled with a 2" depth of clean white sand. Shelves above and below it hold
hundreds of small objects: toys, rocks, feathers, pieces of wood, parts of
machinery, etc. I invited Michael to create a scene in the sand, using any of
the objects he chose (Fig. 5).

On the left side of the tray he placed a figure of a baby surrounded by
nurturance, represented by trees and animals. On the right side he created a
"kingdom of wisdom" with a guru figure guarding "life affirming objects":
rocks, shells and pieces of wood, "once living but now inanimate, finished,
without conflict." Between them was a group of toy buildings, a city representing the business of life, and a toy train about to be set upon by a group of
prehistoric-looking monsters. He said, "The baby knows he can't sit there forever, but he also knows the train will be attacked. He will go to 'the house of
safety,' a castle between the old man and the city, where he'll hang out for
awhile and meet the old man."

In role reversal and dialogues with this old man, whom he named
Akman, Michael talked about issues of spirituality and his early religious
training. He longed to believe in a benevolent higher power, but rebelled

against and feared the punitive God his family had assured him required a perfection he knew he could never achieve. He was disappointed in therapy and angry at my limitations as well as those of his AA sponsor and others he'd risked counting on. He was angry at himself for not being the person he thought he should be. He was afraid he'd be stuck in this anger forever.

As he dealt with these uncomfortable feelings about me he began to focus more on his relationship with his mother, his disappointment in her lack of acceptance of his homosexual life

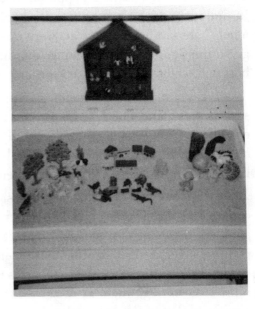

Fig. 5 Michael's sand tray.

style, and his fear that he would never be able to accept himself if she couldn't accept him. He also decided, after much thinking about it, to get tested for HIV. His sense of joy and pride in the Gay Parade and AA celebration, his dream material, and his interactions with me during this period both indicated and further promoted his increasing acceptance of his mother's lack of acceptance of him and his concurrent self acceptance. Despite a disappointing persistent tendency to react to others' anger with a reoccurrence of childhood guilt and an attitude of "peace-at-any-price," his dreams of retaliation, retribution, and subsequent acceptance of his father indicated his capacity to integrate that relationship with his newly perceived strength. He began to think about re-enrolling in the family therapy course he'd dropped and completing the formerly dreaded paper.

Family of Origin

To help him prepare for this I introduced the "Family of Origin" drawing. Asked to draw his family doing something, Michael represented them standing in a row posing for a family picture. He laughed at his appropriate, though unconscious, choice of activity, knowing how important it was to them to make a good appearance. The symbols drawn over their heads represent Michael's metaphors for their personalities.

Through role reversals Michael revealed his perception that all the family members shared an apparent fear of aggressive masculine strength. In dialogues with each figure, Michael expressed his fears of being "too much." He saw how these fears were manifested in the passive postures he'd given the figures in the drawings and in his interactions with family members and others in the past and present, and with me.

He found it much easier to express anger on behalf of someone he saw as weak and needing his protection. When he proudly reported an episode at work in which he'd forcefully confronted a colleague whom he'd observed harassing a subordinate, I led him through visualizations of two earlier occasions in his life when he'd experienced the same feelings.

His drawing of the first occasion shows the family dog hiding under the couch (Fig. 6) after being kicked by Michael's father. The second is a drawing of kittens drowning in a bucket on father's orders. After Michael ventilated the pent-up anger at his father that these memories evoked, I saw an opportunity to help him express this emotion on his own behalf. First I had him reverse roles with the dog, whom we could see was shielded by a protective covering similar to that of the boy under the desk and the cloaked figure in earlier drawings.

He could easily identify with the decision the dog had made to hide and restrain his instinct to attack the man upon whom he depended for survival. Through role reversal with the drowning kittens he was able to own, understand and become more tolerant of his own sense of powerlessness. The acceptance of this weaker aspect of himself was instrumental in increasing his capacity to become his own advocate.

Soon thereafter Michael brought in his finished family paper, on which he got an "A." He had been in therapy for one year. He acknowl-

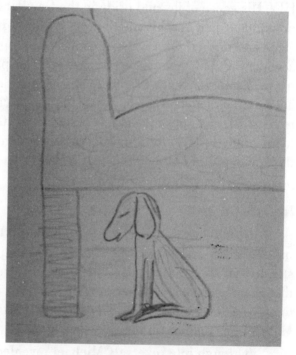

Fig. 6 Michael identified with his dog.

edged the anniversary by realizing how depressed he'd been and how much more comfortable he'd become in allowing himself to feel and express anger and fear. However, he expressed reluctance to lose the standard he had for himself of being "understanding." He had subsequent dreams of hiding things from his mother, of my inability to take care of him, and of himself taking care of his mother.

The HIV Test

Finally, perhaps in reaction to a professor's observation that he took care of others at his own expense, six months after telling me he'd decided to be tested for HIV, he did it. The results were positive. Since his T-cell count was so very low, 45, and he'd been meticulously careful about safe sex since he'd been aware of the danger, he realized he must have contracted the virus at least ten years before. He was afraid of what that meant in terms of his life expectancy.

It was his idea to draw a portrait of his drunk and promiscuous young self (Fig. 7). Sadly he "thanked him for bottoming out" and leading him to the person he had become, and expressed anger that such groping for affection had led to a fatal disease. Next, he drew a portrait of "Super Mike" (Fig. 8): he of perfect health, who worked a 40 hour week, went to school full time, participated fully in AA, and took care of others' needs. This was truly a

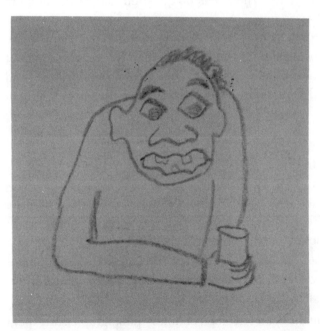

"knight in shining armor," which is how he appears in the drawing; but the protective covering appears stiflingly oppressive and obliterates the identity of the man beneath it.

Michael struggled courageously with the conflict between wanting to be treated specially because of his illness and wanting to be seen as a "white knight" rather than a beggar.

Fig. 7   Michael's image of himself as a young promiscuous drunk.

He expressed anger indirectly through dialogues with his hated pills and directly at me for suggesting he keep a journal. He resented his doctor for not being able to cure him, and was furious at anyone who suggested he quit smoking. He was especially sensitive to any indication that I might be trying to tell him what to do.

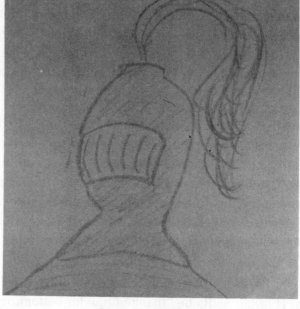

Fig. 8 "Super Mike."

Any suggestions from friends or colleagues that he participate in research, either through lab samples or in answering personal questions, made him angry. He recognized the internal voice that admonished him to be a good sport as the one that had caused him to put up with abuse in his youth. There was no question that he intended to fight that voice with full force now. As his expectations of himself diminished, he reported finding a heightened pleasure in living. At the same time, he was fearful of many aspects of being human, especially of the possibility of dying after a long and painful illness, as he'd seen so many friends do. He had a dream of being pursued by a short-order cook at whom he threw a bag of french fries.

Dream Drawing

When I asked him to re-experience the dream and represent it graphically, he produced two drawings. The first showed a neatly organized arrangement of a hot dog and fries in front of a clock, the nourishment emerging from its containers too late for him to eat it, which was why he'd thrown it at the cook. In the second picture, a pair of strong hands (his own) pulls him over the top of a hill just in time (Fig. 9). Looking at the drawings, Michael remembered his father teaching him to play the piano, and realized he did know what it was to feel needy and good at the same time.

At this time he brought in an envelope of family photographs. We spent several sessions in which he relived memories and integrated new insights

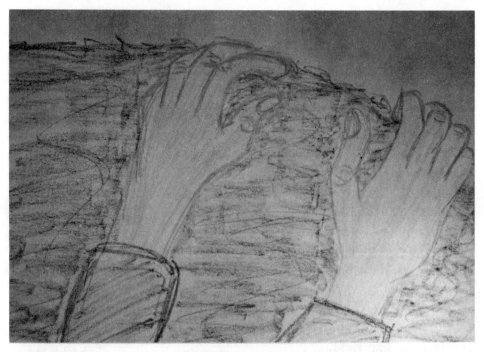

Fig. 9 An illustration from Michael's dream.

through role reversals and dialogues with the pictures of grandparents, aunts and uncles, parents and siblings, and, most importantly, himself.

With the onset of pain, Michael began to express his fears more openly. He began to remember the early religious training he'd received from his father. Not surprisingly, it consisted of confusingly mixed and polarized messages, ranging from how special he was in God's eyes to how much he deserved to be punished for his arrogance.

More Sand Tray Work

At this time Michael created his second sand tray (Fig. 10). On the right side he arranged a family of ten dolls standing in a grove of trees. Lined up in front of them protectively he placed a row of toy soldiers with guns pointing across a space of sand at fourteen monster figures. One of the soldiers was holding a telephone through which he could communicate with the family.

Michael described the family as "a living system." The monsters, he said, were like zombies. The wise old man from the earlier sand tray, whom he described as a spiritual being, sits elevated at the back of the tray, watching. Michael said, "He knows how the battle will come out, but he watches without telling."

Michael began to deal more openly with his anger at his mother for being so passive, protective of his father, rigidly religious, and unwilling to acknowledge emotion in herself or others. He realized that although he would like to be able to feel he was okay whether or not she thought so, he'd always feel a little bit bad about himself. As he began to feel worse physically, he gave voice to an aspect of himself he'd always kept silent: "the complainer."

He found many reasons to complain about me and realized how they reflected complaints he had about his mother and himself. He made a playful drawing of three aspects of himself helping each other out of the woods: one unable to see, one unable to walk, one unable to hear, but all together able to get along. He also connected this with his feelings of guilt and anger at the ways he and his brother had felt forced to deceive and betray each other in order to win their parents' favor.

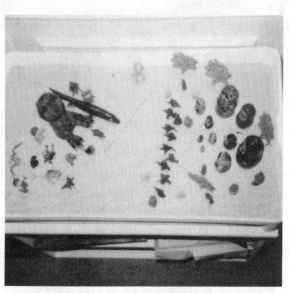

He began to be concerned that maintaining the status quo, not risking a change in his interactions with his family, was a threat to the identity he was so determined to achieve. He still struggled with the need to be right and his difficulty in experiencing anger as we marked our second anniversary of working together.

Fig. 10   Michael communicating with his monster family.

An Update on Self-Image

Before we reviewed his folder of drawings in honor of the occasion, he produced an update of the first art exercise: a drawing representing how he was feeling about himself now (Fig. 11). A sturdy tree trunk rises from strong roots in rocky ground to support a mantle of healthy green leaves which could be said to replace the heavy protective cloak in the first drawing. It appears that the gold sphere has opened to reveal a bright red cock which Michael described as feeling proud but not yet ready to fly.

This brought him back to the internalized voice of his father that said he could do anything, while at the same time admonishing him for having such a high opinion of himself. He feared that if he let himself be all he could be that his grandiosity would be boundless and he would be punished for it. He recognized his old dread of being "too much," which would make others unhappy and he'd get hurt.

This struggle with authority began to take on a spiritual quality. He spoke of not wanting to give God the glory as he felt he should when he performed well, of wanting to be Christlike, but again fearing to be "too much," of resenting having to give God credit for his accomplishments, and feeling guilty about it. Feeling exposed as if under a big white light, he confessed he wanted to *be* the white light.

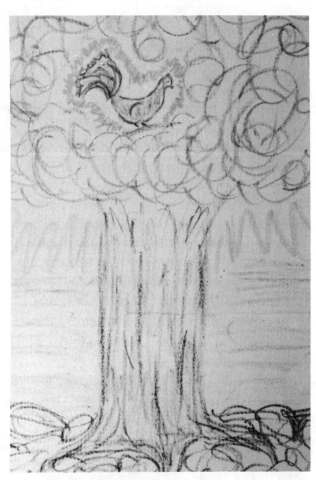

He'd been troubled for some time by his roommate's messiness. Role reversals and dialogues with the representations in drawings of himself, his roommate and the mess revealed his reaction of fear when confronted with a mess and his urge to punish the roommate. Playing the role of the roommate, he identified his own long-held resentments as well as fear of his father. In the role of the mess, his sense of shame for his own imperfections became clear.

Fig. 11   An update on Michael's self esteem.

Through interactions with me and others he became aware that people could acknowledge imperfections and say things they didn't like about one another and still maintain the relationship. He saw how much shame influenced many areas of his life, from being unable to fulfill others' expectations of him to not having enough money; and he saw how closely related shame was to resentment.

79

Working with Clay and Control

In order to deal with the issue of messiness and his struggles with perfection, I suggested Michael spend some time working with clay. Because clay is more difficult to control than the markers he was accustomed to using, it lends itself easily to making a mess. Various manipulations such as poking, slapping, punching. and rolling it can provide a safe avenue for physical and emotional release; and Michael enjoyed working and playing with it for several sessions. He created the figure he titled "Rising Up" (Fig. 12) while talking about how important it was to him that people saw him handling his pain with dignity.

As his illness progressed, Michael felt more depressed. He mourned not only the loss of his father, but the loss of his expectations that surviving family members would make the changes he longed for. Acknowledging and expressing that disappointment here seemed to allow him to accept and enjoy the positive aspects of the relationships and the concerns they did share. The picture of the animals in the forest reflected his growing acceptance of others and the various aspects of himself. He drew it on a day when he said he felt more like drawing than talking. A turtle, a rabbit, a fox and a bird peer out of dense foliage. He described the turtle as slow and therefore the most in need of protection. He claimed to identify most with the turtle, but liked the rabbit best and saw the fox as the most intellectual. He said he put in the bird for color and admired its freedom to come and go and feel "above it all."

He began to cry as he reversed roles with the rabbit, the most "out in the open and trusting." He realized he'd been equating the physical pain he'd been feeling with punishment, and experienced himself as a young child apologizing and promising not to "do it again." But what had he done?

As he dealt with these issues,

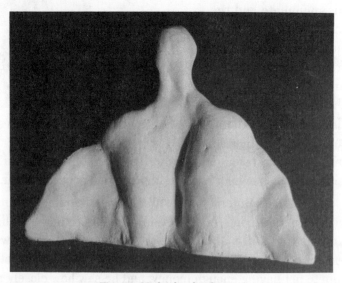

Fig. 12   Michael's clay figure.

including his physical deterioration, he realized he might have to acknowledge rage and separate from loved ones even though he hadn't dredged up all the memories he had thought he would. He felt conflicted over wishing someone else would make decisions for him, and hating to be treated as if he didn't have good judgment. He felt angry at his family for not being able to tend to his needs and guilty over not attending to theirs. He wished his family were here but asked them not to come because he felt he needed his energy to take care of himself. He appreciated their listening to his troubles but felt overburdened if they expressed distress. He felt angry at God but was afraid to say so if he wanted God's help.

During this period he often did not have enough energy to draw. Rather than guide his imagery, I encouraged him to relax, close his eyes and describe his visualizations. After one of them he felt relief from imagining a courtyard garden in which he saw a bust of himself and a statue of the Virgin Mary. A woman emerges from the statue and tells him he's doing very well, that his higher power is pleased. She says she doesn't want anything from him, but transforms into a delightful light show. Then in the form of a woman again, she sits by him and holds his hand for a while before blending back into the statue.

The reflection of his emaciated body was a source of increasing distress to Michael, and as the pain intensified, he feared starving to death. He dreaded becoming too weak to work, both because he loved the work itself, and because he valued the support of his co-workers. Much of the time he seemed as demanding and oppositional as a three year old. He feared his own impulses were the possible root of his nameless terror, just as when he was a child.

After being frightened by a TV program on AIDS that he refused to talk about, Michael drew a picture of a shepherd and his flock facing a glowing obelisk that reminded him of a picture in a Sunday School book he'd had as a child. In role reversal with the shepherd, he described himself, in contrast to the figure in his very first drawing, as standing erect with his energy source exposed. This energy, shown as a golden light, he described as the current manifestation of the gold orb he'd felt he had to hide to protect. It was now enlarged so that it faced forward bravely and expanded above his shoulders, mirroring the radiance of the obelisk, which he described as the source of all energy. The sheep, representing his vulnerable aspects, felt secure enough under his protection to even venture ahead of him on the hill. He talked about how the part of himself that he considered untouchable had so infuriated his father and how intimidated he had been by that fury.

81

Sexual Abuse

This session was followed by a dream in which his father was on top of him and Michael pushed him off, saying, "This is over!" He then was finally able to tell me the details of the sexual abuse he'd experienced from his father, his guilty sense of complicity, the shift of power when he told his father he would no longer participate, and his decision to forget it had ever happened. He felt tremendous relief in being able to recall it now, and feel finished with it. It had been three years and he felt he'd accomplished what he came into therapy to do and what he'd given up all expectation of doing.

During the last four months of his life, Michael experienced and expressed anger at his disease and its various effects on him, as well as the reactions of others that he found disagreeable, especially when they presumed to know what he needed and offered advice. He felt increasingly alone and frightened by his lack of control. He found himself spacing out a lot, but said the worse the news was on his physical condition, the more emotionally stable and reality-based he felt.

He arranged to leave his job with enough notice to participate in the training of his replacement, make the necessary preparations for meals and hospice services, and plan for future care of his cat. He said he felt he'd learned to use his ability to commit himself to others' needs to his own advantage.

Dreams of Closure

He had dreams about getting prepared. One of them was of a butterfly emerging from a cocoon in a cave. He took that drawing home and hung it on his bedroom wall. The last dream he represented in a drawing is shown here (Fig. 13). The tree of life looks much like a crucifix rising out of a flower garden. At the end of one of its arms is a rose in full bloom emitting a golden radiance, while from the other arm hangs a spent flower the color of a bruise. The center post supports an unopened bud which appears to have ejected a small naked human form up into the sky to join the sun, moon and stars in eternal orbit.

Though Michael never felt up to expressing himself through art after that, these last two drawings seemed to inspire subsequent meditations that he counted on to relieve his anxiety and his physical symptoms. Too weak to talk on our last session in his hospital room, he asked me to read to him from a book of poetry a friend had sent. He dozed through most of the hour and didn't wake until I said good-bye. The nurses told me he died in his sleep two days later. I'd like to believe it was the same peaceful sleep.

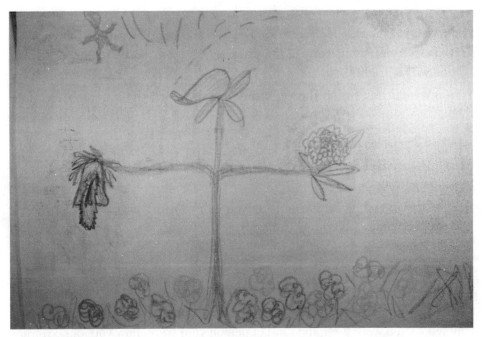

Fig. 13 Michael's last drawing.

Appendix

Exercise 1—How do you feel about yourself in your life at this time?

Materials: I like to have several sizes of paper and an assortment of drawing implements such as crayons, chalks, and markers in a wide variety of colors. I also have scissors and scotch tape available. I find that clients tend to use more as they become more familiar with the process.

This exercise is useful as an introduction, but can be used at any time, and repeatedly with the same client. I say, "Get as comfortable as you can in your chair. You may want to close your eyes so you can focus on yourself. Take a couple of deep breaths and then let your body breathe by itself. The floor is supporting your feet. The chair is supporting your body. Your head is firmly supported by your neck and shoulders. You don't have to do anything but think about yourself. I want you to be aware of how you feel about yourself in your life right now." I pause for few seconds so the client can get in touch with his or her feelings. The first time I explain the process thoroughly, by saying:

"Now, I want you to let an image come into your mind that represents how you are feeling about yourself in your life right now. This may be a representational picture or it may be a symbol, or it may be any configuration of lines, shapes, or colors. Whatever comes to mind, just accept it. When you're ready, I want you to open your eyes and draw that image of how you're feeling about yourself in your life right now. This is not a test of drawing skill. It's simply a new way for you to experience and express yourself to yourself and to me. You may use any of the drawing materials on the table. Whatever you do will be right."

When they finish their pictures I always ask them to sign and date them.

Exercise 2—Childhood Memories

Materials: Large pieces of newsprint and large crayons, like those used in kindergartens.

"Relax, get as comfortable as you can in your chair, close your eyes, and take some deep breaths. Think about the things you enjoyed in your life today." Pause.

"Now think of your life as a movie running backwards. Think back over the past ten years, and let the things that you enjoyed stand out." Pause.

"Think back to when you were about half the age you are now. See yourself as you were then: the kind of person your were, how you looked, what you liked to wear, the people you liked to be with, the music you liked, what you liked to eat, etc." Pause.

"Now let your movie run backwards until you are about half that age. See yourself at that age. What are you wearing? What do you like to do? Whom do you enjoy being with?" Pause.

"Now let your movie run backwards through your childhood to as far back as you can remember. See yourself as a little child. I want you to remember an object that was important to you. It can be anything: a toy, a household object, a piece of clothing, something that was special to you, that you loved. See yourself as a little child with that object, what you did with it, what it meant to you." Pause.

"When you have the object in mind and remember its importance to you, open your eyes. With your non-dominant hand, the hand you do not ordinarily write with, I'd like you to draw that object with these crayons, on this paper. When you finish drawing the object, put your name and the date on the paper, still using that hand." Pause for drawing time.

"Now close your eyes again and think about what has happened to the object since you last saw it. If you don't know what's happened to it, make up the journey it's been on, and then imagine you have the object back with you today." Pause.

"Now I want you to think about giving the object to someone in your life today. Think of who that will be. See yourself giving the object to that person and imagine the person's reaction to it." Pause.

"When you are ready, open your eyes. Share the experience."

Remember to leave plenty of time between suggestions for the client to remember. You may have to add a few more suggestions to set the mood.

Exercise 3—Social Atom

Materials: A sheet of paper at least 8" x 10" and a pencil or marker.

I say, "Imagine a map of your life. Using circles for females and triangles for males, represent yourself on the paper and show the significant people in your life in two dimensions. Indicate their importance to your life by the size of the figures and their emotional closeness to you by the proximity of their figures to yours. Indicate those who are no longer living by a broken line."

Exercise 4—"My Space"

Materials: A sheet of paper, 11" x 15", and crayons, pastels, and felt tipped markers.

I begin with the relaxation induction used in Exercise 1. Then: "You are walking easily along in a place that is familiar, where you are comfortable and enjoy walking. The air on your skin is just the right temperature. The scents that waft over it delight you. So do the sounds. Everything you see is beautiful. Your body moves effortlessly. You're aware as you progress that your surroundings begin to change, and that's okay with you. You notice a mountain in the distance and then are amazed at how quickly and easily you reach it and begin to ascend. Before you know it you have nearly reached the top. There is a lovely flat rock there, and you decide to sit. It's not that you are tired, You just want to enjoy the view.

"You look out over the valley below, and across it to another peak very like this one. Birds are flying back and forth, and you watch them a little enviously. Surprisingly, one of them comes to sit beside you on your rock perch. Magically he communicates to you that if you will just stand and use your arms as he shows you, you'll be able to join him in his flight across the valley to the other mountain peak. You decide to give it a try. Standing, your raise your arms and, following the bird's lead, you are soon standing safely on a rock very much like the one you were sitting on before, but you are, indeed, on the other side of the valley. Things look quite different over here. There are more rocks; and as you explore around a little, you find that two of them flank the opening to a cave. You can't resist going inside; it is a very inviting

85

looking cave. There's nothing forbidding about it at all.

"As your eyes become accustomed to the dimmer light, you see that you are looking down a long hall, with a row of doors on each side. Walking along, you discover that the doors all have names on them, and soon you come to one marked with your name. You try the doorknob. The door swings open, and there, in front of you, is your space, You stand there for a minute, taking it all in, and then you enter, knowing you belong there.

"Take a minute now to look around in this space and see what it is like. When you're ready, I want you to use the materials on the table to make a picture of your space as you discovered it here."

As in the previous exercises, I ask the client to sign and date the picture after finishing it. Then I pin it up where we can both look at it to begin processing it.

Exercise 5—Family of Origin

Materials: A piece of paper at least 9" x 12" and a choice of crayons, pastels or felt tipped pens.

"Get comfortable and think about what it was like to be part of your family of origin. Let an image come into your mind representing you and your family doing something. This may be an abstract image of lines, shapes or color; or in the form of symbols or metaphor, or a more realistic representation. Whatever image comes to your mind, please accept it. Remember this is not a test of drawing skill. Whatever you draw will be right."

When the drawing is complete, I ask the client to sign and date it, and then I pin it up where we can see and process it.

After eliciting the client's initial reaction to the art product, I ask him or her to reverse roles with the figure (s)he is most drawn to first, physically assuming the position of that figure as depicted, and making whatever statement is indicated. Then I ask the client to return to his or her own position and respond.

All of these exercises provide a rich source of self statements and dialogues through which both therapist and client can gain increased access to the client's intrapsychic as well as interpersonal processes, make them more visible and conscious, and therefore more amenable to exploration, understanding and possible change.

These art exercises were originally taught to me by my mentor in art therapy, Harron Kelner, Ph.D., A.T.R. In making them work for me and my clients over the past 12 years, while the art product provides a base of refer ence as a graphic representation of the client's self and all its aspects, I've found the psychodrama technique of role reversal valuable in bringing the art product to life.

References

Fox, J. (ed.). (1987). *The Essential Moreno*. NY: Springer.

Taylor, J. (1984). *The diagnostic use of the social atom*. Journal of Group Psychotherapy, Psychodrama and Sociometry, 37, 67-84.

Kalff, D. (1980). *Sandplay*. Santa Monica, CA: Sigo.

Diagnosing and Treating Children with
Multiple Personality Disorder through Art Therapy
by Patty Churchill, M.A., A.T.R., M.F.C.C.

Patty Churchill, director of Children's Services at Earthwood Center Ventura, California, has worked extensively with sexually abused and multiple personality disorder children for several years. The author of a training manual, Opening the Door: An Introduction to Art Therapy with Sexually Abused Children, *she is currently working on assessment tools for MPD children.*

Art therapy is the tool par excellence for both diagnosing and treating children with Multiple Personality Disorder. Symbolizing is an inherent human quality and from very early on, as we smear our applesauce on our high chair tray or drag a stick through the sand, we are busy creating shape and line and form to explore, organize and claim our world. So both because art therapy meets a deep human need, and because we have yet to bump into a perpetrator who said, "Don't draw about this!" art therapy is a profoundly effective means of working with young victims of abuse.

This chapter is based on two premises:
• the reader accepts the reality of MPD, and
• the reader has more than a passing knowledge of art therapy.

I do understand that may not be the case, but I am starting from here in the hope that if you do not have that foundation, this may intrigue you enough to go and investigate. One of the frustrations in working in this field is the lack of acceptance and understanding of both childhood MPD and art therapy, and so it is important that those who work in this manner share.

MPD is a childhood disorder, even though not listed as such in the DSM-IIIR and even though often misdiagnosed until adulthood. One of the overriding reasons for mis-diagnosis is professional resistance and disbelief of both the severity of child abuse and the reality of Multiple Personality Disorder itself. I once had a psychiatrist tell me it was illegal to diagnose a child MPD! Not so-—if the first split has not occurred before the age of 8, the disorder is not multiplicity. Acceptance of the use of art therapy as a diagnostic and treatment tool is beginning to spread. I know of no other methodology that is as accurate and effective. Because it both plumbs the depths of the psyche and records what is there, it provides a correlation, validation and correction of other history-taking and evaluative measures. It is a way of entering the child's world in a primal way.

If you are working with sexually abused children, be prepared for MPD. Whitman and Munkel (1991) postulate that 25% of severely abused children may have developed multiple personalities. My clinical experience supports this—and this makes MPD not only "not rare" within this population, but relatively common. For a young child who developmentally has yet to acquire many ego defense mechanisms (let alone much ego!), dissociation may be the only way to cope with overwhelming trauma. When dissociation is used repeatedly, as the primary defense mechanism, Multiple Personality Disorder is created. As Braun (1988) states, "Personality fragmentation is a heavy price to pay for the escape from pain and conflict; however, it may be what allows for survival at the time."

Three-P Model

Braun and Sachs'(1985) 3-P Model (Predisposing Factors, Precipitating Events, and Perpetuating Phenomena) clearly shows the progression from abuse and a dissociative episode to full blown MPD. It is important to understand this model and the concept of a continuum of dissociation from normal day dreaming to MPD in working with children. With therapeutic intervention in childhood we have the possibility of pulling in the dissociated events, strengthening the ego, teaching coping and assertiveness skills and supporting the child while s/he learns to live with the tension of having feelings. The goal is an integrated and cohesive sense of self.

One of the issues that becomes vitally important as one understands and utilizes Braun and Sach's 3-P Model is that people with MPD have what may be a *genetic predisposition* to dissociation. In a non-pathological way we see this in families of artists and musicians—the Bach family—since dissociation naturally occurs during the creative process. What this means clinically is that if you are working with a child whose parent(s) has MPD, one of your first tasks is to rule out multiplicity in the child, rather than search for it. I work in a small art therapy-based center devoted to Dissociative Disorders. We have a teamwork approach and the capacity to serve both adults and children within one family. In my practice *75% of children of parents with MPD have proven to have MPD themselves*. There are several factors that facilitate this over and above the predisposition to dissociate.

Often, in a multiple adult, there are several alters who do not own their biological child. Many may not even know the child. This creates intense emotional abuse and abandonment for the child when these alters are out and the parental figure is unresponsive to the child's needs. There is often active abuse to the child, which the child-attached alters may be amnesic about, especially if there are cult alters who have been programmed to initiate, train, or hurt the child.

And even without cult involvement, there is ongoing perpetration in a multi-generational abusive family due to the lack of both parenting skills and a sense of normalcy. Often there is a group of alters within the parent who are attached to the child and serve to protect the child from others within the parental system. They are often very effective, but may be naive or reactive about the outside world. The MPD parent is victim parent who is hyper-vigilant but unable to protect. And we are usually dealing with a single parent household and all the stress that carries with it.

Within an abusive family, MPD works as a functional, adaptive response to family injunctions of "don't see, don't talk, don't feel." Without this coping mechanism to keep the abuse undercover and the existing system intact, the child's options are limited: become psychotic, be killed, or bear the brunt of the chaos that erupts as the family is destroyed. Even children who tell their stories often recant—the threats are real.

Within a family of a multiple parent and multiple child, there is even more encouragement to continue splitting and creating alters to deal with specific events or feelings. A unique symbiosis develops between multiple parents and multiple children. Their child alters may play together, their teen alters may carouse and rebel together, and their adult alters may solve the problems of the world. Often the biological child takes care of the parent's emotional and physical needs. And they are very often "best friends." The MPD parent does understand her/his child in a way no one else can, but is often amnesic about abuse in the child's life.

Assessment for MPD in childhood begins with assessment for abuse: 96% of MPD cases report sexual abuse. With the statistics on child abuse

91

what they are, I believe every child in your office should be screened for abuse, and every abused child for MPD. Thorough history-taking is a must—medical, psychological, and social on each child.

Included at the end of the chapter are drawings from case studies to highlight the importance and use of art therapy in assessment and treatment, and to give you the visual difference in what you might see from a "normal" sexually abused child and a child developing multiple personalities. The major difference is the wide range of developmental stages and styles that will be revealed by a multiple child and the polarities expressed. I allow 3 sessions for assessment and use the following series of drawings diagnostically:

1. Self-portrait— draw a picture that tells me about you
2. Kinetic Family Drawing—you and your family doing something
3. A house
4. A tree
5. Trudy Manning's "Your favorite kind of day"
6. Free drawing
7. Make a world—sand tray activity

These drawings may be done by children ages 4 and up. Two and three year olds I ask to draw self, me and mom, me and dad, etc.—noting the hesitancy or eagerness, quality of line, development of scribble, etc. I introduce these activities fairly casually as part of "what we do here," realizing that any drawing may be too threatening during the first get- acquainted session. I often offer a choice of media.

What becomes strikingly apparent with a multiple child is the variety of responses. A child may do a competent, chronologically age-appropriate drawing at one point, and be able to draw only a straight line the next. When asked to draw "your favorite kind of day," there may be conflict within the child and they may draw two. There will often be different developmental stages expressed on one page—different alters at different ages and stages participated. Pictures of themselves may be floating in air, off the ground-line, perspective may be skewed. Often there is more than one "me" drawn on the page. A silent, self-absorbed child may not be showing autistic or catatonic behavior—"someone else," a proverbial child or infant, may simply be present and need to be acknowledged. Diagnosis in childhood is sometimes missed because we misinterpret what we are seeing: it can be the appearance of younger alters rather than regressive behavior, and abreactive work rather than a psychotic episode.

I think MPD is most difficult to diagnose in adolescence because we expect teenagers to be moody, try a variety of roles and go through regressive stages. Kluft's (1985) list of predictors for childhood MPD is helpful, along with good history taking and corroboration with art work. As with an adult, the bottom line is the presence of more than one personality within the body, and loss of time. With a child, this is often manifested as disavowed behavior and confirmed when you can get more than one alter to draw about a situation or time frame. There may be a designated group of alters who go to therapy, but it is important that everyone is welcome. You will often have a sense of more than one pair of eyes watching you; you are building trust and making contracts not just with the little body in front of you but with the whole inner family! Because children have simply not lived as long as adults and children do not have as much control over their clothing, hairstyles, etc., their alters are often not as well developed as adults, but their uniqueness will show up in their art work.

Having diagnosed a child as MPD, it is important to work within that model. It will give you the framework within which to work with individual issues. As with all hurt children, healing cannot begin until the abuse has stopped. We do not ask children to give up their coping mechanisms when they are still needed. Once safety is established, treatment begins.

Treatment consists of building trust, gathering stories, creating contracts and developing new skills. I do not believe it is fair to offer a choice about integration for a child. They are continually at risk if they are living a split life and they have a right to oneness, everything in place. It is our job to hold an image of wholeness for them, and then allow them to move towards it at their own pace.

Once secure in a safe and consistent environment, the child will generally be quite willing to share stories with you. Structure is important, both in scheduling and within the session itself. The child may be surprised and relieved to hear about his/her multiplicity and the creative way s/he has coped with difficulties and stress. Children wonder if they are "crazy" when they are different from others and will benefit from some discussion about what is happening. Since one of the goals of therapy is "no more secrets," it is important to share with them what we discover as we go along and to accept what each alter shares without judgment. It is exciting for a child to be part of an investigative team working to explore him/herself.

Art therapy provides a concrete means for gathering stories. Alters may first identify themselves to you by favorite color, artistic style, or a developmental stage of drawing. Each session needs to include some directed work as well as free exploration time when the child learns to make choices. Some themes for drawings or three dimensional art projects might be:

- Nightmares
- Wishes
- When I was 2, 3, etc.
- Monsters in my closet
- Voices in my head
- Hiding
- My safe place

As you enter the child's unfolding world the choices become myriad and are sorted out by prioritizing them in alignment with therapeutic goals.

Art Therapy Tasks

Some of the specific therapeutic tasks of MPD are beautifully dealt with through art therapy.

- Children can make Secret Keepers—boxes or containers filled with beans that can be removed one at a time as the children choose to share a secret.
- Sex education can be done by drawing together and labeling nude bodies, front and back—much more fun than coloring books or sex manuals!
- Body tracings and life-size body drawings elicit a great deal of information about guilt, shame and stigmatization and help the child reclaim the body. It is always interesting for a multiple child to discover, through body tracings, that all alters are actually the same size and are really sharing one body—a very foreign concept at first, and one necessary for good self care.

Identifying and developing language for feelings is crucial for health.

- Feeling graphs—draw a line that shows how you felt when you got up this morning, as the day progressed, all the way to right now;
- and feeling analogs—draw a symbol for this feeling—are both helpful to children.

There are also ways to develop co-consciousness:

- Who was feeling that way and why?
- What was going on when you didn't know what was happening?

As co-consciousness develops, you can facilitate contracts between alters to work together, share information, and handle certain situations. The child begins to feel a little more control and has some mastery over his/her life at this point.

Appropriate acknowledgement and expression of anger is a difficult task for MPD children. Art therapy provides a positive means of discharging anger and learning to problem-solve. You can safely put the ugliest things on paper without hurting anyone. You can express your fantasies of revenge by building and destroying clay figures. And you can scribble and tear paper and call it all manner of obscenities until it is all out of you and you can rest. It is crucial that children understand they will not be punished for what is said or done in the playroom and that the bottom line is that no one gets hurt.

When cooperation between alters is established, stories are told and blending begins, integration becomes a topic of discussion. It is a curious concept to children who have no memory of living as one. Chocolate chip cookies is a good analogy—while all the ingredients are necessary and wonderful in their own right, the total is more than the sum of its parts. A band or symphony is helpful to older children: while each instrument is important and unique, it is the blending that moves us. Building, containers and collage work are also helpful. Each child will come up with his/her own image in the end. Integration may be spontaneous or planned, but is always up to the child, not the therapist or caregiver.

Post-integrativeTherapy

Post-integrative therapy is necessary. Children often feel a deep sense of loss and grief and need a quiet time to heal. They are sometimes really surprised by the silence inside and a little unnerved by it. They need stability and support during the first few months and then some ongoing therapy to develop the skills they may have missed. One child multiple was really appalled at what it meant to handle junior high on her own after integration at 12! She'd always had "someone else" to handle difficult situations or hold uncomfortable feelings for her.

But if the therapy has been successful, not only has the child healed, but s/he has learned to draw, write, and tell in order to communicate with others and him/herself. S/he has developed tools that will last a lifetime.

Child A

These drawings are from the assessment series at both the beginning and end of therapy with a 7-year-old boy—a "normal" single incident sexual abuse case. The abuse in this case was a vicious kick in the groin by the school bully which ruptured the victim's penis. The family brought him in for therapy after the reparative surgery had been done and the child had been diagnosed as suffering from Post-Traumatic Stress Disorder.

95

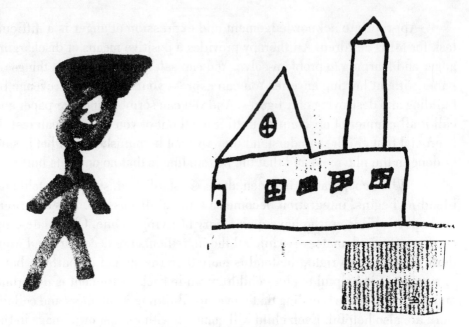

Figs. 1 and 2 Child A.'s art after being hurt in a single incident

His drawings document the sense of helplessness, smallness, isolation, and anger that he felt, as well as the sense of immobilization and threat felt by his entire family.

In the two termination drawings we see the weight lifted off his head, energy moving, and age-appropriate activity with his dad. Please note: this is a child who did not enjoy drawing, nor was he especially good at it. Yet

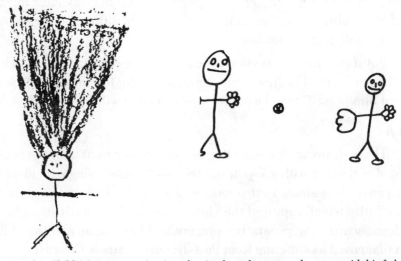

Figs. 3 and 4 Child A.'s art at termination, showing lots of energy and a scene with his father.

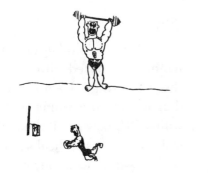

Fig. 5 Two disconnected images of Child B

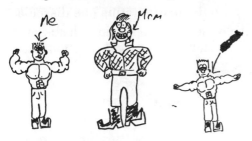

Fig. 6 Child B.'s family picture

the drawings are highly revealing. Much of his work was done through very large paintings and interactive play.

Child B

These drawings are by a 10-year-old male multiple. His mother and younger brother have also been diagnosed with MPD. From a multi-generational cult family, he is currently living in a residential treatment home for emotionally disturbed children run with a heavy behavior modification emphasis.

In the first self portrait containing two disconnected images of self, one can see typical MPD artwork.

The next two pictures are of his family, highly disparate. The last, which matchs none of the foregoing in style, depict a camping trip with grandparents, and we begin to see the emergence of cult themes and images.

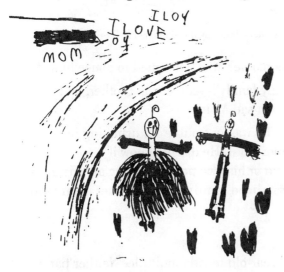

Fig. 7 Child B.'s other family picture

Child C

These are drawings by a 17-year-old male multiple. He was the only son of a female multiple, with whom he lived. These drawings are depictions of two of his alters, drawn by the alters themselves. He had a great deal of conflict with his mother, whom he bullied. They could not figure out how to live together or how to separate—a classic love/hate relationship and typical of the symbiosis between MPD parents and MPD children.

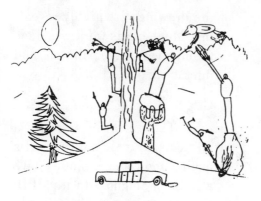

Fig. 8 Child B.'s camping trips

Child D

A 4-year-old boy of a single mother diagnosed with MPD did these drawings. I am careful in diagnosing very young children with MPD, because if their life is stabilized they can heal so quickly. And yet, if, as in this case, the abuse continues and all the secrets are not revealed, you are only incorporating one dissociative event at a time and not changing the basic modus operandi. That is what happened with this child, who did some good work while he was here, but

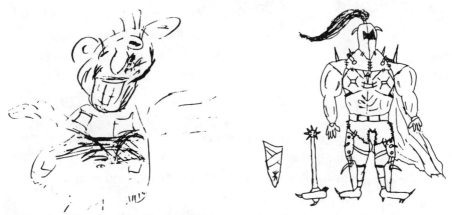

Figs. 9 and 10   Two of Child C.'s alters drawn by the alters themselves

then moved to another state with his mother, who continued to abuse him.

The first drawing is "Me and my family"—me, mom, brother, and "the other me." The second is a portrait of a sad Mom.

The next two were done when he was in trouble for urinating in inappropriate situations and had no memory of it. He did not know if it was something separate (the hose on the ground or his own penis) causing all this trouble. The last drawing shows a normalized family picture—me, mom, and brother.

Child E

These drawings are by an 11-year-old female multiple. Neither parent was diagnosed MPD. Her abuse came from her paternal grandparents and their involvement in a neo-nazi cult. The first example, a feeling graph, is a

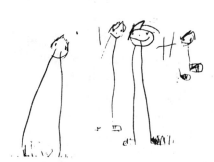

Fig. 11 Child D.'s family

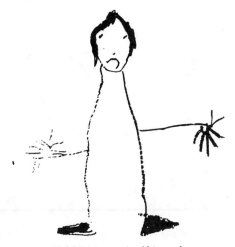

Fig. 12 Child D.'s portrait of his mother

good picture of the mood swings and extremes of emotion experienced by a multiple over the course of a normal day. We had access to 15 of her alters at this point, and they were to work together to tell me about the day.

The second picture, a feeling analog, was obviously done by several alters of different ages with a variety of drawing and spelling skills—calm is included twice, spelled com and clam.

The third drawing is an example of one of her favorite ways to "talk" about the abuse. One alter would draw a scene, another alter would write about it. I would write questions and comments back, all silently.

Not shown are the many regressive, chaotic expressions of feelings around the worst of the abuse.

The self portrait was done when we were working with the feelings around flashbacks. It is her statement

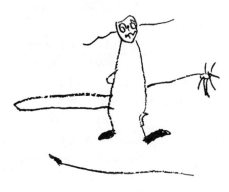

Fig. 13 Child D.'s conflict

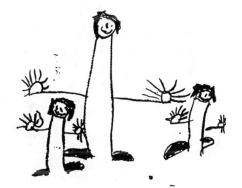

Fig. 14 Child D's resolution

99

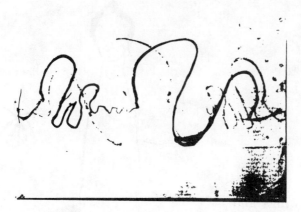

Fig. 15 Child E.'s feeling graph showing many mood

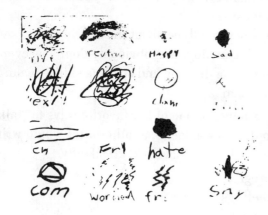

Fig. 16 A feeling analog done by several alters

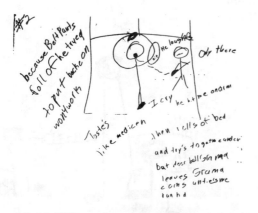

Fig. 17 Different alters working on the same picture

of how she felt as a memory began to surface—it was like "a bubble coming up." We devised a system for living with the tension of the dread/anticipation and what to do with the memory when it hit if she was not in the office.

The next picture is of an event that occurred when she was 5 years old which was very upsetting to all of her alters. It involved a picture she had done at kindergarten as a gift for her parents which her grandparents had taken away from her. There was a great deal of confusion for her about whose child she was—her parents or her grandparents.

She worked at creating a safe place for all her alters so that she could return to school and function better. She had created a lovely home with plenty of room and supplies, surrounded by a moat, for her internal habitat. She even got a wonderful doll house, which she eventually brought to the office, where she could play out again and again all the issues in caring for children. The last is a self-portrait, "All

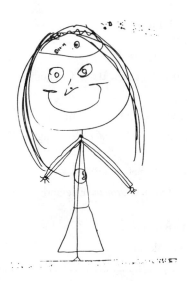

Fig 18 Self-portrait with bubble/memory

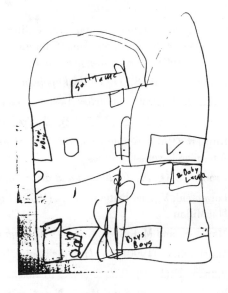

Fig. 19 A distressing event

of Me," as she approached integration. She is crying tears of joy.

References

Belsky, J., and Lerner, R. M. (1984). *The child in the family*. NY: Random House.

Bowlby, J. (1988). *A secure base*. NY: Basic Books.

Braun, B. G., ed. (1986). *Treatment of multiple personality disorder*. Washington, D.C.: American Psychiatric Press.

Burns, R. C., and Kaufman, S. (1972). *Actions, styles and symbols in kinetic family drawings*. NY: Brunner/Mazel.

Cofer, W.M., and Ables, B. (1983). *Multiple personality, etiology, diagnosis and treatment*. NY: Human Sciences Press.

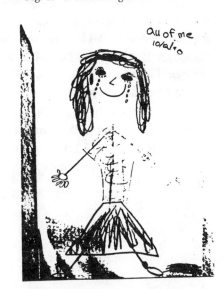

Fig. 20 Self portrait with tears of joy

Cohen, B. M., Giller, E. and LynnW.I., eds. (1991). *Multiple personality disorder from the inside out*. Baltimore, MD: Sidran Press.

Cohen, F., and Phelps, R.I. (1985). *Incest markers in children's artwork*. The Arts in Psychotherapy, 112 (4): 265-282.

DiLeo, J. (1983). *Interpreting children's drawings*. NY: Brunner/Mazel.

Donovan, D. M., and McIntyre, D. (1990). *Healing the hurt child*. NY: W.W. Norton.

Dundas, E. T. (1978). *Symbols come alive in the sand*. MA: Coventure.

Furth, G. M. (1988). *The secret world of drawings*. Boston: Sigo Press.

Gil, E. (1983). *Outgrowing the pain.* California: Launch Press.

———— (1990). *United we stand.* California: Launch Press.

———— (1991). *The healing power of play.* NY: Guilford Press.

Hammer, E. (1978). *The clinical application of projective drawings.* IL: C. C. Thomas.

Kalff, D. M. (1980). *Sandplay.* Boston: Sigo Press.

Klepich, M. and Logie, L. (1982). *Children draw and tell.* N.Y.: Brunner/Mazel.

Kluft, R. (1985). *Childhood antecedents of multiple personality disorder.* Washington, D.C.: American Psychiatric Press.

Kramer, E. (1979). *Childhood and art therapy.* 2nd ed. NY: Schocken

Lowenfeld, V., and Brittain, W. L. (1970). *Creative and mental growth.* England: MacMillan

Magid, K. and McKelvey, C. A. (1970) *High risk.* NY: Bantam.

Malchiodi, C. (1990). *Breaking the silence.* NY:Brunner Mazel.

Putnam, F. (1989). *Diagnosis and treatment of multiple personality disorders.* NY: Guilford

Reed, J. P. (1975). *Sand Magic.* New Mexico: JPR Publishing.

Silver, R. A. (1989). *Developing cognitive and creative skills through art.* NY: Albin Press.

Spring, D. (1988). *Sexual abuse and post-traumatic ztress reflected in artistic symbolic language.* Ann Arbor: UMI Dissertation Information Service, Pub. No. 9002893.

Steinhardt, L. (1985). *Freedom within boundaries: body outline drawings in art therapy with children.* The Arts in Psychotherapy. 12, pp. 25-34.

Terr M.D., Lenore (1990). *Too scared to cry.* NY: Harper & Row.

Wolfe, V. V., Wolfe, D., Gentile, C. and LaRose, L. (1987). *Children's impact of traumatic events scale.* University of Western Ontario, Ontario, Canada.

Whitman, B. Y., and Munkel, W. (1991). *Multiple personality disorder: a risk indicator, diagnostic marker and psychiatric outcome for severe child abuse.* Clinical Pediatrics 30 (7), 422-427.

Reunification with the Adopted Self:
Art Psychotherapy with Adult Adoptees
by Rita Coufal, M.A., A.T.R, M.F.C.C.

On the faculty of the Graduate Department of Social Welfare at U.C.L.A, Rita Coufal has been an art psychotherapy consultant at C.P.C. Westwood Hospital since 1988, working with inpatient and outpatient adults in individual and group treatment. In addition, she has developed and facilitated prevention/treatment programs for at-risk minority youth and their families at the Didi Hirsch Community Mental Health Center. An invited lecturer at universities, conferences and mental health settings, Ms. Coufal is also in private practice in the West Los Angeles area. She was adopted at birth and has been in the process of becoming an adoptive parent for the past three years.

This chapter reviews the author's experience working with adult adoptees (those adopted at birth or in infancy) who enter art psychotherapy with a variety of presenting problems and diagnosis. The common diagnostic impressions are major depression with suicidal gestures and ideation, borderline personality features and substance abuse. Of the individuals presented in this discussion it is significant to note that none of them entered art psychotherapy with the conscious intent to deal with their adoption experience. It was through the analysis of their personal imagery that issues related to their adoption emerged and were subsequently treated within that framework.

NOTE: For convenience, the female pronoun will be used throughout this chapter when making general references. Names and other identifying information have been changed in case vignettes to protect rights of confidentiality. Permission to use the accompanying artwork has been received from each patient.

The graphic and sometimes painful images that developed in the course of individual and group treatment accurately reflect the adoptee's journey from the unconscious to the conscious realm, and illustrate the special challenges inherent in being adopted. Issues and themes that emerged repeatedly in the art products include: abandonment, loss and rejection, guilt and shame, denial, unresolved grief, identity confusion, separation-individuation conflicts, trust and intimacy, and issues of control.

That adoptees are at-risk seems to be more generally acknowledged in the literature, but there is not an overall agreement as to when in the developmental cycle and how to assess for these factors. The available research in psychiatry, psychoanalysis, psychology, art psychotherapy and other mental health professions covering the last 50 years suggests that there are differences in the mind-body experience of adoptees and those of nonadopted individuals, and that these variations may be manifested in some kind of pathology. Most authors agree that adoptees are vulnerable and that the existing structure of adoption is in need of reform (Sorosky et al., 1979).

CASE EXAMPLES

Cindy, a severely regressed 35-year-old woman, was seen individually and in group for 8 months. She was treated for major depression with overwhelming suicidal feelings secondary to Post Traumatic Stress Disorder in response to being raped at gunpoint. She also had a history of being abused and molested, an eating disorder (binge/purge cycles), dissociative episodes and borderline personality disorder.

Cindy was molested by her aunt, and physically and psychologically abused by her adoptive mother. Father was experienced as a "gentle but emotionally distant man" who was unprotective of her. Cindy's "chosen baby" tale was inconsistent, and shrouded with secrecy and badness. She grew up believing that she was "taken from a dungeon" and was chosen by her father, *not* her mother. Her adoptive mother led her to believe that her biological mother was "genetically inferior" and if found by Cindy would only "suck off her" like a poor relation.

The disruptive effects of family chaos and abusive treatment are crystallized in her self-portrait (Fig. 1). Cindy used the art materials as tools to unearth her powerful feelings. She used the paper as a container and a "holding environment," creating a "safe" place where the abandoned, lost inner child could feel held and finally understood by "good enough mothering" (Winnicott, 1971). The creative process and the development of a symbolic language were an integral part of the self-discovery that Cindy utilized so effectively in her healing experience.

Most notable in this artwork is the use of deep, dark intense color and form and its juxtaposition to light, soft flowing color and form, with the distinct central image of a "split merging/separating self." *The affective instability, the polarized themes of goodness and badness, ambivalence about oneself and object representations appear to be consistent in the body of artwork of adult adoptees.* In addition, the marked identity disruption graphically illuminates uncertainty about her self image and her inability to relate and connect with others.

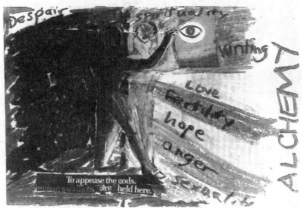

Fig. 1 Alchemy

Cindy grew up with the threat of being rejected and/or abandoned if she did not "do what she was told." In Cindy's family, asking questions about her origins or her genealogical heritage was unacceptable and always considered "ungrateful" and "dirty" behavior. This constant threat of rejection and abandonment was explored in Fig. 2. The punishment for Cindy's basic curiosity was to be harshly scrubbed down by her mother, then exiled to her room. Despite the contained organized appearance of these images, she titled it *Fundamentalistic Overwhelming Chaos*.

This piece of artwork facilitated expression of feelings that were previously denied, repressed and usually manifested in her frantic and chronic efforts to avoid real or imagined threats of abandonment, usually in self-mutilating superficial suicide attempts.

At the time of treatment, Cindy had only received discrediting, devaluing information of her origins. The genealogical confusion and the lack of an integrated sense of self, as well as the history of abuse, is reflected in her painful pictorial worlds of *Alchemy* (Fig.1) and *Chaos* (Fig. 2). Cindy explicitly portrays primitive forms of defense and self protection in attempting to find a magical solution and an "elixir for life."

Art psychotherapy with Cindy elicited powerful countertransference feelings. When carefully scrutinized, they provided me with a deeper understanding and perception of Cindy's unconscious material.

It is a popular and often repeated myth in adoption literature to refer to an adopted child as a "chosen child," or as a "wanted" child. Unfortunately, these terms contrast dramatically with the prevailing reality; the child who is available for adoption is

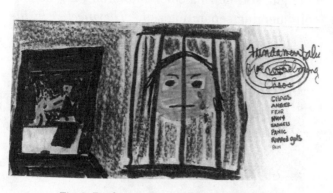

Fig. 2 Fundamentalistic Overwhelming Chaos

unwanted before she ever becomes wanted. Not being kept by one's biological parent is the primary loss in many adoptees' lives. Being given up "as a human sacrifice, to appease the gods" is how Cindy experienced her losses and injuries (Fig.1).

"Chosen Baby" Stories

Frequently, fairytale-like stories, often referred to as the "chosen baby stories," are fabricated to explain the origins of the adoptee/adopter relationship (Lifton, 1988). These tales and the secrecy surrounding them become internalized and appear to contribute greatly to the devalued and distorted sense of self that many adoptees struggle with throughout their lives. Adoptees express life-long frustration and pain over "If I am so wanted, choosable and lovable, why was I given up?" Another plaintive cry often heard is "If I'm so good and lovable, why won't you tell me who my biological parents are?", or, "Why aren't they (biological family) looking for me?"

This missing piece of identity, the state of denial and the double-bind style of communication, significantly contribute to the adoptee's struggle with self-definition and the integration of one's past with the present reality. If the adoptive family can't acknowledge and validate the adoptee's experience, it is then that self-questioning and self-doubt become a way of life.

A multi-media piece (Fig. 3), created in response to the "chosen baby" issue, clearly depicts the open wound-like birth experience entitled *Scard*. Jane, a 21-year-old immature female adoptee poignantly and profoundly articulates the painful memories and fantasies of being born to two families, and the "wonder" she has for some familial identity and sense of connectedness. The misspelled word "scard" when explored by the patient was left uncorrected because she stated, "I have always felt scarred by my differences and scared by the rejection and loss."

This young woman's grieving needs and negative, distorted self image were confronted in her personal symbolic imagery which served as powerful means to overcome the denial and invalidating statements she grew up hearing.

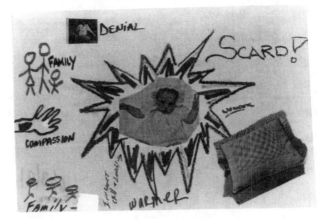

Fig. 3 SCARD!

"In general, it is the policy of the law to make the veil between the past and the present lives of adopted people as opaque and impenetrable as possible, like the veil which God has placed between the living and the dead" (Gaylord, C. L.).

It is this veil of secrecy that must be identified, confronted, and removed so that adoptees may effectively begin to identify, explore, and resolve the conflicts that underlie the struggle in their lives.

In addition to the adoptee herself, there are initial and continuing effects on all members within the adoption triangle. The adoptee, the adoptive parents, and the biological birthparents, are all emotionally affected by the adoption experience. Each member of the adoption triangle experiences ongoing conflict and injury as a result of the issues surrounding the adoption.

Art Psychotherapy: Towards a More Cohesive Self

Art psychotherapy can be an effective modality of treatment for clarifying the complex dynamics related to adoption. The creative process is often recommended as an efficient means of accessing and communicating highly emotional and conflictual material that contains unconscious aspects of intrapsychic injury not readily attainable by verbal, linear language. Providing the patient with a safe holding environment and a space where creativity can take place is recognized as invaluable in the working-through process for adults who experienced a conflicted, or an otherwise unsatisfactory maternal-child fit as infants.

Discovering the lost and hidden aspects of one's self in the creative production, and feeling safe enough to be able to explore complex psychological fears and fantasies, strengthens the adoptee's self concept and ability to formulate a coherent and strong ego identity.

Further, a sense of mastery and the development of healthy autonomous relationships are critical goals for the adopted patient, and are a focus in art psychotherapy treatment.

As the issues relevant in adoption are acknowledged and examined within the art, as the patient's productions are interpreted within a dynamic formulation and the broad psychotherapy process, the individual achieves insight and validation and is able to move towards a complete and well-defined sense of ego identity and begins to resolve major conflicts. I will outline here how a sampling of adoptees have used the art psychotherapy process in an attempt to re-order their representational worlds and effect their impaired object relationships.

Window to my Soul—A Case Study

Samuel was a 50-year-old man who was briefly hospitalized for a major depressive episode, confusion, suicidal thoughts, loss of energy, and disillusionment with his life and work. Initially he presented feelings of hopelessness, helplessness and unworthiness. These emotional states were characterized by isolating behaviors and intense episodes of anxiety and panic reactions.

Samuel was adopted at 6 months old by a mother whom he described as inadequate and a father who was emotionally unavailable. He was an only child with little extended family connection. His childhood was very lonely, and difficult due to numerous learning disabilities, hyperactivity and a lag in growth. Samuel recalls always thinking about being adopted and searching for his *heroes* in extensive science fiction reading. He identified the *heroes* as the idealized good parents that he felt he had lost twice; once at birth and once again in adoption. It was in this world of fiction that he also searched for his own sense of self, unsuccessfully.

Sam's chosen baby tale evolved from being chosen because "you were the cutest baby," to "you were unwanted," and finally the most recent revelation was that "your mother suffered from a severe thought disorder." This knowledge reinforced the *damaged goods* and *bad seed* syndrome suffered by many adoptees.

Sam had been married three times, and felt that he had never experienced a true love relationship. He struggled constantly with trust, intimacy and genuine expressions of love. The most recent marriage was fraught with tension and resentments, the central conflict being Sam's rage at female figures and his idealized fantasy of them. It was his wife's recent threat to leave Sam that precipitated his disintegration and decompensation. Sam's wish for and his fear of closeness was evident in our sessions as well as in the poignant, fragile imagery he created. In his relationships, particularly with female figures, Sam typically felt dependent. Consequently, he experienced a sense of blurred or non-existent boundaries which resulted in a great panic and fear of self dissolution. In his body of imagery there is extreme fragmentation, chaos and, most markedly, a lack of spatial organization.

In our initial session, Sam produced a multimedia expression that reflected his helplessness, worthlessness, shame, fear, and pervasive sense of loneliness (Fig. 4). I provided him with a drawing of a chair and asked him to identify someone in his life that he had unfinished business with, and the feelings and memories associated with that business. He drew in a manner that belied his present state of depression. He evidenced a great deal of rage and anguish, but more significant was the intense purpose—an unidentified resource of energy—from which he appeared to be creating. The slumped-over, crying, line drawing in the chair was identified by Samuel as his birthmother; the black-faced amorphous shape under the chair is Sam—being born "frightened" and "ashamed." The picture of the hands covering the face, preventing the person from seeing, being seen and speaking, became recurring images and themes throughout the treatment process. The art readily accessed unresolved issues related to adoption and subsequent needs that had gone unacknowledged and untreated. Samuel's personal symbolic representations grew and changed as trust developed and a more intact cohesive ego identity was formulated.

As treatment progressed, Samuel's imagery evolved. He felt less

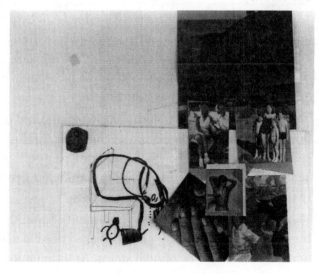

Fig. 4   A reflection of loneliness.

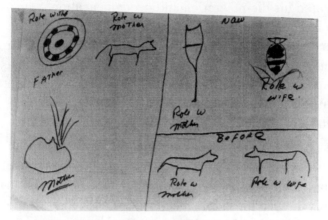

Fig. 5   Family roles.

invisible and increasingly understood on a deeper level than he had previously experienced. In his continued self-discovery process he used the imagery to explore past family roles and present family roles (Fig. 5). The lack of affect and depressed mood conveyed by this piece of imagery reflects Samuel's state of ineffectiveness, helplessness, impotency and enmeshed dependency with his birthmother, adoptive mother, and present wife. The self-depiction as a dog who is unable to see or speak was most remarkable and revealing to Sam. He had always felt like an outsider, so now he leaves himself out. He always felt invisible and unwanted, so now he is the perpetrator as well as the victim. Perhaps the fantasy of being a helpless animal was more acceptable and tolerable than being seen as a helpless and ineffective man.

Ego Identity

Where did I come from? Who am I ? Why am I here? These innocent and frequently-posed identity-related questions take on a more complex and fragile demeanor when the inquiry is made by an adult adoptee like Samuel, searching for a sense of relatedness and connectedness that for others is taken for granted as a birthright.

The sense of ego identity as conceptualized by Erikson (1968) involves the individual's awareness of the continuity of the self. The formation of this self is dependent on the synthesis of the past self, the future self and the present self. The adoptee experiences significant disruption in this dynamically interrelated development of a self.

In the final phase of treatment, Samuel was able to identify his increased sense of control and decreased need to use denial to defend his vulnerable and fragile emotional states. At termination he drew the eyes and the mouth (Fig. 6) that he discovered within himself and indicated with the "golden" tear his attachment to me and "our discovery." The lack of self boundaries continued to be an issue for him. He had through the use of imagery, learned to communicate the losses he had experienced as an infant, child and adult adoptee.

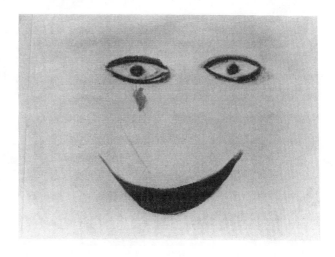

Fig. 6   The "golden tear."

As Samuel so articulately stated, "These images opened the window to my soul." A powerful sense of self had been reconstructed; a feeling of empowerment had been found.

Identity Confusion

Jane's mixed media self-portraits (Figs. 7and 8) depicts the dual existence or the good adoptee/bad adoptee struggle experienced and acted out by so many adoptees in young adulthood (Lifton, 1979). This duality that forces many adoptees to lead a double existence is clearly delineated in Jane's artwork. The surface one in this case is the *Rebellion* identity, and, as indicated in the parentheses, it is a defense, a means to contain and protect her *Scard little girl* self that questions her existence in this far-off distant world that she does not feel related to at this time in her life.

The Birth Process

The adoptee may suffer from the vicissitudes of the interuterine experience as well as from the postpartum disruption. The biological mother's lack of maternal commitment may interfere with the fetus' capacity to feel

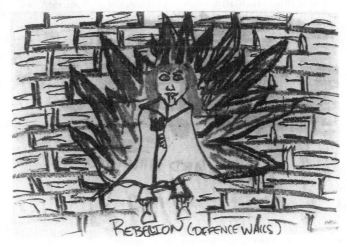

Fig. 7   Study in polarities—self portrait A

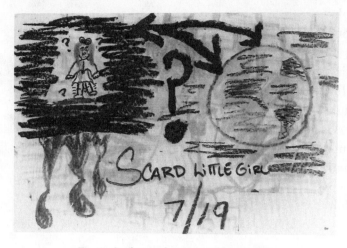

Fig. 8   Study in polarities—self portrait B

containment and a sense of connectedness. Continuity and cohesiveness are disrupted at birth. The devastating and traumatic separation, the interruption of the holding and containing experience and the intense sense of loss and rejection that is felt by many adult adoptees may significantly affect their self and self-object representations (Brinich, 1980).

Due to Cindy's inadequate and ineffective handling by her adoptive parents and the hostile environment they created, she grew up feeling like a *Ragdoll* (Fig. 9), split and fragmented, good and bad, real and unreal. The use of art expression to externalize her internalized conflicts and her fear of self dissolution provides the art therapist with an opportunity to provide containment and symbolic holding.

A Divided Self

The adopted child's understanding and organization of parental introjects can lead to polarized themes of goodness and badness; this splitting mechanism can be seen throughout the imagery of the adult adoptees discussed in this article.

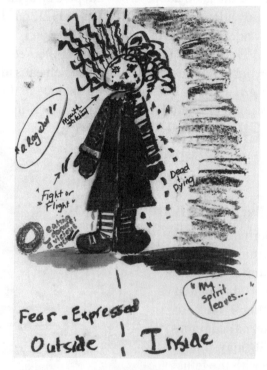

Fig. 9   Ragdoll

The adoptee's task to integrate a polarized sense of self and two sets of parents can create fragmentation and chaos (Figs. 1, 2, 3, 7, 8, & 10).

Unexpressed anger and infant-like rage is evidenced in Cindy's exploration of her self-destructive urges (Fig. 10). This bombastic expulsion and discharge offered a great sense of relief to her. Cindy had grown up believing that if she exposed her real self she would be abandoned again, as she had been originally. Through the use of the concrete images Cindy was able to symbolically gain control and insight into her self-destructive urges. If she could symbolically find relief and a sense of being real, she would not have to act it out as she had in the past.

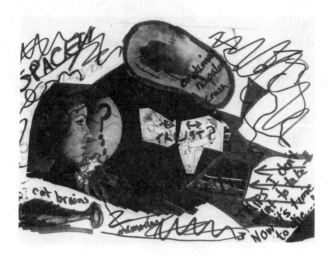

Fig. 10 Unexpressed rage.

The engagement process that takes place between the patient, her personal imagery and the therapist can culminate in a reparative and corrective emotional experience over the course of time. The development of this relationship may ameliorate the original infantile trauma.

Divided Loyalties

Many adoptees struggle with the conflict presented by divided loyalties. This was poignantly brought to my attention while I was seeing both foster parents and their 7-year-old foster child, Earl. The foster parents' own son had died, and their foster child had been separated from his mother and sister. Although he had been relinquished for adoption by his biological mother, and he was "wanted" by the foster family, this bright 7-year-old felt he could not abandon and betray his allegiance to his "real mom." The conflict was acted out behaviorally as the pending adoption grew near; he successfully alienated those close to him and rejected any attempts for emotional contact by becoming violent, and, as he pointed out, "unlovable."

When I asked him to draw what it would feel like to "be part of a Family" (Fig. 11), he drew a picnic scene that included his foster parents with a large basket of "goodies" spread out on a smooth inviting blanket. Off to the edge was the drawing of a small frail image of himself and a woman he identified as his mother, but added, "or maybe it's you, Rita, taking me to the picnic."

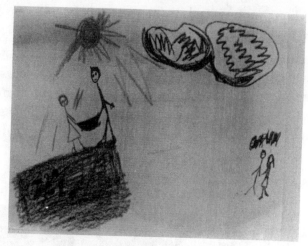

Fig. 11   Part of a family

When the foster parents inquired, "Are you going to join us for some goodies?" he responded with an eerie sense of confidence, "No, not now, ...I'm sorry if that hurts you."

This conflict emerged symbolically in the graphic imagery, and, with the guidance of the art therapist, it was able to be articulated verbally by all parties and processed to a state of completion, There was finality and closure for all, even though there was an intense sense of loss and disappointment. The adoption proceedings were cancelled, and the boy was returned to the residential placement. Because of his age, the severity of his behavior, and the history of abuse, the foster parents gave up their "rescue fantasy" and acknowledged respect for the boy's allegiance to his biological mother. They also were able to confront their own unfinished grief and wish to fill the void that had been created by the death of their only son.

Conclusion

Adoption is one socially approved solution to the dilemma of an unwanted child, and it also is a profound experience that results in reactions with universal themes of loss, abandonment, rejection, identity, and potential vulnerabilities in attachment and the sense of belonging.

A course of events that leads to adoption generally occurs when one or both parents are not willing or not able to provide adequate care for the child they have co-created. Within the adoption triangle, a number of crises have accumulated and as pointed out by Brinich (1980), "...the tragedies, inabilities and failures of both the biological and the adoptive parents are reflected in the adopted child and his psychological development."

The issues and specific needs of this segment of our society have not been adequately identified, addressed or fully understood by many clinicians. That adoption is potentially full of conflicts may be reflected in the fact that "adopted children are referred for psychological treatment two to five times as frequently as their non-adopted peers in countries as widely dispersed as Great Britain, Israel, Poland, Sweden and the United States" (Brinich, 1980).

This is not to suggest that the symptoms born out of the adoption experience are so vastly different from those of other children who have endured early loss and abandonment, but it is the secrecy, denial, and double messages typically shrouding the adoption that leave the adoptee yearning for acceptance, visibility, and validation.

The art psychotherapy process facilitates bringing forth the long-forgotten or repressed experiences of the early crucial developmental years, when so much chaos and disruption may have taken place. It is significant to note that once an adoption placement is finalized, there is a painful and frequently traumatic "waiting period" before it is legal and able to be implemented.

The positive and the negative transference that takes place in the art psychotherapy process is largely unconscious. It is considered a form of object relationship and can be an integral part of the patient's body of artwork. And if we accept that every object relationship is a re-editing process of the original infant attachments, then transference is omnipresent. The healing of psychological problems is partially, if not wholly, a symbolic process in which words and images play the major role. A great deal of the healing process is metaphorical, an "as if" process in which the therapist comes to represent both a series of persons from the patient's past, and also a series of possibilities for her future.

Real improvement and change come about through symbolic interaction. It is my contention that art psychotherapy is invaluable in the assessment and treatment of adoptees and their interpersonal, intrapsychic struggles. It provides depth understanding by unearthing the unique challenges and making real the fantasies internalized by the adopted individual.

Finally, the images that are created in art psychotherapy embody the patient's thoughts, fears, conflicts and feelings. It is inherent in the capacity of art to connect one's internal experience with his or her external reality and also to connect unconscious aspects of the conscious realm. I find this process to be most valuable when the therapist is able to be empathic and intuitive to translate the patient's verbal and non-verbal material into a "directive" or vehicle to be utilized for self-discovery.

There is no prescribed set of exercises to address issues related to the adoption experience. If, for example, the patient tells you of a recent disruptive experience and a subsequent loss and then goes on to report more on a similar theme, I might suggest looking at this issue of "loss" or "disruption" in whatever media you deem appropriate for further exploration. This non-directive spontaneous approach allows for the interplay of primary and secondary processes and ultimately to facilitate the integration and self-actualization sought by the patient in art psychotherapy.

References

Brinich, P. M. (1980). *Some potential effects of adoption on self and object representations.* Psychoanal. Study Child, 35: 107-133

Erikson, E. (1974). *Identity, youth and crisis.* London: Faber and Faber

Gaylord, C. L. (1976). *The adoptive child's right to know.* Case & Comment '81 (article), pg.38

Lifton, B. J. (1979). *Lost and found—the adoption experience.* NY: Dial Press

Sorosky, A. D., Baran, A., & Pannor, R. (1979). *The adoption triangle.* Garden City, NJ: Doubleday

Winnicott, D. W. (1971). *Playing and reality.* London & NY: Tavistock Publications.

Art Therapy with Dissociative Disorder Patients
by Patti Wallace, M.A., A.T.R.

Patti Wallace has practiced art therapy for 19 years in inpatient and outpatient psychiatric settings, and children's and adolescent residential treatment settings. Trained by pioneers Kramer, Kwiatkowska and Ulman, her special interest is the treatment of dissociative and multiple personality disorders, where she focuses on healing, processing and integrating play and art with verbal psychoanalytic work. She is currently a research psychoanalytic candidate at the Newport Psychoanalytic Institute.

> *"I feel that art has something to do with the achievement of stillness in the midst of chaos; a stillness which characterizes prayer, too, and the eye of the storm. I think that art has something to do with an arrest of attention in the midst of distraction."*   Saul Bellow

MPD and dissociative disorder patients were misdiagnosed for years, categorized as schizophrenic because of their fragmentation. It has fascinated me that dissociative disorder patients have always seemed to "take to" art therapy so readily, while the general adult inpatient population adopts a much more well-defended, neurotic "I can't draw" stance. Perhaps it has to do with one's "child parts" feeling more comfortable with a nonverbal tool for expression, or with the developmental arrests caused by the severe abuse that necessitated dissociation as a survival mechanism. Or is doing art work itself a dissociative phenomenon that attracts those who are used to plugging into right brain activity?

I have seen these patients use art to help themselves express therapeutic material, experiences and feelings difficult to put into words. Their art has provided a bridge to understanding and a place to help process information on several levels at once. If dissociating is "to sever the association of one thing from another" (Braun, 1984, p. 171), then the art process can assist the goal of reassociating fragmented thought processes through the power of the visual connection.

Just as it is important how one "teaches" an infant to speak, it is important how one offers art experiences as well. Most patients would prefer to avoid art therapy for fear of replicating early "not good enough" art experiences in school settings and in families where other members were the "identified" artists.

The general adult inpatient population has to deal with the previous traumatic experiences in school and family regarding art expression. Patients wish to avoid repeating such experiences in the present. However, dissociative patients don't seem to have those particular latency-age school traumas. Most were severely traumatized at preoedipal levels and are easily engaged in art activity. Because of the natural suitability of art therapy for dissociative patients, my experience in working with this population has been richly rewarding.

The Art Therapy Process

The art therapy process:
- facilitates the externalization of internal organizational material;
- is a way to process memories on several levels simultaneously;
- gives a more equal expressive potential to the variety of personality alters of different ages and developmental levels.

The art experience by itself is therapeutic but also offers the option of verbally processing the experience and the product as well.

A simple way of summing up the art therapy process is that it allows what is *inside* (feeling states, thoughts or visual images) to be made *outside* (by using art media and "holding" by the art therapist) in order to be taken back *inside* again through seeing the process and created object, so that it may be put *outside* again, but this time, through words shared with the art therapist, who can also process the imagery in relationship with the patient.

To take the inside and make it outside is to be able to take it back inside in a *new way*. An important concept in this process is that of Symbolic Concretization.

Symbolic Concretization

In *Structures Of Subjectivity; Explorations in Psychoanalytic\ Phenomenology*, Atwood and Stolorow emphasize concretization as a structure-maintaining function. One of their clinical illustrations is that of a young woman who would appear to have a Multiple Personality Disorder. Artwork is a major pathway by which symbolic concretization of internal states can occur. Art therapy would have expedited the analytic work with this patient since she presented vivid dream images and symbolic enactments of internal structures.

Art Therapy Evaluation

As close to admission as possible, I do an art therapy evaluation to assess the patient's organization and phase of treatment, and make a recommendation of how art therapy and the art therapist can best be utilized in treatment. For this, I use the Diagnostic Drawing Series created by Barry Cohen and Anne Mills. This procedure calls for the use of 18"x 24" white paper with a 12-color box of Weber Costello Alphacolor pastels.

- The first picture, a free drawing, is elicited by the directive, "Make a picture using these materials."
- The second picture is more structured, and asked for with the words, "Draw a tree."
- The third picture is an abstract feeling picture: "Make a picture of your feelings using lines, shapes and colors."

No one picture is to take more than 15 minutes and so is workable in a one hour block of time. Cohen found that patients often will draw a good representation of their system in either the first or last drawing and that MPDs are usually quite explicit about the meaning of the symbols drawn.

Samples of DDS Drawings

Patient A, a 42 year old female: Spontaneous appearance of a child alter

This first set of pictures shows the personalization of imagery and the spontaneous appearance of child alters during the evaluation, a subtle dissociative style of drawing and an avenue of access to feeling states showing a feeling of being trapped instead of feeling supported.

Fig. 1 shows "My Trunk" done in black outline, and filled in anxiously. There is no foundation for the trunk. The patient say she hid there as a child to get away from scary things and people. Although a "Safe Place," it serves as a refuge but not a solution to environmental childhood trauma.

The second picture, Fig. 2, "Mr. Sanders," is the tree drawing done in a mature drawing style but executed fairly quickly. The same anxious coloring of the tree trunk in brown with black cutting strokes shows the same ambivalence as in the first drawing. It was said to be a particular tree on the way to the therapist's office. The patient became full of vitality and gleefulness as a *child alter*, to tell about the tree and how it came to be named after the tree that served as Pooh's house in *The World of Pooh.*

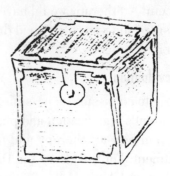

Fig. 1   A "Safe Place"

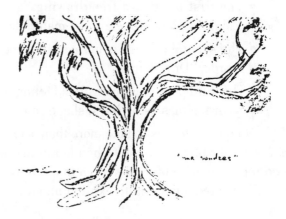

Fig. 2   "Pooh's house"

The third drawing, Fig. 3, is of a central black square surrounded by a red square, surrounded again by a light blue square. Black fragments are then slashed around the page. A thinner trail of red "blood" around all four sides of the paper and six large tear drops are added to express the "Pain." The tiny stick figure in peach in the center of the black square, representing the patient's feeling of being lost in depression and surrounded by "darkness, blood, tears and pain"

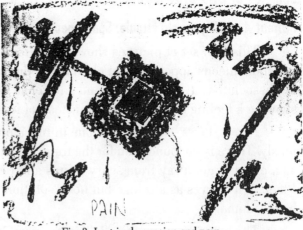

Fig. 3   Lost in depression and pain

was added last.

Patient B, a 42-year-old female: Eating Disorder

The second set of drawings is the work of a woman with an eating disorder. Fig. 4 shows a predominantly black and purple area of color filling most of the page in a cave or mouth-like shape with several tooth-like shapes descending. Delicate, multicolored fingerprints inside the dark area represent "all of the parts, that I barely know about, inside of the cave." Although this powerful devouring image was done by the bulemic patient substantial dissociation and multiplicity were uncovered later.

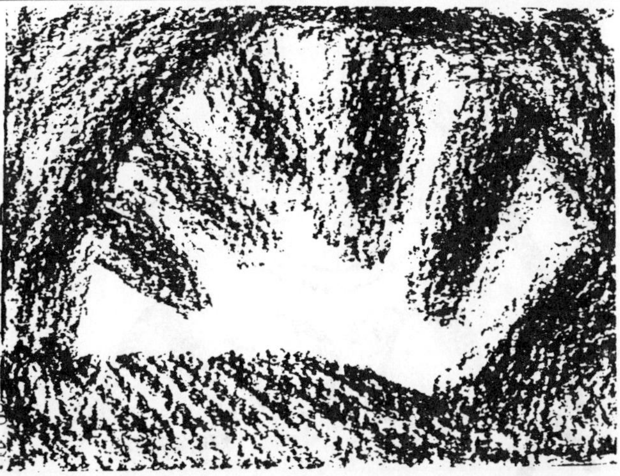

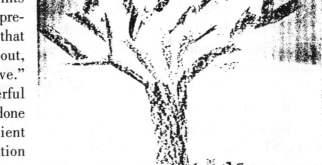

Fig. 4   Patient with an eating disorder draws a cave/mouth

Fig. 5   Same patient's bare tree, in contrast withher cave

The second drawing, Fig. 5, shows a hastily done sparse autumn (leafless) tree centered and resting on the lower edge of the paper. The trunk is straight and broad with the branches drawn in what I call a "dissociative style" where they barely touch the main branch revealing a literal disconnection in the drawn line. The emptiness of the second image is contrasted to the enclosing, devouring first image and replicates the patient's bingeing and purging cycle.

The third image, Fig. 6, was of her present state of feeling somehow "broken," "missing something," "sad," "depressed," "scared," "in lots of pieces," "losing time," "getting lost," "leaving my body," identifying herself with her fragmented and empty drawing.

Patient C, a 34-year-old female: Ritual Abuse

The third set of drawings shows a 34-year-old female patient in the

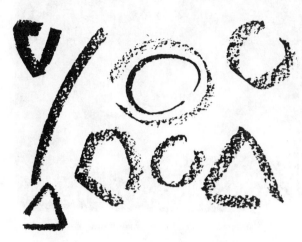

Fig. 6   An image of a fragmented inner state

midst of feeling over-whelmed by uncovering traumatic memories of ritualistic abuse as represented in Fig. 7.

Many intersecting repetitive diamond shapes are drawn to the left side in multicolors followed by a similar pattern of overlapping repetitive circular shapes on the right side. The two large multicolor groupings reflect "all the pieces inside." The picture is divided diagonally by a black line.

The patient said the central black and red area represented a ritualistic ceremony and reminded her of "candles," "people watching and groups of people in configurations." The two sides represented her internal response to the central scene with "internal parts" all moving around and feeling "scared" about the scene.

The second picture, Fig. 8, is of a tree which is also drawn in a divided way in black and brown, "dead," with no leaves and with a superimposed double window, emphasizing the already split-in-two tree.

The last picture, Fig. 9, is of feelings of "anxiety" and "needing to cut" and "trying to make connections in therapy" where the multicolors are used again in a fairly compulsive way. All of the three images are floating with no attachment to any side of the paper. A complex of multicolored, interconnected and layered representations of a complicated but split off internal organization is portrayed.

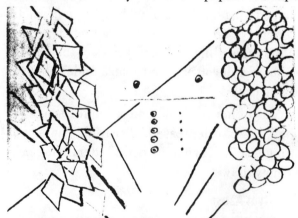

Fig. 7   A drawing recalling a scene of ritual abuse

As you can see from the illustrations, the dissociative style is sometimes quite subtle and sometimes quite obvious. Multiplicity may be shown in an array of fragmented, disconnected images or in the collec-

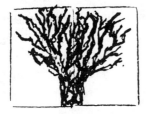

Fig. 8 Ritual abuse patient draws a divided tree

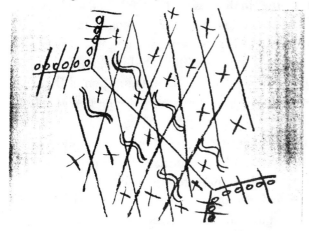

Fig. 9 An abstract disconnected anxious drawing

tion of repetitive color patterns and groupings. The pictures are most helpful when observed as they are being drawn and linked with the art therapist's seeing and hearing the associated words and behaviors that do not necessarily imprint themselves on the created product. An evaluation is formed via the combination of intuition, observation and the relationship between the patient, the art materials and the art therapist.

I use the DDS as an evaluative procedure as well as to introduce the patients to art materials and the art therapist as a resource during their hospitalization.

Working with the Patient

I also see patients in a mixed population group art therapy setting in Free Expression Time and Directed Theme/Issues groups, and in individual art therapy sessions to allow them to work on processing material from sessions with the psychiatrist or work of their own choosing.

A useful opening in working with dissociative patients is "Drawing A Safe Place."

The theme first appeared spontaneously when patients were encouraged to "draw whatever comes to mind." Since others could relate so well to this theme, I began using "Drawing A Safe Place" in those group sessions where I supply a directive. Many dissociative patients see this as a place they can go to in their minds to hide and be safe. I ask the patients to draw their safe place and embellish it. It seems to be a positive manifestation of their dissociative skills. Expressing feelings about safety is the most important factor to be established in working with the severely traumatized patient.

123

After they express their feelings about safety, they frequently become open and even playful.

Most often I simply offer a range of expressive art materials to the patient, hoping to touch upon an area that will allow them to put outside into an art form the inner turmoil that has brought them to the hospital. I allow the patient to work spontaneously in order to show me where he/she is so that I may offer different media, or suggest a specific feeling or subject focus when they feel blocked. I have magazine pictures for collage and rubber stamps for those who feel incapable of direct use of art supplies. I also encourage the patients to do journal writing as well to facilitate expression and increase internal communication.

One patient's painting had the written message, "Even in the chaos, there is order. If you recognize the order in the chaos, it not only becomes recognizable, but manageable." The patient has been able to look at the splits through the imagery produced by stamping separate images with rubber stamps as well as use art materials to create more integrated images of phases of her treatment. Art therapy is only limited by the imagination of those who are creating at a particular time. Be open and your patients may teach you some new ways that are helpful.

In our program, we ask the patient to draw a "Map" of their system (Ross, 1989). After supplying the patient with art materials, I encourage them to help the treatment team understand how they are organized inside. They are aware of this organization and may inquire "within" to get assistance with where different "alters" are, and to whom they are close.

Play Therapy

I also run a Play Therapy Group for the Dissociative Disorders Program which includes art materials, toys, sand tray, structured leisure time and socialization skills and tasks. There is definite need for play because of the fear and anxiety some of the child alters expressed. They apparently had been hurt and/or had rigid rules about "staying clean," "being a good girl, " and "doing it right" followed by fears of punishment for playing or having fun.

Theme Ideas for Dissociative & MPD Patients

- Make yourself a blank journal notebook to allow everyone to have a place to communicate in drawing and writing.
- Draw a safe place.
- Create a secure place to keep memories.
- Create a safe room for alters to rest and play in.
- Use both hands to write and draw a dialogue with yourself.

- Draw an internal bulletin board for important messages.
- Draw your anger in a safe way.
- Draw the child parts (little ones) playing together.
- Draw how you experience your internal system.
- Draw the part that is having a problem right now.
- Draw arguing inside.
- Draw negotiating inside.
- Draw everyone working together on a project.
- Draw oneness and separateness.
- Draw/collage images that nurture the child/children within.
- Draw/sculpt the nurturing parent within holding the child in a caring way.
- Create a unified symbol to represent everyone coming together.
- Draw the importance of feeling understood.
- Draw something about understanding yourself.
- Draw yourself and your connection with your mother, father, both parents, together.
- Draw pictures about how you learned to talk, to think.
- Draw a picture of how you think you learned about feelings.
- Draw a picture of how you feel about your body.
- Draw a picture of how your mind and body work together.
- Make an image of how your mind and body work against each other.
- Make a picture of how you feel about words.
- Make a picture of trusting and trust.
- Make a picture about hiding.
- Make a picture about secrets.
- Draw a picture about "making up stories."
- Make a picture about being believed.
- Make a picture about feeling relieved.
- Draw your multiplicity: past, present and future.
- Draw a picture about how dissociation feels in your body.
- Draw a picture that tells a story about how you "go away inside."
- Draw a picture about "leaving the body."

Duality Drawings:

- Draw evil and good and their intermingling.
- Draw dangerous and safe and their relations.
- Draw sick and well and how you tell the difference.
- Draw north, south, east and west and how we need them all.
- Draw up and down and how they work together.

I use Lucia Capacchione's *Recovery of Your Inner Child,* a most helpful resource in increasing dialogue within the system. It is valuable in integrating the dissociative patient in a group with other diagnostic categories of patients, where all are encouraged to utilize the metaphor of the "inner child" as a way to beginning recovery.

For those clinicians interested in early analytic writers, I would encourage the reading of the Hungarian psychoanalysts Ferenczi and Balint who used the internal child metaphor in the 1920's and '30's as they spoke of regressive phenomena. Another related early source recognizing multiplicity is Fairbairn's *Psychoanalytic Studies of the Personality* which contain the clinical papers, *Notes on the Religious Phantasies of a Female Patient* (1927) and *Features in the Analysis of a Patient with a Physical Genital Abnormality* (1931), which touch upon the ubiquitous theme of "good and evil" so often present in Multiple Personality Disorder patients, especially in those who have experienced ritualistic abuse. Marion Milner's *On Not Being Able to Paint* and *Hands of the Living God* are wonderful sources for the crossover of art and psychoanalysis. I recommend D.W. Winnicott's *Psychoanalytic Explorations* where he writes about the essential relationship between mother and child. These books serve as the background for my theoretical beliefs in working with patients.

Refereences

Atwood, G. and Stolorow, R. (1984). *14 structures of subjectivity: explorations in psychoanalytic phenomenology.* NJ: The Analytic Press.

Balint, M. (1968). *The basic fault : therapeutic aspects of regression.* NY: Brunner / Mazel.

Braun, B. G., ed.(1986). *Treatment of multiple personality disorder* Washington, D.C.: American Psychiatric Press.

Capacchione, L. (1989). *The creative journal: the art of finding yourself.* North Hollywood: Newcastle Publishing.
————— (1991). *Recovery of Your Inner Child.* NY: A Fireside Book, Simon and Schuster.
—————(1984). *Wellbeing journal: the art of self care.* San Diego: Lura Media.

Dalley, T., et al. (1987). *Images of art therapy: new developments in theory and practice.* London and NY: Tavistock Publications.

Fairbairn, W. R. D., (1952). *Psychoanalytic studies of the personality.* London, Henley and Boston: Routledge & Kegan Paul.

Gilroy, A. and Dalley, T., ed. (1989). *Pictures at an exhibition: selected essays on art and art therapy.* London and NY: Tavistock / Routledge.

Kluft, R. P., (1989). *Playing for time: temporizing techniques in the treatment of multiple personality disorder.* American Journal of Clinical Hypnosis.32 (2).

Landgarten, H. and Lubbers, D., ed. (1991. *Adult art psychotherapy: issues and applica-*

tions. NY: Brunner / Mazel.

Langer, S. K., (1957). *Problems of art: ten philosophical lectures* NY: Charles Scribner's Sons.

Milne, A. A., (1926). *The World of Pooh: The complete Winnie the Pooh and The House at Pooh Corner.* NY: E. P. Dutton.

Murphy, E. F., (1978). *The Crown treasury of relevant quotations.* NY: Crown.

Putnam, F. W., (1991). *Recent research on multiple personality disorder.* Psychiatric Clinics of North America. 14 (3).

Ross, C. A., (1989). *Multiple personality disorder: diagnosis, clinical features and treatment.* NY: A Wiley Interscience Publication.

Rubin, J. A., ed., (1987). *Approaches to art therapy: theory and technique.* NY: Brunner/Mazel.

Winnicott, C., et. al., ed., (1989). *Psychoanalytic explorations.* Massachusetts: Harvard University Press.

Art Therapy with a Left-Hemisphere Post-Stroke Patient
by Angeline Leonard, Ph.D., A.T.R., M.F.C.C.

Angie Leonard has been a registered art therapist, licensed marriage, family, child counselor and certified hypnotherapist for over ten years. In addition to teaching in the San Fernando Valley College art department for 25 years, she holds a master's degree in clinical art therapy, a Ph.D. in clinical psychology and has engaged in private practice for many years.

Art psychotherapy presents many advantages as a modality in treatment of the left hemisphere post-stroke patient, especially one with aphasia.

A cerebral vascular accident is defined by the National Stroke Association as damage to the brain through disruption in the flow of blood to one or more areas and is caused by a blood clot, hemorrhage, aneurysm, tumor or head trauma. Hemiplegia often accompanies a CVA: a weakness or paralysis on the side opposite the affected side of the brain.

Although cognitive functioning may be intact, aphasia frequently appears when damage from a CVA occurs to Broca's area in the left cerebral hemisphere. Aphasia, here, refers to loss or impairment of verbal and/or written expressive communication. With such an occurrence, comprehension can be fairly clear yet the ability to express thought clearly through speech is damaged.

Art psychotherapy can be a powerful and effective tool that helps the stroke patient improve function in the damaged brain, and can help the undamaged brain assume functions of the damaged brain. The intact right cerebral hemisphere is nonverbal, but accessible through graphic expression of art therapy. Art psychotherapy can help the patient communicate feelings of loss, anger, helplessness and depression. And art therapy can supply motivation to communicate verbally about the artwork, and so spur a patient to regain damaged speech skills more quickly.

In describing the characteristics of right and left cerebral hemispheres, art therapist Evelyn Virshup writes, "The right hemisphere is intuitive, able to abstract, wordless and imaginative. It processes our orientation in space, it recognizes forms, and works relationally, acoustically, simultaneously and more holistically than does the left hemisphere. The left hemisphere appeared to be the logical, verbal part of the brain. It analyzes and processes information in a rational, linear, sequential way" (Virshup 1979).

For a person whose speech and writing skills have been impaired, drawing pictures and working with collage and clay are methods of creative communication, of mind travel when physical travel is limited, and a safety outlet through which to express overwhelming emotions appropriately. Strength for a patient's improvement resides in the abilities of the right hemisphere.

Art therapy accesses and activates right cerebral hemisphere abilities to work to support the healing. We think in pictures before we formulate words. When the ability to express words is damaged, the mental filing system relies on the stored system of images for expression. Myra Levick, art therapist, writes, "Infants develop a storehouse of images upon which language is built. Infants can indicate by behavior that they recognize objects before they respond to names of those objects." Object constancy, the ability to keep an image of an object in mind after the object has disappeared from sight, precedes language development. One who has lost the ability of verbal speech through stroke can, through art therapy, begin with pictures to rebuild the foundation for clearer speech.

The post-stroke patient may feel powerless and resent having to depend upon health-care givers, family and friends. Art therapy aids in diminishing the power of dependency fears by exercising development of remaining abilities. It empowers the stroke patient by providing control within his or her range of abilities, and assists in developing confidence through teaching the patient to make use of even a stroke-impaired hand to weigh down the paper being drawn on. The paralyzed hand assists the undamaged hand to support supplies when carried to the art table, and it can be traced around as a way of being included instead of denied, both cognitively and emotionally. Helen Landgarten, art therapist, writes of its benefits: "Symbolically the art therapy session proves to the patient that dependency (regression due to the need for care) and independence (taking responsibility) can coexist during the period of rehabilitation" (Landgarten 1981).

Often a patient will resist following directives because of feelings of inadequacy or depression. It is essential that the art therapist explain to stroke patients that simple art tasks and discussion of the artwork will help them through their difficult time. An explanation of the objective benefits of participating in art therapy as a path towards healing is not only helpful, but is sometimes the key that leads to action. "The nonverbal visual aspects of this modality give the patient an opportunity for communication, self expression and interpersonal exchange which otherwise might not be possible" (Landgarten 1981).

Memory is stored in the body as well, as clearly explained by the writings and work of Deepak Chopra, M.D. (Chopra 1989). Each cell plays a part in healing the whole system, and can be influenced in many ways by feelings and thoughts. Carl Jung sums it up when he writes, "Often the hands know how to solve a riddle with which the intellect has wrestled in vain" (Jung 1960). Art psychotherapy activates the mind/body connection in such a way, bringing to conscious awareness memory, insight and capability that stroke trauma may have rendered inactive.

A Case Study

The following case study illustrates the dynamic use of short term art therapy with a 67-year-old male who was four years post-stroke. His name and some specifically personal information have been changed to insure confidentiality.

James suffered a left hemisphere stroke four years before working with me. Before the stroke, James, a college graduate, had been an athlete, actor, and successful businessman. Afterward, he experienced partial paralysis of the right hand and leg, slow shuffling gait, speech that was almost incomprehensible, and an expressive aphasia. Recently he had developed severe depression, shortened attention span, and increasing agitation with episodes of physical violence. Although he denied any feelings of anger, he had frequent violent physical outbursts at home, one of which had resulted in a broken front door, and a black eye to himself and a family member. His wife, afraid of his physical outbursts of aggression and unable to cope with the depression, sought help for him at a day treatment center.

Starting day treatment care in a hospital in Southern California, James was admitted to the low functioning group. At this time, he was able to walk by himself. He could use his right hand to grasp objects, and would hold them in front of his body like a shield. He had been right-handed, but was now able to write with his left hand and draw with it. Though he was generally active and helpful, he experienced episodes of agitation and depression that rendered him nearly incapable of sitting through a session.

James was referred to art therapy. It was thought art therapy might be beneficial as an aid to communication, for emotional ventilation through the artwork, and as a means for more appropriate social interaction.

For two weeks James was placed in an art therapy group. Fig. 1 shows a response to a non-threatening directive designed to allow the patient the most control in volunteering information to the group: "Choose a photo from the collage box that tells the group something you want them to know about you." Aphasia is evidenced in the left-handed writing James included on his collage, where he describes growing up on a place where there were cows, and he had to milk them..

After two weeks, James began individual art therapy. We met privately for an hour once a week. My major objective for James was to stimulate his feeling of autonomy and promote his ability to exercisee control in his life rather than feeling help-lessly dependent. A further goal was to assist him to own feelings of anger that had become destructively expressed and allow them appropriate expression through the artwork.

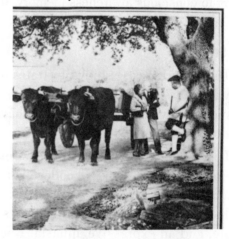

Fig. 1. Collage of early memories

Methods used toward accomplishing those goals

1) James *role-played* feelings expressed in photographs assembled into collages in order to decrease discomfort in acknowledging feelings.

2) His *voice was recorded on cassette* during the first part of therapy and later at the end of therapy to demonstrate progress in verbal communication.

3) Directives were formulated about making marks or shapes or doing a *drawing with the right hand* in order to exercise it to improve its use and fine motor dexterity.

4) To promote decision-making and self-esteem, he was directed to use the *art therapist as secretary* for dictation of memories in order to encour-

age positive life review. Dictating provided a valuable aid for him, as it reminded him of his business experience when he employed a secretary.

5) At the end of each session he would be asked to *help clear up materials*, sort pen colors into sets, put them in containers and carry some. Even though he was handicapped, he was noticeably pleased to know that he could be of service.

6) *I would not offer help unless he asked for it.* He experienced difficulty with tasks that required fine motor control, such as cutting paper shapes with scissors. Fiercely independent yet agitated and depressed by loss of physical skills, he had not been able to ask for help from staff. However, through an agreement that I would not offer help unless he asked for it, and when he did, he would consider the request as one of empowering himself, he became able to ask for help after a couple of sessions.

7) By my asking him to choose magazine photos and indicate with a finger where he wanted the paper cut, he was reminded again and again that he retained control.

8) He was encouraged to talk about his artwork.

9) He was encouraged to write on and about his artwork.

Individual Art Therapy Begins

Session One.

The first art therapy session was spent in getting acquainted, discovering our similarities and differences and patterns of communication. Much of the time was spent in my asking James to repeat the few words he spoke. He would gesture with his hands and amplify with facial expressions in efforts to clarify verbal speech. I asked questions about his responses to treatment at the hospital, about his family, about his life and changes after the stroke in order to weave a framework on which to design the treatment plan. Most of his replies were incomprehensible, and his patience was enviable as he calmly repeated, gestured and searched for other words that might be more clearly understood. His verbal pattern was of one- or two words.

He selected pictures from a collage box that represented family members (which would be used in later sessions). As a means to develop the relationship on a more equal level, where verbal communication would not be an issue, I suggested a dual drawing and James eagerly assented. A dual drawing can be verbal or non-verbal, between clients or therapist and client. It is a means to gauge interactions between two people (or more), to further a connection (as between therapist and client) and to provide support at an unconscious level. It was a way to go beyond the obstacle of works and connect directly on the paper. After a short review at the end of the session, I asked James if he was interested in continuing art therapy and he nodded his head emphatically. Smiling, he began to return the colored markers to their boxes and to assist in straightening the room.

Session Two

James was waiting in the hall outside the art therapy room, for the second session and seemed in a hurry to get started. Fig. 2 was in response to the directive to "Pick a picture about something you would like to deal with here in therapy." Chosen was a color photograph of a right hand apparently gnarled and limited by arthritis. James' right hand had been partially paralyzed by the stroke. Fig. 3 was in response to the directive, "Select a picture that symbolizes or represents your self." James chose a picture in grey of a man in a wheelchair and titled it, "Sad, handicapped man representing self." It was an opening of the window to his feelings of inadequacy.

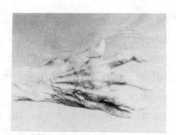

Fig. 2 James' concern in therapy

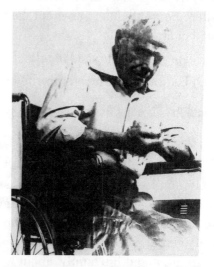

Fig. 3 How James saw himself symbolically.

Session Three

In the next session, physical issues were addressed immediately by his dictating a list of impairments from the stroke and improvements since the stroke. He was asked to illustrate the lists by making pictures of the impairments and improvements (Fig. 4). One goal was to heighten his awareness of feelings and encourage expression of them through the artwork rather than through violence.

James was asked to pick the colors with which I wrote and he drew. On the left side of the page he chose black, which he identified as "angry" and with blue as "sad." On the right side of the page he chose red, which he identified as a "happy" color for him.

Note the drawings and compare for a dynamic view of the unconscious at work. The drawing of the arm on the right (improvement) side is thicker, indicating muscle development. The mouth on the right side drawing is larger, possibly indicating clearer speech. As the conversation progressed in regard to improvements, James

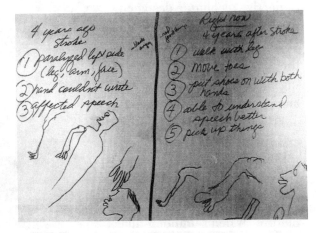

Fig. 4   Impairments and improvements

spoke longer sentences, using phrases like, "The stroke affected my speech," instead of his customary use of one or two-word responses. It appeared that as he gained confidence by being positively reinforced for his drawing, the confidence spread to include speech efforts. When it was pointed out to him he had listed three impairments and five improvements and that positive gains outnumbered the negative list, he agreed, surprised and smiling. It seemed to be the first time that his gains had been brought to his attention in such a way.

Next, James was asked to dictate a contract to increase verbalization from one word to several in a sentence, and develop more confidence in himself. He dictated that he would try to "improve speech, move leg better, work on hand, be more happy, less sad and safely express anger."

Another picture he made that session was an "Emotional Vocabulary." He chose colors from the box to represent various emotions, made representative marks with each, and we labeled each mark so that in the future when he used a color it might serve to identify what he was feeling when he made a picture.

Session Four

In the third session, he was able to acknowledge rage and fear that had been previously denied. His method of dealing with the subject of anger when it came up in the sessions had been to deny that he felt angry. He would admit to feeling frustrated, worried, and concerned. The directive in Fig. 5 was to "Choose from three to five pictures (pictures of angry people) and make up a story about each one," a projective technique designed to focus his awareness on anger, to express—through the artwork and story—feelings and attitudes about anger, and to work on a previously stated goal of "safely expressing anger."

At first he could not make up stories about the three angry persons in the picture. When reminded that he had been an actor and was asked to role play what each person in the photographs was doing and feeling, he smiled at the memory and energetically portrayed the emotions expressed in the pictures: anger by hitting, fear of being hit and anger by frowning and holding feelings in.

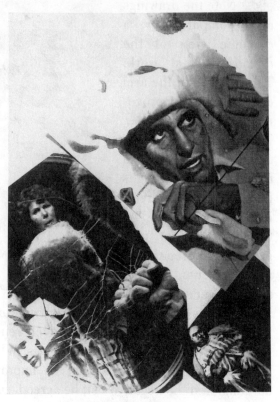

Fig. 5 A collage of angry people

James volunteered it was not good for the man to hold his feelings in, and it is better to hit something, like the man in the photo was doing, (like James had done at home). The last part of the session was spent discussing alternative, appropriate methods of releasing angry feelings without harming self or others: e.g., hitting a punching bag, making marks on the page, pounding clay.

Session Five

James was directed to trace around each hand with the other, and was reluctant to do so, fearing failure. In the previous two sessions, he had maintained that he was incapable of doing so. In Fig. 6 the right hand (drawn by the left hand) was done with a stiff, rigid line. The left hand (traced by the impaired right hand) is larger than the other and the line is actually more fluid, with a sensitive adherence to actual contours of the fingers. This was pointed out to James in the form of positive support. After he finished, he tried to fill in spaces by drawing with the more familiar left hand, and was told that the drawing was fine as it was, and that it had been the "right hand's turn to draw." When asked, he said he had never done drawing with his right hand since the stroke, that he liked doing it and would like to do some more next session.

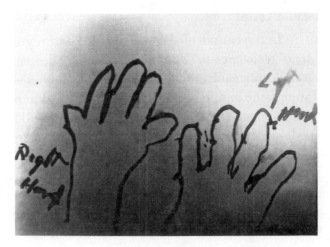

Fig. 6 Hand tracings

Session Six

The sixth session began with another exercise for the right hand. I asked if he wanted to make something with his right hand. He said he couldn't draw with it, but would try (customary willingness to comply with directive, coupled with

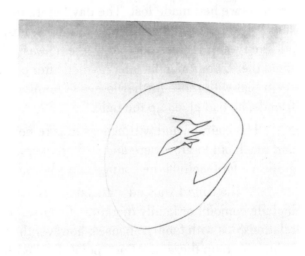

Fig. 7 James gives himself a star.

stroke-impaired short term memory). I showed him the right-handed drawing from the previous session, reminding him he had done it and asked him to make a circle (easiest form to draw, since the hand moves in a radius). He drew one slowly, was encouraged, then repeated the circle, on another paper, moving his hand faster. He was told to draw freely with the right hand and give his picture a title. Fig. 7 presents a drawing that appears deceptively simple. The shape is again a circle. James drew it with his right hand. He chose the shape to draw, and drew it the first try on that sheet of paper. I complimented him on his ability to accomplish it the first time, and he then added the shape in the middle which he identified as a star. Perhaps it was a star he bestowed upon himself for accomplishment; perhaps it represented a symbol of himself as a star. He appeared very pleased.

137

Gains & Losses

In the course of six weeks, gains and regressions were experienced. James' resistance to dealing with his anger decreased somewhat. His speech became noticeably clearer, both to me and other staff on the treatment team. Towards the end he did not have to be asked to repeat every sentence. His speech broadened from one word answers to full sentences. The steps were small—yet meaningful in comparison to the improvements in the four years preceding art therapy. Record of progress can be traced through the modality of art therapy. In this case, art therapy provided a valuable means of communication and interaction to a man who had all but lost his ability to communicate verbally, and through the process he discovered and developed abilities which helped him feel better about himself.

Unfortunately, the sessions were terminated prematurely, and the progress we had made lost. The day before the seventh art therapy session James was transferred by his wife to another hospital, where he was placed on a locked ward. He was not told where he was going, or that he would be confined there. Four months later he died after contracting pneumonia. It would seem that with those further losses of familiar surroundings and new-found friends, he had given up the fight.

His courage and willingness to take new risks in therapy, help others and reach out to grow were and still are inspiring to me, and to him goes my gratitude for teaching the courage to go beyond the trauma of stroke.

At the time I worked with James, the day treatment program did not include conjoint or family therapy. Of course, patients would talk about their relationships with family, spouses; however the treatment was geared to individual or group therapy. At one point, I asked James' primary psychiatrist if James' wife could be seen conjointly with him, or if family members could be brought in. The wife refused to attend, and I made no further requests. In the course of art therapy, James became more in touch with his anger and could outline alternative choices rather than hitting someone. It is of interest that he moved from living at home and attending day treatment, to a locked facility, and that no one—not day treatment staff nor James himself, was told of the move until after it was accomplished.

Appendix

Directives:

• Choose a photograph that tells the group something about yourself you would like them to know.

- Ask for help when needed. It is available, not mandatory.

- Indicate with finger where I should trim or glue a photograph.

- Pretend I am your secretary and dictate information for me to write.

- Select colors that represent different feelings. Make marks to represent those feelings, and label the marks.

- Choose a photograph that symbolizes what you want to deal with in therapy.

- Choose a photograph that represents your self.

- Make a list of the goals you want to accomplish.

- List impairments from the stroke and post-stroke improvements.

- Choose from 3-5 pictures of angry people and make up a story about each one. Paste them all on the same page.

- Trace around each hand with the other one.

- Make a circle.

- Do a free choice drawing. Give it a title.

References

Chopra, D., M.D. (1989). *Quantum healing: exploring the frontiers of mind/body medicine.* NY: Bantam.

Jung, C. G. (1960). *The structure and dynamics of the psyche:* collected works. Vol. 8. NY: Pantheon.

Landgarten, H. B. (1981). *Clinical art therapy: a comprehensive guide.* NY: Brunner/Mazel.

Levick, M. (1984). *Imagery as a style of thinking.* Art Therapy. 1 (3) 119-124.

Virshup, E. (1979). *Right brain people in a left brain world.* Los Angeles: Guild of Tutors Press.

Group Art Therapy Intervention with Bereaved Children in the Elementary Schools
by Thelma Z. Kornreich, M.A., A.T.R.

Thelma Z. Kornreich is a registered art therapist at the Belmar Child and Family Center and the coordinator and a facilitator of adult bereavement groups at Temple Isaiah in West Los Angeles. For a decade, she worked with emotionally disturbed children, adolescents and families at the Centinela Child Guidance Clinic in Inglewood. She conducts Separation and Loss Art Therapy groups in the Los Angeles Unified School District elementary schools for grieving children.

A six-year-old boy with a forlorn-looking face glanced up from his drawing and explained in a low voice, "My father killed my mother and then killed himself." After a pause, another first grader responded with, "My Daddy got shot dead by people driving by in a car," as he looked at the first little boy, his eyes filled with tears.

These two children were in an art therapy group in an elementary school, in the Los Angeles Unified School District (LAUSD), part of a Separation and Loss Group Art Therapy Program under the sponsorship of the Belmar Child and Family Center, located in West Los Angeles. This effort has been directed at children who have lost or were separated from significant caretakers. Not all the children in these groups experienced the violent death of a parent—some parents have died of natural causes, some caretakers deserted their families and some children were separated from one or the other parent by divorce.

One of the goals of this program has been to help such children begin to work through their grief and achieve acceptance of their loss. A second goal has been to help the children feel better about themselves.

Mourning Conditions

Bowlby states that infants and children exhibit instinctual attachment behavior toward caretaking individuals. When death or separation interferes with the relationship, the infant or child usually becomes grief-stricken, and displays feelings of anxiety, sorrow and anger. It has long been thought that parental loss in childhood is a devastating experience and contributes significantly to adult psychopathology (1980, p. 38).

Bowlby believes that children's responses to loss are influenced by the following favorable variables:

- The child has enjoyed a secure relationship with the parent before the death.
- The child is given prompt and accurate information about what happened.
- The child is allowed to ask questions.
- The child is allowed to participate in family grieving, including funeral or memorial rites.
- The child receives comfort from the surviving parent or a parent substitute.
- The child is assured that the relationship with the remaining caretaker will continue.

By acknowledging the children's grief through our group art therapy intervention, and encouraging the children in drawing and talking about their losses, our program helped in their healing processes and probably reduced the intensity of their future grieving.

Method

We treated and evaluated 40 students in seven groups of six children (two students moved after the first or second session) aged six through twelve in racially and ethnically mixed Los Angeles elementary schools, who have lost, by separation or death, significant caretakers, either through violent or non-violent means. School children targeted were those who would not normally have access to a psychological treatment program dealing with children's individual responses to grief and loss. The program was funded through private grants and has been free to the school and the children served.

142

At each school, the principal was approached and, if approval was gained for the program, the school psychologist became involved as a co-therapist. The teachers, school psychologist and principal selected the group members, and written permission was requested and given by the children's parents or guardians. The groups were as homogeneous as possible concerning age, grade and sometimes gender. It was difficult to gain proper group cohesiveness with some fifth and sixth graders, if the group contained both boys and girls. Much cooperation was needed and received from school personnel, school psychologist co-therapists, principals, teachers and office secretarial staffs.

Many of the children who participated in the group meetings were severely emotionally disturbed, were not doing well scholastically or socially, and/or may have been learning disabled. All had suffered loss and trauma. Teachers were given the shortened version of the Burks' Behavior Rating Scales (1968) and were asked to rate the child they had recommended for the group.

The shortened version, for elementary school children, of the Burke's Behavior Rating Scales (1968) was useful in determining specific emotional and behavioral states of these mourning children. Three areas of individual behavior considered in this scale are vegetative-autonomic, which concerns such behavior as hyperactivity and restlessness, perceptual-discriminative, which may reflect confusion in following directions, and social-emotional which concerns such behavior as frequent crying.

Parents were informed about the group and were asked for their written consent for treatment and for the anonymous use of the drawings and case material by the therapist in her publications and lectures. In all seven groups, only one parent refused to give her consent, saying the child was not in need, although the teacher felt otherwise. Forms were filled out on each child, stating pertinent information needed for group work: for instance, address, phone numbers at home and at work, who else lived at home, and how the child did scholastically.

Eight sessions completed the group work. The children's significant caretakers and teachers were always interviewed during the course of the group sessions, and attempts were made to help them deal more appropriately with the grieving children. After the first session with the children, the children's teachers and parents were all interviewed, and the interview recorded. After the seventh group session, feedback was provided to the parents and teachers, and the teachers were again asked to fill out a Burks' form. The comparison between the first and last rating has been helpful in determining change. Progress notes and a summary were written about each child.

Goals

Our goals for the children were:

- To reduce feelings of anxiety, anger, sadness, isolation and fear by providing a safe and caring environment where these emotions may be shared and worked through
- To empower group members through adult and group acceptance of the child's feelings and thoughts
- To help the caretaker improve supportive parenting behavior
- To provide the means to develop confidence in abilities, stimulate creativity and increase self-esteem and self-image
- To help children improve scholastic achievement
- To develop more social relatedness.

In order to achieve these goals, the first task was to form a therapeutic alliance with these children. As their trust developed they became freer in both verbal and art expression, and their feelings of grief and loss became more accessible.

Description of the Eight Group Art Therapy Sessions
Session One:

Becoming acquainted with each other, the rules, the purpose and completing a Diagnostic Art Interview.

The children and the therapists sat around a large table. When the six children first assembled, many did not understand why they had been chosen for what they perceived was a special art class. We discussed the reason they were there, to draw about and discuss their feelings of loss (disclosure was neither encouraged nor discouraged at this juncture), acquainted them with each other (children printed their names on stand-up folded paper and these identifying signs remained in front of the child on the table at all times), went over some group rules stressing confidentiality, and administered the *Diagnostic Art Interview,* which helps determine a child's emotional state and developmental stage.

(The only time this procedure was not followed was during the height of the American war involvement with Iraq and the Los Angeles civil disturbance of 1992. At both of these times, coincidentally, groups began on crucial days involving the war and riots, and it seemed appropriate to deal with how the children felt about those issues immediately (Fig. 1).

The children were given three papers, 12" x 9", one at a time, along with a number two pencil with an attached eraser and were instructed to draw *Draw-A-Person (DAP), Draw-the-Opposite-Sex (DOS) and a Kinetic-Family Drawing (KFD)*. The first two pictures (DAP, DOS) were drawn with pencil; colored felt-tipped markers were used by the children to draw the KFD. The children were asked to discuss their pictures in the presence of other group members and therapists. The group leaders asked the children some leading questions, such as:

- How old is this figure?
- What sex is she or he? (if this was not apparent)
- Where is he or she going?
- Will she or he meet someone?
- Is this person happy or sad?
- If this figure could talk, what would he or she say?

Comments were recorded by the therapists and, later, progress notes were written which contained an analysis based on the children's characteristic drawing traits, such as line quality, structure and placement and the content of their stories. Some time during the course of each session, usually at the end, the group members were treated to some cookies.

Session Two:

Constructing a Life Line Graph

If the children hadn't finished the Diagnostic Art Interview, the work was completed during the second session. The group was then asked to construct a Life Line Graph, representing the children's life in time from birth until ten years beyond their current age.

White construction paper was pre-cut to 6" x 18" dimensions, and the children were asked to fold the paper horizontally in half and then each section was folded again horizontally. Each child was given colored felt-tipped markers and asked to write along the left vertical edge the name of the *most significant people in their lives*, each name written with a *different color.* They were asked to use *one of these colors to write their own name (this points out the most connection and identity the child feels)*. At the top center of the sheet of paper, they wrote the word *"happy,"* in the middle in the center *"okay,"* and on the bottom center *"sad."* They were also asked to indicate the numbers of *0, to 10 years beyond their actual age, across the top of the page,* creating a simple graph which not only was divided into years, but measured their emotionality and showed the important people in their lives. They were asked to indicate their happiest, saddest and earliest experiences concerning events and people in their lives at different ages. (Wolff [1975] in group work also asks for the earliest memory in order to stimulate disclosure and intimacy.) With the device of 10 years hence, hope for the future was injected into the process by having the children focus on a future envisioning them possibly more in control of their lives and environment.

The construction of the graph was an emotionally difficult task for most children, and the therapists provided a great deal of empathy, support and individual attention. The group shared the information, although if some children indicated they were uncomfortable talking about their graph with the group, this was honored. Such a child was taken aside and worked with individually, but not outside the group room.

Session Three:

Drawing the Earliest, Saddest and Happiest Memories

Session Three further focused on the graph material. The children were asked to illustrate their earliest, saddest and happiest memories on 18" x 12" sheets of white construction paper and colored felt-tipped markers. A child was never given more than one paper at a time, as this could be overwhelming. During this session the children were encouraged to draw memories of the individual they lost; the circumstances of the illness, death, divorce or abandonment, as appropriate; and the details of the funeral, if experienced. The therapists were very active in clarifying, supporting and noting the various issues presented. If the artwork was not completed, it continued the next time, and the drawings were shared and discussed with the other members in the group at the end. It seemed best to start with earliest recollection, progress to the saddest and end with the happiest. The children at this point were familiar with each other and the therapists and understood they shared a commonality of loss with the other group members.

Session Four:

Painting a Self-portrait

In session 4, the members of the group were asked to draw their own portraits. They used 18" x 24" white construction paper, watercolor, paintbrushes and individual standing mirrors. The art therapist briefly demonstrated the properties of the paint and how to go about drawing a self-likeness. The children were also given the option to use other art materials such as felt-tipped markers or crayons. Most opted for the paint in combination with other art material. It seemed important for the therapist to encourage the children and help avert failure.

Watercolor, although fraught with peril because of its flowing hard-to-control properties, is still a satisfying solution in portraying skin color. The art therapist needs to be active in briefly teaching some basic watercolor techniques such as painting washes, blotting with tissue and allowing washes of skin color to dry before painting facial features.

Most children have found this an exciting experience, since few had done this before. The aim was to allow the group members an activity which focused on themselves, increased their pleasure of accomplishment and expanded their sense of self.

Session Five:

Designing Self-badges

Children were given three pre-cut circles of paper about four inches in diameter. We talked about how people wear buttons describing who they are and what they believe in; how T-shirts and car licenses address personal issues. The group was asked to draw circular badges of self-interest (Jeppson, 1982) with colored felt-tipped markers. These paper badges were positioned anywhere on the portrait and glued in place. Self-identity was the focus in this session, helping the children explore and feel good about who they were.

Session Six:

Drawing Together in a Group

In the sixth session, the children created a group community on paper. Each member chose a different colored felt-tipped marker and took turns drawing. The paper was passed around the table; all children focused on the artist of the moment, and usually discussed the things to be included in their community. Group drawing, more than any of the other activities, demonstrated social relatedness, how children interacted and felt about one another. The group effort further helped the children feel supported, and focused on the experience of being a part of an intimate school group which understands and encourages sharing their feelings and thoughts.

Session Seven:

Saying Good-bye

In the group session addressing closure, the children were given scissors, glue, colored felt-tipped markers, and paper and, using these materials, were asked to say good-bye to each other and the therapists. At the same time, the activity also was used as an important opportunity to say good-bye to their beloved lost parent. Some of these children had not been able to say good-bye and their inability to do so remained emotionally draining until addressed.

Session Eight:

Reviewing the Children's Artwork at a Good-bye Party

Closure was again provided during the last session for the children. In a group, all the artwork was reviewed and discussed, a cathartic and strengthening experience. The therapists underscored certain issues concerning better adjustment to loss. Children were counseled to engage surviving parents or caretakers in conversation when they feel sad and need comforting. Also they were reminded that although the group had ended, they could still interact with other group members and the school psychologist. It was explained that they had shared their feelings in group and they needed to continue to do so at home. Contact with the caretakers and teachers served as a way for these adults to gain insight and be receptive to a child's attempts to gain a closer relationship and more support.

Separation and Loss as Seen in the Children's Drawings

These children lost significant caretakers in various ways. A small number of the children experienced an early death of a young parent, or abandonment by unmarried fathers. The majority endured separation from a significant caretaker because of parental divorce, with or without issues of abandonment. The losses varied in severity from the impossibility of having the relationship again, to an ambiguous and indefinite separation of the caretaker and child.

In examining the records of the forty involved children, 15% experienced the loss of a significant caretaker. Of these, 5% were violent deaths and 10% were deaths of natural causes. The remaining 85% of children suffered separation in varying degrees: by parental divorce with neither parent abandoning the child (45%); by parental divorce and abandonment by one parent (30%), and abandonment by one unmarried parent, 10% of the children.

The Artwork—Figure 1

Fig. 1 was drawn in one of the first sessions after the Los Angeles riots. In it, a boy drew Joe's Market burning down. Joe is seen in the doorway of his market yelling, "Oh, no," and the fireman is trying to extinguish the flames on the left side of the drawing, while a man on the right side of the page is dumping gasoline to ignite the flames. The boy has made a judgment in the upper left hand corner, "This is not right." He clearly identifies with Joe and his horror of the situation.

Diagnostic Art Interview and Portrait

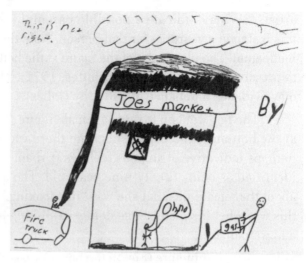

Fig. 1 Joe's Market, burning down

A handsome, racially-mixed, twelve-year-old boy in the sixth grade, whose unmarried father had abandoned him and his mother when he was a toddler, usually appeared angry and was combative with his classmates, and defied authority. He was failing scholastically and appeared generally unhappy. His teacher and principal were constantly involved with him because of his explosive nature. The mother of this boy was completely bewildered by his fury and anger and was at a loss about how to mother him. She had admitted that she had gotten into a habit of avoiding him. She disclosed how she suspected him of gang involvement and felt powerless to stop him.

He drew an obviously angry, snarling man identified as thirty-five years of age (Fig. 2). The boy was uncooperative and gave little information about this figure and would not explain why the illustrated person was so angry. Machover (1949) feels that when the drawn figure is much older than the

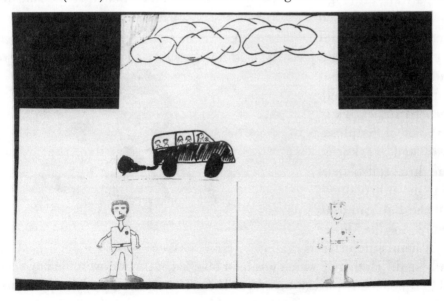

Fig. 2 Diagnostic Art Interview

149

artist, this may indicate a possible parental identification and perhaps in this instance a yearning for that person. Note that the arms appear weak and ineffectual. The placement of the figure at the bottom of the page may indicate depressive feelings (Machover, Jolles, 1971). The wide stance of the figure may evidence a defiance of authority (Jolles).

The boy went on to draw a female figure (Fig. 2) which was also placed at the bottom of the page. This time there was more shading and erasure, perhaps indicative of anxious feelings (Urban, 1963/1981). This female was identified as being twenty-nine years old. The only information he supplied about the female was that she was "just looking." It occurred to me later that this was what his mother was doing, exhibiting anxiety and just standing by and watching.

The last picture (Fig. 2) the boy was asked to draw was of all the members in his family, each doing something. He drew his family out for a drive with his mother driving the car. He explained that he was the second figure on the left riding in the car (this face has a mouth drawn in a straight line, which appears unhappy). The car is belching forth very black exhaust fumes and clouds partially cover the sun. Klepsch and Logie suggest that when clouds hide the sun, "there is a possibility the child is not receiving parental love" (1982, p. 45).

Fig. 3 shows how he drew a self-portrait and self-badges during the fourth session. There is a similarity between his thirty-five-year-old man and his portrait, although the self-portrait shows no evidence of the snarling mouth and exposed teeth. He has cut off his figure at the knees, and the arms appear thin and weak, both perhaps indicative of feelings of helplessness and weakness. The three self-badges were never explained, but the Bart Simpson figure in the lower right hand side origi-

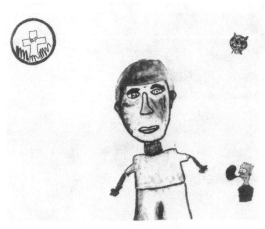

Fig. 3 Self Portrait and Badges

nally said, "Hi there," which was later blacked out. It was as if the boy needed to squelch any pleasant gesture. The self-symbol in the left upper hand corner may refer to gang involvement and membership; also, it seems reminiscent of a cemetery marker.

Even before I had a chance to talk to the teacher and the mother, the *Diagnostic Art Interview* provided insight as to how the boy felt and functioned. Attempting to hide his bi-racial inheritance, by denying his mother's background and emphasizing his father's racial characteristics, he appeared angry, aggressive, sullen and quite ready to explode. He constantly challenged and fought with the other children. When the children discussed the reasons for attending the group, he said, "I don't live with my father, but that's okay, because I get to see him every Sunday," and also stated, "I'd like to live with him!" Later, I learned there had been absolutely no contact with the father for many years.

A defiant, oppositional and aggressive boy, he said very little in the beginning of the group experience, except to argue with and attack the other children, but by the fourth session during the self-portrait activity, he admitted that he really liked to draw. It was apparent this task offered him a measure of pleasure and an opportunity for self-respect.

I talked privately with this boy about his wish to be with his father and indicated that I knew there was some difficulty with this happening. During this conversation he said, "Other kids have fathers who see them and live with them, it's not fair." I told him I understand how much he wished his father was in his life and how sad and angry it must make him not to have this a reality. I empathized and agreed that what came our way was not always fair, but we have it in our power to make life different and more suitable, particularly as we get older. My purpose was to lend him support and empower him. This conversation could never have taken place if the boy had not participated in the art activity and learned to trust me. The art activity enabled him to express his needs.

When the mother was told, we suggested that she take the boy to a child guidance clinic, where he could obtain further help. I also stressed that she needed to be involved in talking to the boy about his feelings and assuring him of her affection, if not her understanding. Although this boy was more disruptive and uncooperative than most of the children in the groups, he still managed to use the art therapy to ventilate some of his emotions and finally talk about his abandonment by his father. He also gained some pleasure in exhibiting his artistic ability, influencing his sense of self in a positive way. When youngsters are this hurt and angry, they need long-term treatment.

A Life Line Graph Evokes Sad Memories

During the second session the children were requested to construct a

Life Line Graph. A nine-year-old in the fourth grade had recently lost his father, who had died of a sudden heart attack while lifting a heavy piece of equipment on a construction site. The boy was shocked and traumatized by his father's sudden death. He looked sad, cried easily, slept poorly, suffered gastric disturbances and was irritable with his friends, whereas before the parental death, he had been amiable, cheerful and popular. He was considered a bright, congenial, high-achieving youngster by teacher and mother. Recently his scholastic effort began to slacken, and he seemed preoccupied all the time.

He identified, with colored felt-tipped markers, the members in his family on the left side of his graph. He used the same color to write both his mother's and his own name, showing his close connection to her. He also listed an uncle and two cousins.

He indicated on his graph that his earliest recollection was playing ball with his father at one year of age . His saddest memory was when he learned his father died and he went to his funeral. His happiest memory was when he was eight years old and his father took him places. He drew himself standing close to the father in the casket (Fig. 4) at the funeral and verbally described the details of the funeral and how sad he felt to see his dad so quiet, without life. He had always had a good relationship with both his mother and father and his emotions seemed close to the surface and known to him.

The boy was a great facilitator in his group; he always seemed to lead the other children into disclosure because he himself disclosed so matter-of-factly and seemingly without effort. Many times this boy drew huge raindrops falling in overwhelming amounts on himself. Later we will see his large raindrops in a group drawing. Rainfall is thought to be "associated with depressive tendencies" (Burns and Kaufman, 1971, p. 250). He sought comfort and support from his mother and received it. His teacher reported at the end of the group sessions that his mood, manner and scholastic effort had improved.

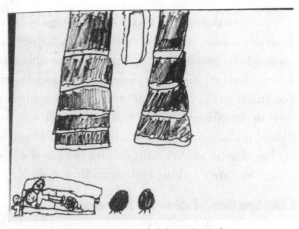

Fig. 4 Memory of father's funeral

A Life Line Graph and a Good-bye Drawing

Two six-year-old children, previously mentioned, had lost their fathers through violent means. The first little boy lost both parents when his father shot his mother and then himself. His parent's violence and instability in no way prepared this boy to withstand such horrible trauma as their deaths. He was in the school principal's office daily, exhibiting angry, aggressive and uncooperative behavior. He had a caring maternal grandmother who had become his guardian. This woman was the sole support of four children and, since she could not break away from her job, my co-therapist and I went to her office. The boy showed a very different behavior pattern at home—he complied with the household rules, and the grandmother was amazed to hear about the aggressive behavior from the principal, teacher and now us.

He constructed his Life Line Graph (Fig. 5) and said he remembered his toy vacuum cleaner at one year of age, that at age 6, now, he was happy when he swam, and was very sad, mad and scared at age four when his mother and father died because of his father's violence. He used the opportunity in the seventh session, when the children were asked to say good-bye on paper to their loved ones, to draw himself saying good-bye to his mother and father. The self-figure is without legs, which may reflect his feelings of helplessness and lack of support (Urban).

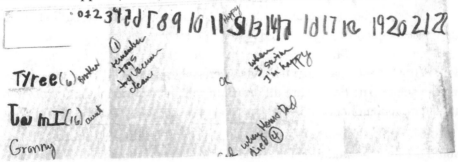

Fig. 5   Life Line Graph

We talked to the grandmother about the details of the family history and how the boy might respond to intensive individual psychological treatment. We tried to help her understand some of the ramifications of the child's suffering and and how he might fantasize that she might send him away if he was a "bad" boy at home.

Sad Memories

The second little boy responded to the first boy's story with his own disclosure about his father's violent street death and spontaneously drew a representation of his father's funeral (Fig. 6). He illustrated Daddy's friends carrying Daddy in a casket and all the family members looking sad, but close to one another. The child seemed visibly comforted by sharing his memory with children and adults who could understand and care. This boy had a sup-

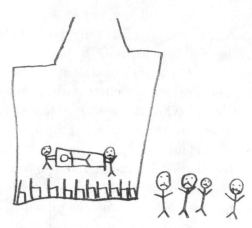

Fig. 6 Another father's funeral

portive mother and a close-knit family with siblings, grandparents, uncles and aunts. The positive family relationships acted as an emotional buffer for this child. He, like the nine-year-old boy, was able to draw and talk easily about his feelings in connection with his father's death. His mother reported that his mood seemed improved as the group experience ended.

More Sad Memories and a Creative Good-bye Drawing

When asked to illustrate a sad memory, one eleven-year-old girl in the fifth grade, drew a picture (Fig. 7) of her father being shot in the chest by a woman firing a gun. It showed her at age seven, at the top of a flight of stairs, holding her doll, in front of the apartment building where she lived with her parents, observing the scene. The details are all drawn in red and brown colors; the blood of her father is prominent on his chest.

She talked about how scared she was and frightened that her father would die and she would be left alone and how the am-bulance came and took her father to the hospital. She felt the need to draw a second picture, this time of a courtroom where her mother and father divorced, shortly after the father recovered from his wound. He disappeared from her life and she felt very angry at him.

An amiable girl, well thought of by her peers and teacher, with average ability, she was not performing well academically. She had been functioning according to her skill until the shooting and the divorce of her parents. She rarely talked about these occurrences, even with her mother, but shared with us that she thinks about these unhappy events quite often. The group and art provided this girl with a means to express secret thoughts which plagued her and she tried to suppress.

The mother was advised to share some of her own feelings and thoughts about the father with the girl and to encourage her daughter to talk about what she was thinking and experiencing emotionally, in order to find some resolution, in spite of the ambiguity of the situation.

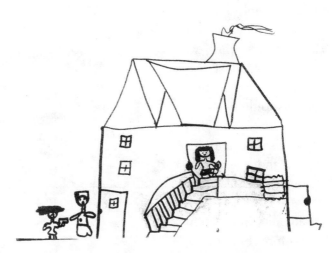

Fig. 7 Witnessing father's shooting

Many weeks later, during the good-bye session, she was very creative when she drew and cut out a decorated teapot and carefully constructed eight triangles upon which she wrote all the names of the group members and the two therapists. She placed the triangles into the top of the teapot. It was a cheerful expression of togetherness, warmth and comfort. It was apparent by her pleased look that she felt happy about her creation and the people represented.

Two More Sad Memory Drawings

Another ten-year-old boy, a hyperactive and impulsive fifth grader, in the same group as the previously-mentioned girl, also responded to the divorce of his parents and the abandonment by his father when the father went to live in New York, with much sorrow but no visible anger. The boy appeared good-natured with the other children, and had a very close relationship to another ten-year-old boy in the group who was born in Israel. This youngster found himself in the group because his parents had recently divorced; he lived with his mother and had contact with his father.

When the children were asked to draw their saddest memory, the boy drew himself crying big tears, titled the drawing "Dad New York," and in a speech balloon wrote "wa wa wa wa" repeatedly (Fig. 8). The drawing not only indicates sadness, but perseveration concerning the drawing of the tears and the wa wa's, which was a symptom of his impulsivity.

When it became time for group discussions, he began laughing as he showed the others his drawing. His Israeli friend looked at him and said, "Sometimes when we are the saddest, we cover it up by laughing because otherwise we would cry." This boy was wise beyond his years and seemed to understand and sympathize. The boy fell silent and drew another picture (Fig. 9), his mother and father

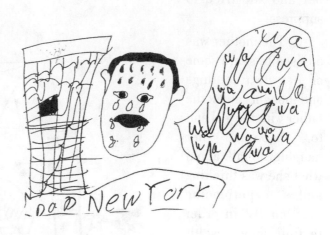

Fig. 8   Father in New York

yelling at and arguing with one another, and he said, "This is what it was like." The second picture reflects a calming of impulsivity.

A Happy Memory of a Pet

In another group, a ten-year-old fourth-grade girl, from a country in the Near East, was described by her teacher as a dreamy, sad, withdrawn, underachieving child. The parents were recently divorced. The teacher felt that the parents were always very busy with their lives and paid little attention to their daughter. The child had been sent back to the mother's sister, but something unknown happened and she was returned to the United States, where the girl now lived with her father. The teacher felt the child was closed off from other

children and could only relate to her drawings and her pet cat, Lucky. The girl was an extremely gifted artist and would draw mermaids in underwater scenes filled with sea creatures when she should have been working on math problems. She responded to the *Diagnostic Art Inter-*

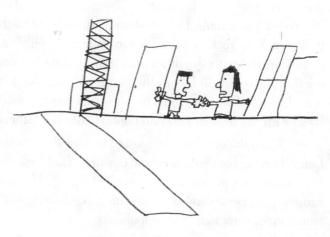

Fig. 9   Parents arguing

view by drawing a girl leading a horse and a boy leading a horse and a dog; of course, this last drawing should have reflected her family doing something. When she was asked to draw her saddest memory, she drew her mother giving away her dog to a man, the self-figure tiny and forlorn-looking. There seemed to be a connection between the lost dog, the drawn dog and her family. Perhaps she felt more involvement with the dog than with her mother and father. As a happy memory, she drew herself with her cat Lucky (Fig. 10) and titled it "When I Got My Cat, Lucky."

Her talent was unusual and she was very much admired in the group for her artistic skill. She used the art to tell us her story, and the telling may have been helpful to gain catharsis, if not resolution.

We held several conversations with the father, trying to make him understand how withdrawn and isolated this child appeared to us. He tolerated her poor academic achievement and felt she was fine because she was never troublesome and "didn't she love to draw pictures."

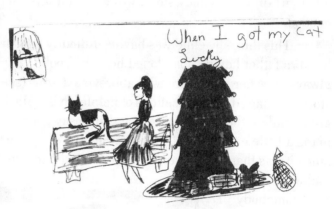

Fig. 10 "When I Got My Cat, Lucky"

A Group Good-bye Picture

Each group was asked to draw a picture together creating their own community. They were excited about this project and cooperated with one another. Many became invested in seeing that their community had all the features that were important to them. In one group were a nine-year-old boy, whose construction-worker father died suddenly; another severely disturbed boy, also nine years old, two eight-year-old girls and an eight-year-old boy.

In general, the children were friendly with one another and enjoyed their group involvement. The troubled boy didn't participate in group activities a few times. Once, he sat most of the session with his head buried in his jacket; another time he did the same without the jacket. He was invited to stay, but also given the option to leave, and he always chose to stay. He was a child of divorced parents and lived with his father but saw his mother. Although he was absent when the children created their drawing of their community (Fig. 11),

157

upon his return the following week, they all encouraged him to add to their group world. He added the sky to the picture and seemed pleased to be included.

The group's environment consisted of two buildings, a representation of an historical house and a candy store, plus play equipment in a park, and an ocean scene. One of the girls drew her version of an historical house, which she had visited. Her enthusiasm was so contagious that I went to see the house myself. She was so pleased that she had influenced me so much. The other girl drew the candy store, which the children felt was appropriate and needed.

This thin, shy child was having difficulty adjusting to a new stepfather, her own father having abandoned her. She spoke very little in the group and always drew her self-figure with abbreviated arms (seen in front of the candy store), perhaps denoting feelings of helplessness (Machover, 1949). When the group ended, the children were asked to say good-bye. In compliance, she made a little card (Fig. 12) for me. She drew a picture of a Christmas tree, since it was that time of year and wrote on the inside, "I had a good day you make me feel like I'm somebody. I love you good-bye." Apparently the art therapy intervention increased her feelings of self-worth.

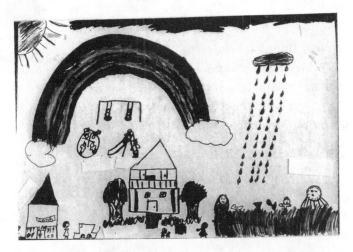

Fig. 11 Group good-bye picture

The eight-year-old boy drew children engaged with play equipment at a park. The boy who lost his construction worker father drew the ocean with himself and his mother swimming with fish. They are threatened by an octopus and large raindrops pour from a cloud. The octopus is so much larger than the two human figures that they seem in danger. The boy had been sad and anxious since his father died. His symbols, the octopus and rain may relate to these feelings.

The children took turns creating the rainbow which ended in two clouds. They used all the colors to draw the rainbow which Raymer and McIntyre (1987) believe is a symbol for creating order. At the end of this activity, the children seemed happy and pleased with themselves, having formed a creative and cohesive group.

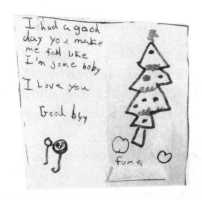

Fig. 12 A good-bye note

More Sad Memories and Good-Bye Pictures

One of the group participants was a ten-year-old boy who had recently moved from another state. His parents were divorced and he had been sent to live with his biological father. Somehow, the boy wound up living with his paternal grandfather and grandmother for two years where he took care of his dying grandfather. When his grandfather finally died, he moved back to California to live with his mother, stepfather and younger half-brother. The mother claimed she could not retrieve her son until she threatened the grandmother with legal means. He had been referred to the group because he was mourning the death of his grandfather.

The boy's teacher complained about his behavior: his inability to sit still, his lack of attention and his difficulty in following directions. In group the boy looked depressed and exhibited all these behaviors. It was thought he might have hearing problems, but after testing, it was found that his hearing was within normal range.

When he was asked to graphically describe his sad memory, he drew his grandfather lying upon his bed for two years, attached to machines nearby. He described how he took care of him, brought him his food and the M&Ms his grandfather enjoyed. He was traumatized when he died, because he was unprepared for the event. He looked utterly despondent as he talked about his loss. He was asked to say good-bye to Grandpa, and he responded by drawing a self-figure crying and saying, "Good-bye Grandpa, I love you a lot."

Toward the end of the group sessions, there was a remarkable change in his behavior. He heard directions the first time, he stopped getting up every five minutes and walking around the room, his art work appeared more colorful, and he smiled a little and socialized more with other group members. It appeared that his artwork had helped him to express his grief, and calm him. His teacher reported a similar change of behavior in the classroom.

The Last Good-byes

The last two good-bye drawings are by a girl whose father had died suddenly of a heart attack, and by a boy whose dying mother sent away her children to live with her sister in the United States. Both children were eleven years old, attractive, friendly, pleasant and well-liked by their peers and teachers.

The girl seemed quite enthralled with the boy; he was very shy toward her. He did poorly in language but had above average achievement skills in mathematics. He suffered from mood swings, appearing anxious, uneasy, and sad one moment and good-humored the next. As he became comfortable in the group, he disclosed how he suffered guilt because he felt he and his siblings had contributed to his mother's death by being bad and troublesome for her. He said he had a heavy heart because he never said good-bye properly to her since he didn't know he would never see her again. He experienced feelings of guilt about his mother a lot of the time.

He and his siblings had been left out of the rituals and ceremonies concerning the loss, creating much unfinished business for this boy. Bowlby (1980) and others believe it is important for children to participate in family grieving, including funeral or memorial rites. Kubler-Ross (1983) has made us aware that children often feel guilt for believing they caused parental death. We talked about the nature of cancer, how children cannot cause a parent to die even when they misbehave, and how much his mother must have loved them to want to spare them pain. He talked about some family history and he drew a happy memory of riding through a grove of trees with his younger sister on the way home to his mother. When it came time to say good-bye to his mother, he did a very careful drawing (Fig. 13) of his mother in bed with him close by and touching her. He titled this "Good-bye, Mom, I love you." His aunt was a warm woman and she seemed to provide solid and loving support for her sister's children.

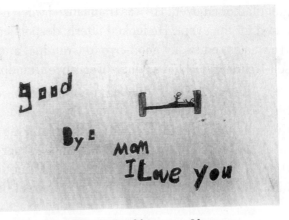

Fig. 13 Good-bye, mom, I love you

160

The girl felt grief for the recent death of her father. One day, her father left for work with his briefcase and never returned because he suffered a fatal heart attack at his office. She was a pretty, popular girl and put great value on education, and she tried very hard to succeed in all her activities at school. Her teacher reported that she looked sad and daydreamed since her father died.

She drew her memories of her life with her father. One picture concerned him holding her newborn baby sister. She loved her two-year-old sister and it was touching to watch her carefully wrap up the cookies she received in group to save for the baby. She drew her father lying in the church (Fig. 14), and she wrote, "Good-bye I love you, Dad. Thank you for teaching me things." The picture is colorful and carefully executed. Her hearts and balloons, Raymer and McIntyre (1987) point out, may be a common graphic theme in bereavement art, possibly referring to the deceased entering heaven. When the group started, it seemed as if her early memories were blocked. As time went on, however, she recalled more and more good times she had with him.

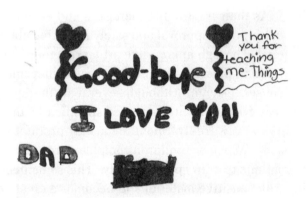

Fig. 14 Good-bye, I love you, dad.

Discussion

The parent and teacher reports and the Burks' Behavior Rating Scales concerning the success or failure of the intervention indicated the following change at the end of group involvement.

- At least three of the six children in each group responded quite positively to the treatment, two children in each group responded a little and one child remained unchanged.

- Individual psychological treatment was recommended for eight of the children.

- In three instances, the caretaker immediately followed this recommendation; it isn't known if the rest sought help, since there was no follow-up.

Drawings Are Keys

The children's drawings are keys to unlock what they may feel are shameful, painful and/or guilty feelings. The drawings are important because not only do they help the therapist understand the child, but on several levels they help the child face his or her truth on paper and experience catharsis, and closure. Discussion becomes easier after the children draw what they have been contemplating secretly. The permission to draw promotes courage to address sometimes forbidden subjects, fears and unspoken thoughts. Some children talk sparingly about what they have drawn, others talk a great deal and some not at all, and all this is accepted by the therapists.

The children are able to talk and express through art their feelings about the lost significant caretaker, parent, foster parent or grandparent. They express appropriate anger, anxiety and sadness about their loss, correct misinformation, share experiences, develop new understanding, create emotional bonds with new friends and explore their fears of the future.

As their trust in the therapists and each other grows, they experience mutual support, approval and safety in talking about perhaps formerly-hidden material. Through appropriate art tasks, group members have the opportunity to gain in pleasure concerning these achievements and increase their feelings of self-esteem. Although several art therapy directives are designed to address grief and self-awareness specifically, the children also have opportunity to draw freely. Spontaneous art productions appear throughout the sessions. Whenever children complete directed art tasks they are encouraged to continue to draw spontaneously. This sometimes provides relief from dealing with sensitive material and becomes a creative opportunity giving satisfaction and increasing self-worth. The children often use this means to work out their mourning issues even further.

Most of the children benefit from group art therapy experience to some degree. The majority are able to talk about their feelings of grief and loss. Their capacity for verbalization of emotions increases as the group progresses. The group members appear to find relief in graphic and verbal expression of their sadness, anxiety, fear, guilt, anger and isolation and begin to work through separation and loss issues. The children gain understanding about their situation and cope with their emotions and thoughts better.

The *Diagnostic Art Interview* functions as a projective test, but also stimulates self-disclosure. It serves to focus the children on themselves and one another. The six children who come together as strangers are less so at the end of the first session.

The *Life Line Graph* leads the children into the purpose of the group, to deal with their feelings of separation and loss. It is interesting that, many times, the sad events listed in the Life Line Graph are different in content from the pictures later drawn illustrating the graph issues. Sometimes children can't tolerate disclosing their saddest feelings in the beginning and only later, when they feel supported, more familiar and comfortable with each other, can they deal with sensitive issues.

The early *sad and happy* pictures are helpful in understanding how the children feel and what their concerns are. At this point, the heart of the grief work begins and continues with the good-bye effort and the review of the art production.

The *portrait with self-badges* and *group picture* helps them deal with issues of self-awareness, self-esteem and social relatedness.

Kind and severity, that is, whether the children suffer a sudden violent traumatic loss or the natural non-violent demise, abandonment or separation of a caretaker, in varying degrees, is not as helpful to acceptance of loss as the surviving caretaker's behavior and acceptance of the child, the child's previous family experience, the child's basic emotional and intellectual makeup and the child's involvement with the family mourning rituals and ceremonies. When children are kept separate or sent away to avoid their unhappiness and death involvement, and/or the caretaker is self-absorbed, the grief seems more difficult to reconcile.

Surviving parents and teachers gain insight, feel supported and seem better able to help the children during this difficult period. (An adjunctive parent group is recommended to increase positive results.)

Many of the children gain in self-worth and improved self-identity, as seen in group and reported by caretakers and teachers. As the groups progress, an emotional cohesiveness with other group members helps individuals reach out to other children and therapists, as seen in the good-bye statements and the help extended by the children to each other.

Raymer and McIntyre (1987) used a creative arts team to work with bereaved children in a hospice facility in Michigan. They found art therapy to be an important process in grief expression and believe that feelings which "may have been repressed in other kinds of communication formats are freely expressed in a protective environment utilizing the arts" (p. 29). They list some common graphic themes which they found in the children's bereavement art:

• Monsters (perhaps reflecting child's feeling of lack of control)

163

- Rainbows (creating order and color suggesting emotional phase of grieving)
- Balloons and birds (referring to upward movement, perhaps deceased entering heaven)
- Roads and time (searching for the deceased)
- Dead trees (damaged self)
- Fire, lightning, explosive sun, storms (angry feelings)
- Lack of hands and feet (helplessness)

Many of these images appear in the artwork of these children. The art therapy process seems effective both when the children are temporarily separated from their caretakers or permanently lose them through death. All the children evidence unhappiness and stress and the same art therapy techniques appeared to serve all the children. The art therapy directives do not have to be tailored to specific cause of loss, since the children do this themselves in art and verbal response. The art emphasis seems to supply the proper element of distance and protection for the children. It helps initially to avoid too direct and premature disclosure. The art serves as a critical factor to distance the process when appropriate, to illuminate issues, to help to gain in self-awareness and bring satisfaction of achievement to the young participants.

I am grateful to Verna Suarez, Lynette Gonzales, Frances Baskett and Kim Sneider for their expertise as co-therapists. I wish to thank the two elementary school principals, Michelle Bennett and Shirley Kouffman, for their dedication and Bella Schimmel, M.D. for her constant support and encouragement.

References

Bowlby, J. (1980). *Loss: sadness and depression.* Attachment and Loss, Volume IL NY: Basic Books.

Burks, H. F. (1968). *Burks' behavior rating scales.* El Monte, California: Arden Press.

Burns, R. C. (1982). *Self-growth in families, kinetic family drawings.* (K-F-D) Research and Application. NY: Brunner/Mazel.

Burns, R. C. and Kaufman, S. H. (1972). *Actions, styles and symbols in kinetic family drawings* K-F-D, An Interpretive Manual. NY: Brunner/Mazel.

Di Leo, J. H. (1973). *Children's drawings and diagnostic aids.* NY: Brunner/Mazel.

Furman, E. (1974). *A child's parent dies.* New Haven: Yale University Press.

Hammer, E. F. (1958). *The clinical applications of projective drawings.* Springfield, IL: C. C. Thomas.

Hulse, W. C. (1951). *The emotionally disturbed child draws his family.* Quarterly Journal of Child Behavior, 3, 152-174.

Jeppson, P. M. (1982). *Self-symbols.* Lecture at California State University, Northridge.

Jolles, I. (1971). *A catalogue for qualitative interpretation of the House-Tree-Person*

(Revised). Los Angeles: Western Psychological Services.

Klepsch, M. and Logie, L. (1982). *Children draw and tell, an introduction to the projective uses of children's human figure drawings.* NY: Brunner/Mazel.

Kranzler, E. M. (1990). *Parent death in childhood.* In L. E. Arnold (Ed.), Childhood Stress (pp. 405-421). NY: John Wiley & Sons.

Kubler-Ross, E. (1983). *On children and death.* NY: MacMillan.

Kwiatkowska, H. Y. (1978). *Family therapy and evaluation through art.* Springfield, Ill.: C. C. Thomas.

Machover, K. (1949). *Personality projection in the drawing of the human figure.* Springfield, IL.: C. C. Thomas.

McElhaney, M. (1969). *Clinical psychological assessment of human figure drawing.* Springfield, IL.: C. C. Thomas.

Piaget, J. (1952). *Judgment and reasoning in the child.* NY: Humanities Press

Raymer, M. and McIntyre, B. (1987) *An art support group for bereaved children and adolescents.* Art Therapy Journal of the American Art Therapy Association, 4 (1), 27-35.

Rubin, J. A. (1978). *Child art therapy, understanding and helping children grow through art.* NY: Van Nostrand Reinhold.

Schimmel, B. F., and Kornreich, T. Z. *The use of art and verbal process with recently widowed individuals.* American Journal of Art Therapy, in press.

Speece, M. W. and Brent, S. S. (1984). *Children's understanding of death: A review of three components of a death concept.* Child Development, 55, 1671 1686.

Ulman, E. and Dachinger, P. (Eds.) (1975). *Art therapy in theory and practice.* NY: Schocken Books.

Urban, W. H. (1981). *The Draw-A-Person catalogue for interpretive analysis.* Los Angeles: Western Psychological Services. (Originally published in 1963).

Wenck, L. S. (1977). *House-tree-person drawings: an illustrated diagnostic handbook.* Los Angeles: Western Psychological Services.

Winnicott, D. W. (1977). *The squiggle technique.* In J. F. McDermott, Jr. and S. I. Harrison (eds.), The Psychiatric Treatment of the Child. NY: Jason Aronson.

Survivors of Sexual Violence
and the Process of Art Therapy
by Donna Heider, M.A., A.T.R., M.F.C.C.

Donna Heider, consultant for the Survivors of Incest Unit in a major Southern California hospital, supervises graduate and post graduate students of Loyola Marymount University's Clinical Art Therapy Program, from which she graduated several years ago. She has a private practice in the South Bay area of Los Angeles.

While my work with survivors of incest has been very rewarding, I have often been frustrated by the little hope that the traditional medical model or psychological theories have to offer my clients. Much of the existing literature and the assumptions behind clinical practice seem to suggest that my clients' tragic starts in life have forever doomed them to be "damaged goods." My work with survivors has not borne out conventional psychological wisdom. I have developed and am constantly evolving a tried and changing, growing formula, an eclectic blend of theories and experience. One thing clearly known from my experience is that many survivors are far from defeated by childhood trauma, but are truly survivors who want help in reaching a full resolution of thoughts and feelings about their childhood experience.

The reasons that bring survivors into therapy are diverse. Most often, they are not the immediate recognition of childhood sexual trauma but are specific problems relating to important developmental issues. These include commitment to an intimate relationship, decisions about having or raising children, struggles with an authority figure at work or school, death of a parent, and the ensuing depression about the inability to resolve their thoughts and feelings that these events evoke.

This chapter is based on my personal search to find a treatment framework that integrates psychological theories and the practice of clinical art therapy. It is a non-empirical and descriptive random study of female adults whom I have treated. It is an overview of the intricate individual treatment of survivors. All of these adults have used art therapy techniques in their struggle on the road to health and understanding. In the description of my treatment framework, therapy is directed towards the development of a relationship from which the survivors can rework the trauma and integrate the self. In each phase, I will give examples and some imagery directives. The treatment does not move along in a linear direction, but progresses by stages, with frequent regressions and setbacks along the way. The treatment is highly individualized for each survivor and follows the process of re-experiencing and integrating the trauma.

The art therapy directives cannot take the place of establishing a relationship and following the individual patient's process—what works for one may not be appropriate for others. There is no formula one can follow. Being with the client, offering support, containment and a safe trusting environment in which they can explore their trauma is what fosters the capacity for integration—not specific directives. Without first establishing trust and camaraderie, plunging in with art directives may even be counterproductive to the individual's process.

Stage One—Presentation and Gathering the Ingredients

During the initial stage of treatment, you may not hear or see any disclosures. For many adult survivors, disclosure is blocked by feelings of alienation, guilt, badness, inadequacy, "craziness," and helplessness. Approximately half of all survivors who seek treatment do not disclose their incest history during the initial phase. The most common presentations and their reasons are (Courtois, 1988):

• *Lack of awareness about having been abused.* The trauma has been contained by developing a number of ego defenses.

• *Naivete or ignorance about abuse.* Abuse was imbedded within patterns of "normal" family behavior and interaction, so it clearly served a positive purpose, or it was presented positively by a favorite adult who did not use pressure or coercion.

• *Age and chronicity of symptoms.* Many older survivors have experienced severe and chronic mental health problems for which they have undergone years of treatment. Unfortunately, their problems were treated without awareness of or attention to sexual abuse. *The symptoms were treated but not the cause.* Consequently, many of these women "never got better." It was not unusual for them to have received multiple diagnoses and to be labeled as chronic with little or no hope for improvement.

• *Intimidation as a means used to silence the survivor.* The type and degree of intimidation used to silence the victim is closely linked with the ability to disclose at the time of the incest or years later. Many survivors continue to fear reprisal years later if they violate the instruction to "keep our secret family rules" and patterns, such as intense family loyalty. Shame, denial of problems, enmeshment, mistrust of others, and closing ranks to outsiders, also serve to reinforce silence. When you have established a trusting relationship, you might ask your patient to *"draw how you feel about secrets?"*

• *Previous negative experiences with disclosure.* If early experience(s) of disclosure has been discounted and denied, there is a reluctance to retell the memories. *"Draw how you feel about not being believed?"*

• *Feelings of stigma.* Having been involved in a taboo activity creates feelings of shame, guilt, low self-esteem and stigma. At this time, they might draw *"what it feels like to be me today. Where do I put my feelings of shame, hurt, anger and embarrassment?"*

• *Silence as protection.* The daughter involved in role reversal learns to take care of the needs of others at her own expense and is rewarded in the family for doing so. Silence often serves as a way to keep the family intact or to protect certain family members from the pain of knowing about the incest. At an appropriate time you might suggest they *"draw a family secret."*

• *Mistrust of others.* Survivors may resist disclosing their history due to mistrust of non-survivors and authority figures. They may believe that only another survivor can accept or understand them.

During this stage of treatment, I ask very specific questions and educate the client on *what constitutes abuse.* I am aware of what is being said, as well as what is being put down on the paper. I often expect the polarities of overcompliance, eagerness to please, a need to gain my approval and rigid resistance. The presenting symptoms and after-effects of incest correlate directly with the concerns for which survivors seek treatment. At this point, I become very clear about what treatment will involve and what the client's expectations should be. Examples of these issues are *the longevity of treatment* and *feelings of being worse before getting better*, which is most likely to bring up depression and in turn will affect all areas of function.

Establishing Boundaries

Many survivors have been violated by so many people they need assistance with establishing physical boundaries. I reassure them that no touching (hugs, handshakes, etc.) will happen without permission. The therapist needs to find out specifically "how close is safe," and then assure them that no touching will happen without asking first. I tell them what *confidentiality* means and what the reporting laws are.

During this initial phase, what may show in the artwork/imagery is again wide open, but most assuredly, lacking appropriate affect. My directives are structured and clear, emphasizing trust-building techniques. *I am careful not to use words like "sexual abuse, incest or victim," unless the client mentions them first.* My directive may simply be *"Either with drawing or collage materials, show me what it was like growing up in your family."*

This allows the client to depict a wide variety of situations and behaviors and gives her the opportunity to control what she wants to discuss. It is important to keep in mind that any remembering process may be very difficult, particularly when memories have been unconsciously repressed. The inability to remember actual childhood in general or specific details can be very frustrating. When some of these memories emerge, they may be so distressing that they cause the woman to doubt her sanity or to regret she ever remembered.

Even when the survivor talks and addresses imagery of incest openly, she may have difficulty discussing more than the superficial disclosure. It is imperative that the therapist make explicit that:

- the survivor's story is believed
- she is safe
- she is and will be supported
- she will not be rushed

The survivor needs the assurance that her experiences, whatever they are, will receive validation and not be subject to further suppression. *It also must be made explicit that disclosure does not mean resolution but rather signifies the beginning of the working-through process.* During this phase of treatment, the therapist should sensitively present her observations with the aid of the imagery produced. The fact that incest therapy is complex and it takes time for the survivor to develop a strong therapeutic alliance should be addressed. I explain that the *exploration of working through abuse can cause disruption in all areas of her life and that she needs to learn to process her reactions and imagery at a pace that is tolerable to her without feeling overwhelmed and re-victimized.*

Stage Two—Mortar, Bricks and Barbed Wire.

In this stage, it becomes extremely clear that the client has had a fundamental disruption of trust due to early childhood experiences and traumas. The transference barriers and countertransference issues surface during this phase. The therapeutic relationship is instrumental in providing the survivor with the necessary support to address and work through the trauma while modeling a healthy, non-exploitative relationship. *Remember slowness and patience.*

Transference, Countertransference and Trust

The imagery begins to clearly and concretely show many aspects of the incest. Now, the family experience and individual personality style are brought to therapy and projected onto the therapist. Imagery and verbalizations center around the survivor's compromised ability to trust, due to her experience of betrayal in her most significant relationships. In remembering Erikson, we recall that *building basic trust is the earliest developmental task* and the foundation on which all others are built. Failure at this initial stage impairs identity development, the ability to form healthy and mutual relationships and the ability to be intimate.

The imagery may address these trust issues by portraying you as an authority figure (albeit disguised or veiled). Expectations or questions of your availability and caring surface. On some level, the client tells you to abuse them in some way. *Be consistent and reassuring and do not take trust for granted.* Throughout the course of therapy, the client may engage in *testing* behavior to set up the therapist and reinforce the belief that no one will be there for her. *Be very careful not to personalize this testing or any accusations the survivor might make.* Here, often, a crisis presents itself, a time when anxiety concerning abandonment is at a peak. This crisis may provide an opportunity for you to prove yourself trustworthy by remaining available, caring and consistent.

Some survivors have another trust problem—*that of trusting their own perceptions and experience.* During this time, the imagery may be repetitious and fragmented. The survivor might constantly call her memories and emotions into question and doubt her sanity. The therapist's task is to assist the survivor in reframing the abuse and encouraging the identification and development of the genuine self through the expresssion of previously unacknowledged parts of the self (the good vs. bad parts). The therapist must continuously strive to create a safe environment and to provide a reliable and trustworthy relationship. *Be clear about the possibility of missed phone calls and*

appointment changes and clearly explain reasons for exploring painful mater-
ial contained in imagery. The ability to trust others allows for secure detachment. Such connections set the stage for healthy ego development and a positive self-concept. A significant number of incestually abused children come
to believe that something about them, something inherently wrong with them,
caused the incest to occur. The imagery may begin to contain pictures of
unlovable bad children with verbalizations and written words that address
issues regarding the unlovableness and unworthiness of "this bad child." The
survivors project their shame onto their therapist, expecting the therapist to
hold them in the same contempt they have for themselves and to behave as
disrespectfully as their families did. The imagery provides an opportunity to
concretely change the picture and paint a new one. At this time you might
suggest a drawing of *"your latest unresolved conflict. What were the best and
worst things that happened to you?"*

Anger Management

This stage of therapy can last a very long time. The work and imagery
can become repetitive and increasingly graphic. The survivor begins to feel
her anger and rage. Oftentimes it is necessary for the therapist to introduce
anger management techniques and activities or directives geared towards
positive and healthy discharge and at times, containment. The survivor must
learn that feelings of anger and rage are appropriate considering what happened to her and that anger is not an inherently bad emotion. The therapist
will support her anger and her right to it, but not support expression which
is indirect or aggressive. Through the imagery, the art therapist can assist
the client in "dosing" her anger and devise and provide means to discharge
it in healthy ways.

Directives such as *"How do you take care of yourself when you are
happy, sad, or angry?"* and *"Put your rage on the page. Where in your body
does it exist?"* can help the patient express the anger safely and open new
areas to explore.

Loss and Grief

In conjunction with experiencing and feeling the depth of their rage
and anger, feelings of loss and sorrow are expressed *throughout* therapy. *Loss
and grief will need to be confronted and worked through in order to appropriately mourn and move on.* The most common losses include:
- lost childhood
- lost innocence and trust
- lost identity

- lost potential
- lost good family and good parenting

Victims may have more idiosyncratic losses to mourn as well. Grieving, a necessary therapy component, brings to the surface feelings of sadness, depression and anger which must be encouraged and supported by the therapist. At this point, *a therapy or self-help group*, as well as individual therapy is instrumental in the mourning process, since the survivor is often able to acknowledge and accept her own losses only after she has identified and empathized with the losses suffered by others. At this point, in a group setting, I might ask the group to draw their losses.

Important to the process, as I have mentioned, is awareness of *countertransference reactions and issues*. We, as professionals, have no immunity to the dominant societal attitudes concerning incest. These may be projected, along with more personal reactions onto the client and onto the therapeutic process. *The reactions to be aware of are dread, horror, denial, avoidance, shame, pity, disgust, guilt, rage, and more idiosyncratic reactions.* Be aware of your own processes and your absolute need to take excellent care of yourself as you work with survivors.

Alice Miller (1984) states, *"Only therapists who have had the opportunity to experience and work through their own traumatic past will be able to accompany patients on the path to truth about themselves and not hinder them on their way. Such therapists will not confuse their patients, make them anxious, or educate, instruct, misuse, or seduce them for they no longer have to fear the eruption in themselves of feelings that were stifled long ago, and they know from experience the healing power of these feelings."*

In closing, many issues are brought to the therapeutic process. We, as therapists, must always take special care to respect the client and not cause further shame. We must remember that many issues are brought to the therapy process by both the survivor and us. Incest inspires strong emotions in everyone, eruptions which neither the survivor and therapist can avoid. We, as good clinicians, must strive to arrive at a balanced perspective within the treatment. The survivor must be encouraged to present information about her past; then both the survivor and what she divulges must be accepted.

It is possible for the survivor to disentangle the present from the past and to live free from the effects of childhood incest. Be gentle and respectful, go slowly, watch and listen. Healing and health come from the deepest place in the heart.

173

References

Bass, E. and Davis, L. (1988). *The courage to heal: women healing from child sexual abuse.* NY: Harper & Row.

Courtois, C. A. (1988). *Healing the incest wound, adult survivors in therapy.* NY: W. W. Norton.

Miller, A. (1984) *Thou shalt not be aware: society's betrayal of the child.* NY: Farrar, Strauss, Givous.

Art Therapy with Families Who have Experienced Domestic Violence
by Shirley Riley, M.A., A.T.R., M.F.C.C

Shirley Riley received her M.A. in Art Therapy in 1975 from Immaculate Heart College in Los Angeles, became a registered art therapy in 1976, and a licensed Marriage and Family Therapist in 1979. She has practiced family art psychotherapy at a community mental health center and been a faculty member of the Loyola Marymount University Master's program in Marriage and Family Therapy (Clinical Art Therapy) since 1979.

Having taught family art therapy in university programs nationally and internationally, presented papers at conventions and published articles in art therapy journals, Ms. Riley received the 1990 American Art Therapy Award for outstanding clinical services to families. She has been a board member involved in many committees of the American Art Therapy Association.

Families who have experienced violence often seek treatment through outpatient clinic services where the focus moves from crisis intervention and case management to longer term therapy. The primary issues addressed often are those dealing with post-traumatic separation and loss, single parent family structure and rethinking old patterns of gender assigned roles. In addition, socio-economic concerns enter into the field of therapeutic goals. Art therapy can address these difficulties and provide a positive therapeutic experience for parent and children.

A Personal Construct of Art Psychotherapy

The way I practice art therapy derives from my belief that visual memories cannot be separated from the emotional/behavioral recollections and verbal explanations of events. For example, our earliest sense of self begins with the ability to retain a pictorial image of "mother." This talent for imagining, or imagery, is integrated with all our thoughts whenever we describe a series of actions or interactions. When we talk about a situation we also attempt to convey the "picture" of the environment in which the behaviors occurred. The emotional quality of behaviors becomes more clear when expressed as visual metaphor: "He was as big as a bear," "Her eyes flashed red with anger," are examples of the ordinary use of visualization.

The art psychotherapist is a clinician who has developed the skills and sensitivity to help the narrator visually illustrate the actions he sees in his mind. In addition, often the second level meaning of the behaviors emerges in the art task. Through these art expressions the art therapist is better able to comprehend the unique view of the speaker and move into his/her world. When imagery is turned into art expressions that can be talked about, the client/family and therapist can more easily enter into a shared world reality. The synthesis of verbal communication with visual images made concrete through art expression, together with a knowledge of therapeutic theory, is the essence of art psychotherapy.

It is no accident that children turn to drawing rather than words to tell their stories. Pictures are "closer" to their thoughts than words.

This concept of art psychotherapy reflects also a social constructivist view of "knowing" our created realities. The art therapist assists in making "real" the vision of events that are meaningful to our clients, and, in turn, we are able to help them build a better world than the one they bring to therapy. The ability to appreciate in a non-judgmental manner the emotional, physical and social environment of families who have lived with violence is essential to successful treatment.

The desired goal is to establish a therapeutic relationship with clients which is enhanced by the creativity of the clinician as artist/therapist who is trained to utilize the entire palette of transactions that we call art therapy. The therapist enters into the client's picture of his/her world and makes use all of the components of creativity, language, theory and art expressions. There is no division between the clinical treatment plan and the integration of that plan with the art therapy modality. The art expression is fused with appropriate theory and responds to the therapeutic necessity of each case.

Introduction to Treatment

As an art psychotherapist engages in treatment of a client family that has experienced abusive violence, the first issue to be considered is their natural reluctance to expose their weaknesses, their mistrust of outsiders and the loss of dignity they experience when impelled to ask for help (therapy). This distress must be addressed early in treatment, since the primary concern of the therapist is to begin to view the family's world and problems through their lens.

Introducing informal, non-structured drawings, collage, and family group drawings gives the family an opportunity to express pleasant and less pleasant memories and to begin engaging in treatment in a non-threatening manner. Central to the therapist's ability to understand their unique reality is the skill to be able to see, through the art, how they perceive their environment and hear the language they use as they relate their family myths and personal explanation of events. In the process of the clients' overt interpretations of their images, the art therapist attends not only to the information offered verbally but also to the non-verbal messages embedded in the art. The meta-message often moves the therapy in useful directions since the conventional words struggle with revealing issues of "don't tell," shame and painful repressions. Understanding their unique circumstances as the family relates their stories helps restore dignity and invites the trust necessary to establish a therapeutic alliance.

When this first and most important step has been accomplished, the more challenging creative process of therapy may begin.

Domestic Violence: A Broad Overview of Treatment

A high percentage of families who have suffered abuse in the home enter treatment at an outpatient clinic subsequent to an interim stay in a shelter for battered women. During this time the degree of shock, from the abuse, from the flight and from the loss of the familiar surroundings, has insulated the family from experiencing the full meaning of this move (Malchiodi, 1990). The shelter offers the protection and support needed to cushion this dramatic change of life circumstances. However, the crisis treatment is brief and all too soon the single parent and the children must find housing, financial aid and schools; they must pick up the routine of living. The challenge of living alone, making all the requests needed for social services and continuing to avoid contact with the abuser is a very heavy burden for the woman. These anxieties and fears are transmitted to the children as they, too, face new schools, new housing and the threat of being reunited with the perpetrator without adequate protection.

Immediate Treatment Goals

These reality circumstances call for a treatment plan with goals that are basically supportive and utilize the case management skills of the therapist.

At this point, the need for communication and understanding between family members is particularly poignant. However, the cognitive and development gap between parent and child may very well stand in the way. Art therapy provides a therapeutic vehicle for communication and understanding that is eminently appropriate since the process of art compensates for the verbal and conceptual skills available to an adult in contrast to those of a child. The art therapy at this point should mainly be group tasks that focus on the family's strengths and support the mother's parenting skills.

The initial goal of group art tasks and group sharing is to enhance the abilities of the family to communicate with each other. The pleasure of creating an expressive product as a team can be very rewarding and a skill that was inhibited while living in fear and shame. Violent homes restrict the experience of pleasure and freedom of speech.

A minimal search for dynamic or behavioral change is appropriate—the disruption of the life circumstances is enough to deal with at this time. Collage tasks that review past coping skills and positive moments when the family functioned well are recommended for the initial period of therapy.

Second Treatment Goal

Therapy with a family that has experienced violence, battering and subsequently separation, moves through many phases of treatment. After the family has secured lodging, entered schools and found some financial support or job, the basic needs are met and the therapy can begin to look at past and present issues that call for attention.

The recovery phase (or mid-phase) of treatment may be defined as the period that follows after the family has dealt with the initial loss, mourning and flight from the abuser. It is introduced by observing that the family has gained sufficient strength to consider going back into the world of relationships and inter-gender negotiations. It is time to regain socialization skills with an increased sensitivity for self-preservation. A treatment plan is implemented that emphasizes strengthening their skills and expanding a destructively narrow world view. In addition, we co-create a new meaning to relationships, gender roles and the right to live safely in a difficult world.

Case Example
History

Nora, a young mother with two children, a daughter of nine and a son of five, sought outpatient treatment at the local community mental health center after having just terminated a ten-year marriage. It was necessary for the police to rescue her from a violent domestic battle with her husband. He was hitting and choking her and kicking their children to keep them away. The argument began when Nora refused to get an abortion, and he became enraged. The little boy had attempted to defend his mother with his toy sword, and the girl had risked harm by dialing the emergency number and calling the police. Subsequent to this trauma, the family requested outpatient treatment.

The modality of art therapy was used from the start of treatment and greatly facilitated the grief work necessary to reconstitute this family of three as a single-parent family. The father refused treatment at the clinic. His contact with the children was limited to brief monitored visits bi-monthly. By four months, the family entered the mid-phase of therapy.

Working Through a Metaphor: Art Therapy Task #1

The therapist asked them to decide on and then create their favorite fairy tale. They chose Little Red Ridinghood. The art expression of this classic story took the form of a plasticene and construction paper three dimensional scene of Red Ridinghood in the forest. As they recreated it, Grandmother stood in the doorway of her home, the wolf was in his "doghouse" and the woodsman bravely defended Grandmother (Fig. 1). It was fascinating to observe Mother identifying with Red Ridinghood, the character who, as she said, "foolishly goes into the woods knowing that it was dangerous." The daughter created both Grandmother and the wolf. As the parenti-

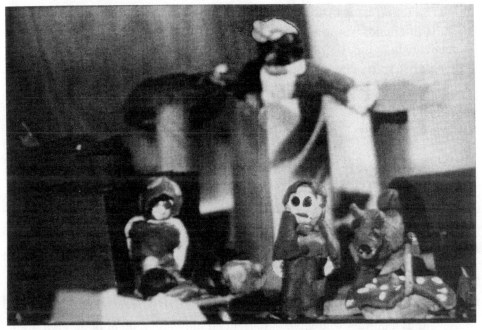

Fig. 1 Red Ridinghood (in center), grandmother and the wolf on either side with protective woodsman in the background. Plasticine and paper construction.

179

fied child she expressed in this choice both her matronly role, the jeopardy she had been through, as well as her strength to contain the wolf through the metaphor of the doghouse. The little son created the "mighty" woodsman who saved Grandma and killed the wolf, just as he had bravely rushed into the fray with his toy sword.

The therapeutic value of this construction was powerful. The drama and the trauma were channeled into a fairy tale where the familiar story allowed these family members to re-enact their roles in a mythical setting. The mother, through Ridinghood, could caution herself and her children "not to go back into dangerous places when it is clearly indicated that harm will befall you" (reinforcing her newly-gained ability to see that the old sequence of harm-forgiveness-harm of her marriage was a repetitive pattern). The little woodsman was encouraged to transfer his role to a real "big man" (adult/therapist), who would protect him and his mother, and he could start being his five-year-old self. He had learned to trust the help available to him through social services and the therapy. The daughter could relinquish identifying with "grandmother," who was delegated to "take on" the villain (wolf/father), and who, in that role, had been triangulated into a partnership of violence with her parents.

The family also enacted the drama, adjusting the fairy tale to their own needs and providing a new/safe ending to their own violent tale. The children understood; the mother understood the projection of reality into the fairy tale. The therapist was able to suggest modifications to the legend of Little Red Ridinghood, which if made directly to the family, may, perhaps, have been overwhelming. Using a fairy tale, a story that has retained symbolic and universal significance over many generations, provides the therapist with a secure metaphoric base from which the transition from mythic to personal interpretation is more readily available for the family. Adding the illustrative quality of art forms created by the clients allows opportunity for further projections. The ancient fairy tale becomes a modern metaphor for their situation.

Following this expressive construction and a period of further self-observation, a series of repetitive patterns emerged in the art expression indicating a need to bring the father into the therapy hour. The challenge was how to do this in a safe manner. Including the abuser in session may be undesirable because of the fear his presence evokes in the children, and often it is impossible (as in this case) because of court restrictions; however, he/she may safely become part of the therapy by using the art.

Facing the Abuser: Art Therapy Task #2

Many families who have experienced only one type of male character, a man who resorts to violence to win his argument, have a very limited appreciation of the broad variations in the male personality. Every man does not fall into the stereotype of this man with whom they lived. (Goldner, Penn, Shienberg, Walker, 1990).

Limited as they are by their singular view, battered families have a tendency to feel more "at home," more comfortable with another person who reflects these same abusive traits and abilities. This return to what seems "normal" explains the redundant patterns of abuse so often observed in abused families. This statement is not meant to convey the same meaning as the outdated notion of a woman who "plays the victim" or retains a masochistic drive for suffering. It merely states that behaviors that we know well and have grown up with do not seem strange or foreign. We have to learn how to live in new environments. Therefore, it is of the utmost importance for the therapy of damaged families to introduce broadened concepts of relationships and the possibilities of mutual respect. It is a vital safeguard for the mother to reassess what type of mate she might find attractive, and it is essential that the children find a healthy male model before she establishes a future relationship.

A technique that has been very useful as an introduction to an exploration of this vital issue is to ask the family to "invent a man who would suit this family." This is a task where the mother and children can create a husband/father who fulfills their fantasies of the "good man." This creative expression also allows the therapist to observe their stereotyped expectations in the male/female relationship and the parent/child association. Both family and therapist assess the mother and child's ability to discard old unsuccessful patterns in relationships. Later on this same task is repeated and the family is asked to "bring in" the abuser (on paper) and tell him their feelings about issues they have repressed in the past and say "good bye."

The art therapist draws a big man on a 6 foot piece of paper. The outline is not definitive except for a recognizable male physical shape. The family is invited to fill in this figure with collage pictures of what they would like from a "good man" (Figs. 2, 3 and 4). The parent is put in charge of working out where to put various images; for example, they may choose nurturing, protective functions placed around the chest near the heart, financial support pictures posted on the upper torso, near shoulders and arms. The family is urged to write explanatory statements, and often the art therapist becomes the youngest child's scribe, writing the words for the little one. Here the fantasy of a "new" mate/dad comes into the consciousness of the session.

This family filled in their father/husband collage man with very healthy images. There were desires expressed for fun as well as support, sports as well as love, intellectual challenge as well as relaxation. In particular, the therapist admired how the mother was helpful and generous with the space and pictures, but still maintained her own territory and her own adult needs. It was encouraging to see that the collage images chosen were well balanced with reality. The issue of safety was spontaneously discussed and the possibility of that "nice" man, like this "paper man," really existing in this world was talked about at length. The mother and children also discussed what was not there, the behavior and traits that they left out because they led to unhappiness. The final aspect of this task is important. Constructing their own male-friend was fun, and, for the first time, they could be playful and disrespectful in the presence of a man and enjoy it. The man co-created by the children and the mother was significantly different from the man from whom they had fled.

Discussion

The longings for safety and caring from a supportive partner do not go away just because the real man had failed to meet these

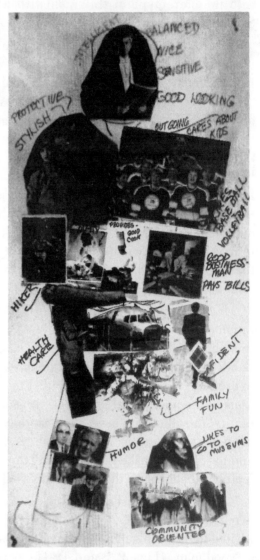

Fig. 2   Collage of the "Good Man" 6'x3'

expectations. These wishes are acknowledged and turned into a creative art task. The ensuing family discussion turns toward a direction which opens up questions around old patterns in gender defined roles, old patterns of reciprocal support and respect in the woman/man designated functions, old patterns of parenting and discipline delegated to male or female parent, all the major areas where men and women are conflicted over power and control.

Clearly the family doesn't solve this complex issue through one collage, no matter how grand its size. Making the drawn man "real" and "big" lends a sense of reality to this construction; however, on paper he doesn't threaten and is a "man" that the family can tailor to their needs. Another useful aspect of this task is that it makes apparent the "ghost" that is present but unacknowledged in the session. This absent father cannot be brought into the therapy, but his presence and all the love, hate, drama and authority that he once possessed are still real for his relatives. Through this art expression the family actively engages in a task that invites a safe confrontation of violent actions, the inequalities of power and domination and the fear that this patterned relationship will occur again. The guilt that many women feel is often activated through this collage. When this occurs, the therapist can begin to alleviate the guilt by helping her rebuild a more reasonable understanding of the life events that led up to this marriage.

In addition, the violent relationship is not solely a violent one. The partners have other times where love and passion are dominant. To ignore these positive moments, no matter how few or how brief, is to discount the capacity of the woman (and the man) to love, a denial that turns her into a masochistic puppet. There are aspects of romantic love present in these long enduring painful marriages, minuscule in most cases, but the therapist must honor the woman and acknowledge that she has the power to love or she will feel dehumanized. She must be joined in separating out the circumstances that

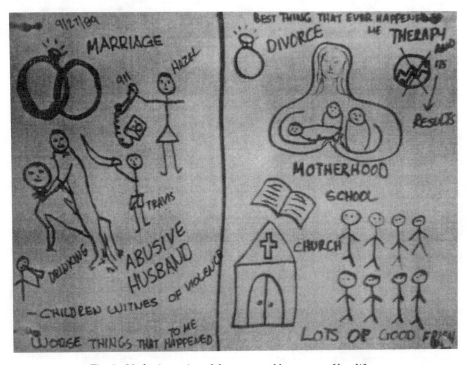

Fig. 3 Mother's version of the worst and best parts of her life.

made her love endure such danger and learn to use this most treasured human capacity in a manner that could result in safe affection in the future (Goldner, 1992).

Moving Toward Termination: Art Therapy Task #3

Now therapy turns to "family of origin" work. It becomes clear, in many cases, that the partners share similar childhood backgrounds of abuse which made violence more tolerable for them than it is for other persons.

The abusive family background often will have been ignored or denied by the clients. The source of the belief system that encourages over-tolerance for abusive behaviors is most easily addressed by helping the mother develop a family tree with the assistance of the children. Adding art therapy to the process greatly increases sophistication. For example, through collage, the members of the family can be shown with their gender, affect and behaviors, and by adding color to the connective lines that demonstrate relationships, the emotional temper can be color-coded. Tracing violence (if it exists), from generation to generation can give a clear picture of the abusive socialization these persons experienced. The less restricted the client feels about "how" to do a genogram, the higher the chances that it will be personalized and the greater the amount of information will emerge.

If there is opportunity to create a similar genogram of the husband's

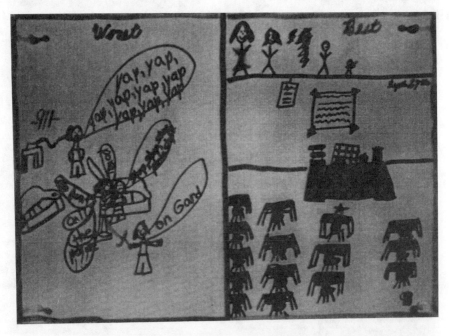

Fig. 4 A portrait by daughter of the final fight resulting in her calling 911 and her brother defending mother with toy sword. On right side, she portrays herself at school as star student.

family, the similar patterns of violent relationships often are observable. Thus the powerful force that influenced both mother and father to interact in this passionate/harmful manner is better understood. For example, the majority of persons, male or female, who tolerate violent relationships have come from families of origin where male/female stereotyped roles were exaggerated. Individuating from the family of origin will be greatly enhanced through subsequent art tasks based on these family maps. It is a time when the mother can help her children understand the circumstances that surround this "secret" behavior from the past and introduce a new set of values for them. As the parent teaches the child, she teaches herself! There cannot be lasting change for this client until she perceives herself through a new lens that recognizes her value as mother, worker, companion and citizen, and supports the right to be an active voice in society.

Termination: Art Therapy Task #4

The next phase of treatment is when the family becomes involved in inventing a future, a new reality (Watzlawick 1984).

Drawings and collage of "what it will be like in one year, 10 years, etc." are the vehicles for viewing change and the preparation for a new interactive life in the community. This invented reality and projected future does not ignore hard facts of life and the therapist swings back to an earlier mode of semi-case management. Finding support groups, after school activities, memberships in community service groups or church are all important re-entry steps. Simultaneously, helping the family acknowledge but let go of the lingering desires to repeat the old life and look more clearly at the past is the continuing task of therapy. When the family of origin is accepted realistically and their inadequacies seen as human, the magic and power of the family mythology diminishes and are seen merely as family legends. At this point, parent and children are ready to start on their own journey, plan their future and exercise their own identity (Fig. 5).

Every step of this process can be recorded and amplified by the art therapy expressions; tasks can be worked on and molded to introduce a broadened world view to these restricted families. Each art creation is one that brings the therapy closer to termination. The record of their work and reviewing their artwork produced in therapy will illuminate the progress as well as the remaining difficulties.

Termination will be a challenge, but having experienced the concrete experience of making decisions in a therapy that provides kinesthetic, verbal and visual engagement in the process of growth keeps these families on the path of change and offers a new ending to a sad tale.

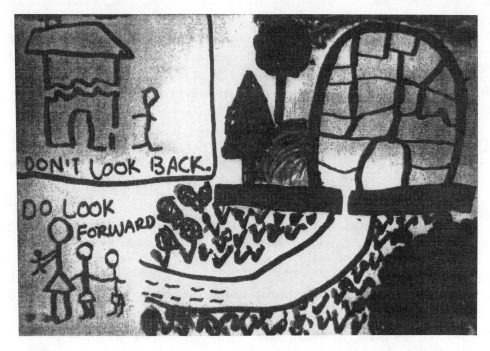

Fig. 5   Mother sets the goals for the future.

Conclusion

There is no "correct" formula for conducting art psychotherapy. The examples provided here are suggestions for treatment that are open and flexible and leave room for individuality. No families are alike, no family circumstances are identical and all families have their own legends and worldviews. Each experience of violence hurts the family in a unique manner and cessation of that behavior is experienced by each member in their own way. Therefore, it follows that the art expressions must also be elicited and explored with the respect and appreciation for individual differences. Clinical issues are projected into visible tasks that illuminate the therapy by the therapist's creativity as he/she finds appropriate expressive art suggestions that parallel the client/family's desire for change.

Art therapy continues to be the therapy of choice. This expressive therapy lets the client take a self-observing stance and through that distancing, understand the context of the art product and process, enabling her to co-create with the therapist a more satisfactory reality for herself and her family (Goodrute, Rampage, Ellman, Halstead, 1988).

In summary, the treatment of families who have elected to deal with extricating themselves from volatile relationships falls into four general phases. The first is protective, nurturing crisis intervention, at a shelter or elsewhere. The second is a recovery phase that introduces the opportunity to rework old attitudes, beliefs and gender assigned roles both in a primary relationship and in society. The third phase occurs as the family regains its self-worth and readjusts to new living circumstances and terminates family treatment. The last phase is individual therapy for the woman, if she elects, to explore the remaining areas of discomfort in their life (Pittman, pgs 284-290, 1987).

As with all problematic and potentially life-threatening situations that are brought to therapy, the issue of domestic violence must be handled with care and caution. The art therapy expressions are safeguards that help the therapist divert potentially dangerous actions and destructive behaviors and somewhat temper the difficulty of treating these clients.

Family art therapy is a recommended choice for successful resolution in domestic violence cases.

References

Byng-Hall, J. (1988). *Scripts and legends in families and family therapy*. Family Process, 27:167-180.

Coleman, K.H. (1988). *Conjugal violence: what 33 men report*. Journal of Marital and Family Therapy, 6: 207-213.

Efran, J., Lukens, M., and Lukens, R. (1990). *Language, structure, and change*. NY: W. W. Norton.

Gilligan, C. *In a different voice*. (1982). Cambridge: Harvard University Press.

Goldner, V. (1985). *Feminism and family therapy*. Family Process, 24:31-47.

Goldner, V. (1992). *Making room for both/and*. The Family Therapy Networker, 10 (2), 54-61.

Goldner, V., Penn, P., Shienberg, M., and Walker, G. (1990) *Love and violence: gender paradoxes in volatile attachments*. Family Process, 29:343-364.

Goodrute, T. J., Rampage, C., Ellman, B., and Halstead, K. (1988). *Feminist family therapy*. N. Y.: W. W. Norton, 169-172.

Hurtado, A. (1989). *Relating to privilege*. Journal of Women in Culture, 4 (11): 834-846.

Landgarten, H. (1987). *Family art psychotherapy*. NY: Brunner/Mazel.

Malchiodi, C. (1990). *Breaking the silence*. NY: Brunner/Mazel.

Penn, P. (1985). *Feed forward: future questions, future maps*. Family Process. 24: 299-310.

Pittman, F. (1987). *Turning point*. NY: *W.W. Norton.*

Riley, S. (1990). *A strategic family systems approach to art therapy with individuals*. The American Journal of Art Therapy. 28 (3): 71-78.

Riley, S. (1991. *Couples therapy/art therapy*. Art Therapy Journal of the American Art Therapy Association. 8 (2): 4-9.

Segal-Evans, K. (1988). *A general heuristic model of batterer's treatment* (unpublished). Los Angeles.

Watzlawick, P. (1984). *The invented reality*. NY: W.W. Norton.

From Entrapment to Empowerment—Family Art Therapy with Battered Women and their Children
by Gayle M. Callaghan, M.A., A.T.R., M.F. C. C. and Mary Rawls, M.A.

Gayle Callaghan, a 1989 graduate of the clinical art therapy master degree program at Loyola Marymount University ,is a clinical art therapist, and marriage and family counselor, working through the Children's Program at Haven House, a shelter for battered women.

Mary Rawls, M.A., Director of the Children's Program at Haven House shelter, also teaches parenting education for court-ordered parents and provides counseling services in her private practice. She is currently completing requirements for her doctoral degree in theology from Union School in Monrovia, California, on the topic, "The Reprobate Mind."

Introduction to Haven House

Haven House is a shelter and recovery program for battered women and their children. The battering partner is frequently also a substance abuser, adding co-dependency to the family's characteristics. This recovery program includes a 45-day stay which offers residence, food, clothing and personal needs, as well as counseling (individual and group) and support groups for the women and children. From five to nine families can be serviced at any one time, including up to 25 children from infancy through adolescence. Shelter residents come from a variety of cultures and ethnic groups. Bilingual counselors service Spanish-speaking families, while volunteers offer translation for some Asian languages and an interpreter for the deaf is available. In addition, Haven House is one of the few shelters which accepts teenagers of both sexes.

As a safe house, there are restrictions on women returning to the area of their battering partner, contacting him or persons who may reveal the location of the shelter to the batterer. Except for emergency services (police, fire dept., social services), the address of the shelter is kept confidential.

Haven House also offers outreach services for former residents and community clients. Outreach services cover a full spectrum from individual, group and family counseling to supplies for the home, participation in social events, and even holiday presents. Although individual outreach counseling is usually limited to ten sessions, services may continue in some cases for extended periods.

Because of state requirements, school age children in residence must attend school. Since there is no classroom on grounds, the children attend the local public school. Counselors help families with transference of school records and to prepare the children to enter mainstream education. Precautions are taken to protect the anonymity of the shelter's location. The inherent problems are addressed as children cope with adjusting to a new school while in residence at Haven House. Children coming from a low income, abusive and often chemically dependent household inherently carry a higher risk for developmental and learning disabilities. When appropriate, families are given referrals for psychosocial testing and support services so that provision for special education is expedited.

Crisis Intervention Plus

Family art therapy at Haven House basically follows a crisis intervention model with one major exception. Rather than restoring the family to a pre-crisis level of functioning, the therapy is geared to offering the mother *insight to her behavior and relational patterns so that she avoids getting involved with another batterer*. Her poor self-esteem and lack of confidence are countered by helping her get in touch with inner strengths, present, though often unrecognized by the recovering family members.

In addition, the families receive housing and financial aid information, alcohol education, co-dependency awareness, parent education, "Mommy and Me" activities, and self-esteem groups, plus participation in weekly Alanon groups. If the mother is in recovery from addiction, she is also referred an appropriate 12-Step program. Her privilege to remain at Haven House is contingent on her participation in that recovery program. This combination of services creates a more holistic approach to the family's recovery and promotes positive movement in the time available.

Meeting the Family

When the art therapist meets a new family, the first session is essentially verbal. The family learns about where they are and what they can expect during their stay. Often, the mother has not explained to the children that Haven House is a battered women's shelter and a temporary refuge (45 days). Safety rules and limits of confidentiality (child abuse reporting) are explained, terms are defined, and questions encouraged. Commonalities are emphasized to the family members, particularly the fact that all of the women in the shelter have been battered and all of the children have experienced having a battered mother and frequently have been abused themselves. They acknowledge grief over possessions and loved ones left behind, as well as loss of hope for a relationship which went badly, perhaps after several years of attempting to "fix" it.

Client Attitude Problems

The initial meeting generally sets the stage for a working therapeutic relationship, if indeed the family members are ready to work on changes. If the family came to the shelter in response to a child abuse report made on her partner, the mother may have been threatened with removal of the children by Children's Protective Services (CPS) should she choose to remain with the batterer. This mother may arrive at Haven House with a resentful attitude of the system which would "dare" to interfere with her life and plans. Entering the program with such an attitude precludes openness to alternative and healthier behavior. In the case of a client attitude problem, the narrow possibility for a therapeutic connection can be broadened through alignment with the mother by empathizing with her frustration with the "system." Following this, the therapist can help the mother consider how to avoid a repeated involvement with that same system, thus empowering her for change.

Family Art Therapy

Family members have a choice of whether they wish to meet with the art therapist individually, in sibling or peer groups, and/or as a family. Usually, a combination of meetings each week includes both children's therapy and family therapy. Although children's sessions are offered to those age four and above, family therapy includes all members, whatever the age. There is currently no funding for art therapy services to women as individuals or in groups at Haven House. We hope in time to expand the services to include adult sessions.

Introduction Through Collage

Validation of individual experience, clarifying family member roles, and communication between family members are the thrust of the beginning art therapy sessions with a new family.

A collage created by each person in the family about themselves serves as a good introduction to the therapist. Each member selects what color construction paper background to use, then selects precut pictures from a basket. Comments about the colors chosen and how the family resolves sharing the picture basket can offer the therapist information about family dynamics even before they begin to create their collages. Since clients often feel the need to perform and "look good" for their therapist (and others), we see a tendency to "split" by their representing only the positive traits along with something about their position as "victim."

In order to get a clearer picture of their psychosocial makeup, the therapist asks *the members to include a polarity of pictures showing both things they like and do not like,* or good memories and bad memories, perhaps three pictures of each. As mentioned before, each member discusses his/her collage while others are encouraged to listen. How well the family is able to adhere to the guidelines, plus their comments made about each other and their art, offer a wealth of information about family dynamics.

In addition, a *conjoint family drawing* generates further information about family dynamics and roles played by each member within those dynamics. While one member is explaining a collage, others are discouraged from simultaneously doing art work or speaking to one another. A *listening stance* is established in the family, perhaps for the first time. Blaming, teasing and frustration with other family members can be gently confronted and explored. By addressing each person as an individual, this exercise helps get past many defenses and splitting often present in dysfunctional family communication. If conflicts are revealed, questioning may clarify behavior patterns. While this first exercise is deceptively simple, it can offer a wealth of information to and about the family. The mother is often surprised by her children's awareness and insight.

Fig.1 shows a section of a typical introductory collage. This nine-year old boy shows what it was like for him at home when his father was abusing alcohol and becoming violent. The mother in this family had admitted that since she was the only person battered in the household (not the children), she thought she had managed to hide the abuse from her three sons. This collage confronted the mother with the children's awareness of their

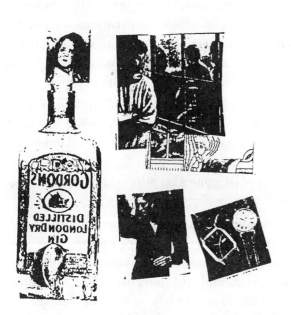

Fig. 1 Nine -year-old's view of living with domestic violence

mother's suffering, and her denial of their pain. At this point, the children's suffering was also acknowledged, and the mother had the opportunity to express her sorrow in response to her children's pain.

Following individual collages, a verbal or non-verbal family drawing can offer additional diagnostic information about member roles and patterns of interaction. Family members are encouraged to express their experience of the activity and what each "noticed," as the therapist feeds back observations.

In the family session, it is helpful for each family member to draw what he or she thinks is the most important family problem to work on while at Haven House. Mothers are frequently surprised when confronted with their children's priorities in the concrete (and undeniable) form of their art. Children are often blunt about their feelings toward the battering partner and their desire to return or not return to him. Their confused and anxious feelings about the batterer can be normalized and partially defused.

A Safe Place in Plasticene

A large percentage of mothers are concerned with finding a new home and with getting their children to "listen" to them. The children are also wondering about a new home and decreasing conflicts among family members. A logical art therapy response to these defined goals is for the family to create a "safe place" for themselves, encouraging the mother to be the "boss" of the project. An eldest, parentified child may vigorously resist the mother's role as "boss." However, with the therapist's support and occasional reminders of who is truly the head of the house (freeing the child to be child-like), the response is usually positive.

Family members use plasticene, plastic figures, construction paper, craft sticks, and other media to create their "safe place." A construction of this type may continue for two or three sessions. During the family's process of creating their product, the art therapist offers observations on issues revealed, and congratulates members on effective problem-solving and role-appropriate behavior. Family members are frequently delighted with their new-found skills of cooperative effort toward a successful end product.

Plasticene modeling clay, along with figures, is one of our most popular media for exploring sensitive issues through metaphor. A variety of small figures to chose from is offered from a basket, along with assorted colors of plasticene. The client is instructed to chose three of the figures, then to create a "place" for the figures using plasticene and other materials (sticks, pipe stems, stones and paper).

The use of three figures at a time lends itself to projecting personal dynamics, based on the Bowenian theory of relationships existing in triads within family systems. Plasticene is used because of its permanent pliability, which allows for change, correction, and additions over time. The non-hardening clay's capability for repair, no matter how severe the damage, is metaphorically a positive message for these traumatized families.

Clients are encouraged to "story tell" about their figures. Acceptable expressions of aggression, problem-solving and role shifts are explored within the sanctuary of the metaphor of their stories, before trying these new behaviors in real life. This same plasticene and figure directive can also be used with conjoint family projects, where each member chooses one figure to represent the self in *a shared space*. A piece of cardboard approximately 12" x 18" (one side of a cardboard box or a tray) offers a base.

Opening the Treasure Chest

If a client is having difficulty creating a story, it is sometimes suggested that a "treasure chest" be constructed and included. A small block of plasticene (1" x 2") with a slice from the top to serve as a lid is often enough to act as a catalyst to creating a story. A bit of glitter or small paper representing a map or a deed (ownership) may serve as a treasure to be placed inside. Frequently, this treasure will metaphorically represent some highly defended part of the client's self. Speculating with the client how that treasure might be used and providing for its protection can encourage self-nurturing through creativity.

These often overly serious families are encouraged to be playful together while working toward their family goals. Improved communication skills, self-esteem building, and healthier interaction between family subsystems may be "practiced" in the process of creating (achieving) a successful art product.

Art Therapy with the Children

In the children's art therapy sessions, directives are given based on the developmental level of the child, plus the issues presented by each. In addition to validation of experience in younger children, art activities are geared for self-esteem building through achievement. Both individual and group projects are accomplished to validate, build self-worth, and to encourage socialization skills.

Figures 2, 3 and 4 are examples of validating a child's experience. Figure 2 shows a 7-year old boy's experience of *what it feels like when his parents punish him.* Paying attention to the proportion of the popsicle stick's size compared to the figures, the drawing speaks for itself of how painful corporal punishment can be when the impact has literally lifted the child from the ground. This drawing led to a child abuse report and improved parenting skills in the mother.

Figure 3 shows a 10-year-old girl's experience of walking the fine line between honest communication and remaining mutely withdrawn about her pain. Describing her drawing, she stated, "I try to keep the anger (red) locked up inside (the black cage), but sometimes it gets so big it explodes out." She added that her sadness (purple) also "spills out like tears." The blue is the calm she attempts to keep on the surface. Following such a drawing, the therapist encourages the client to explore appropriate ways of expressing

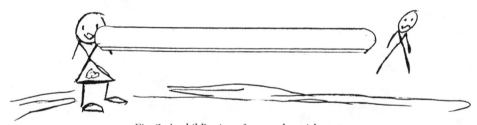

Fig. 2 A child's view of corporal punishment

these "normal" emotions, ways which she would find acceptable, thereby alleviating some of the need to repress.

Figure 4 shows a 14-year-old girl's anticipation of talking to a social worker and a detective following a sexual abuse report that was filed on herself and her sister. Her fears about the consequence of revealing, her rage at feeling trapped by the interview, and her nervousness are represented. How to set boundaries with others (even determined caseworkers) when interaction becomes unbearable was discussed. The art therapist offered to be the child's advocate during the interview. The child was encouraged to give the therapist a "signal" when things were getting too uncomfortable for her during the

questioning. Follow-up drawings served to further demonstrate this child's experience.

Adolescent Issues

Adolescents often have
a particularly difficult time
with the transitions of moving
from friends and familiar surroundings to a place like
Haven House, which may or
may not have other teens.
They may lose many freedoms
because they must be supervised at all times by adults.
The age-appropriate tasks of
adolescent separation and
individuation become difficult
when an adolescent is "stuck"
in a cottage with the mother
and siblings.

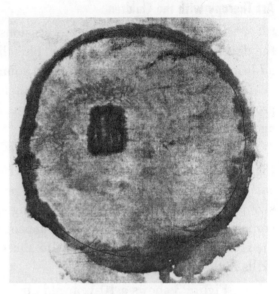

Fig. 3 The inner cage cannot contain
the feelings of this 10-year old child

Offering teens individ-
ual and peer group sessions,
rather than sibling sessions,
encourages individuation from
the family and identification
with issues specific to the age
group. Since many of these
teens are parentified to the
role of primary caretaker, the
art offers an opportunity for
them to be both creative and

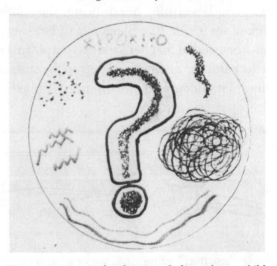

Fig. 4 A teen's mixed and anxious feelings about a child
abuse report and anticipation of the CPS work interview.

"playful" with the materials. The teen is encouraged to get in touch with and
nurture the inner child who may have been suffocating beneath layers of
defense mechanisms in order to survive in the battering family.

Expressing Rage Playfully

Media such as splatter painting and torn paper collage offer ways to
express frustration and rage in a non-destructive and even playful way.
Experimentation and creativity also inherent in adolescent "work" are

196

encouraged through unconditional acceptance of client artwork by the art therapist.

A Locking Diary for "Secrets"

In addition to separate sessions for teens, *a locking diary* has been found to be a welcome possession, and the staff at Haven House attempt to keep them on hand. The therapist may help teens to work out a "secret code" using symbols and images for their diary, in case some overly curious and determined sibling finds a way past the lock. Art directives can address what the teen believes might happen if his or her secret was revealed without actually revealing the secret. Keeping the teen client's work in a separate folder further encourages respect for privacy.

In-betweenness

In dealing with families in transition, we believe it is essential to address their very "in-betweenness." Directives geared to this issue are particularly helpful when a family first arrives at Haven House *and* as they have to move on from the program. Often the mother's self-esteem has deteriorated in response to living with the abusive partner, and she is often unsure of herself in the role of "single parent" (although frequently she was already struggling in that role). A large percentage of the women came from an abusive family of origin, with low self-esteem already firmly established in their psyche. The children's exposure to the abusive partner's attitude (that the mother was inadequate and valueless) takes its toll on their confidence in the mother as leader, protector and provider.

Figure 5 shows an 8-year-old boy's house drawing when he arrived. Although this child was severely abused by his father, he was deeply worried about what would happen to his father after the family left. The boarded-up windows, lack of inhabitants and stormy weather all reflect his difficulty with the transition of leaving home and coming to a shelter. He stated that the solitary blue bird did not mind being alone, and has a home in the tree which protects him in spite of the harsh surroundings. Close observation, however, reveals that the access to the tree "home" appears blocked, preventing the resident from returning as effectively as a locked door. There is no safe way to return to this "house."

The Inside/Outside Box

The *inside/outside box* is a valuable directive for defended clients and for adolescents, due to separation issues. A covered box with a lid (a shoe box works well) is offered along with the collage basket. The client selects pictures representing the self he/she shows the outside world for the outside of the box, while some for hidden characteristics are placed on the inside. Inside pictures *are not glued* to allow for outside placement or removal should the "hidden" change, or be revealed. Issues of trust and respecting others' privacy may then be explored.

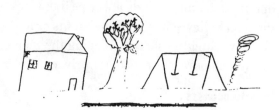

Polarities through Drawings

Throughout the recovery program, directives to use polarity drawings can be beneficial. By presenting multiple views to avoid client "splitting," polarity drawings defuse client anxiety about revealing

Fig. 5 An eight-year-old's picture of being in transition

personal experiences. For example, if a family member shows both what he/she loves and dislikes about what the batterer does, the member's mixed and complex emotions about the battering member may be defined as "normal" (not "crazy") and thereby are acceptable. *Advantages and disadvantages* of staying within a relationship can also be clarified to support decision making. Most experiences explored in the sessions lend themselves to this approach. Some polarity drawing topics are:

- What did you like about coming to the shelter and what is hard for you about coming to the shelter?

- What do you miss about not being back at home, and what don't you miss?

- What do you like about your relationship with your parent(s), and what do you wish would change?

- What would you like to tell your parent, and what would you like to know from him/her?

- What is your relationship to your child like, and what was your relationship with your parent like when you were your child's age?

- What have you found helpful in the program, and what do you wish was different?

Whatever issues are being addressed in the sessions, from the family's arrival through their leave taking, "polarity" directives can be invaluable in drawing out and illuminating the problems.

Bridge Drawings

Bridge drawings, *then vs. now,* are also useful in exploring *what members left behind, where they are now, and where they are headed.* Unrealistic family goals can be gently confronted and clarified, while appropriate and attainable goals can be encouraged and congratulated. Again, losses and grief are acknowledged, while the family's support network is defined and plans made to access that support (church, family, friends).

Outreach

A week before the family finishes their program, members are introduced to the outreach counselor who will be helping them. The outreach counselor acts as a buffer in obtaining financial, housing and material necessities as the family prepares to make the move to a new home. When appropriate, the outreach counselor can make referrals to other shelters and counseling services to ease the transition.

Because many families' experience of art therapy is a positive one, they frequently request that art therapy continue on an outreach basis. We offer it on a limited basis to some families who remain in the area for as many as ten post-residence sessions.

The Significance of Good-byes

Also relating to transitions is the potent issues of termination and good-byes. At Haven House, a good-bye session addresses *current and past good-byes* for each member. Family members are encouraged to create a *polarity drawing reflecting both what they found helpful in the program and what changes they might wish to make to improve it.* Opportunities are planned to resolve any conflicts with staff or other residents whenever possible, in direct contrast to many of clients' past experiences, where conflicts are left unresolved, good-byes often unsaid, and "business" left unfinished.

This final session is often a difficult one for clients; the therapist should be wary of transference and counter-transference influences. While some clients find the last session so painful that they refuse to say "good-bye," others embrace this as an opportunity for growth and healing. *A good-bye party for departing residents* offers further closure for families as they prepare to move on. Because of their shared experiences (the traumas of battering), groups of clients quickly bond to each other and their therapists. The termination session offers an opportunity to express that bond by allowing clients to create "tokens of friendship" to give each other as gifts. Tokens may be as simple as a friend's hand or thumb print in clay or a more elaborate construction. Many clients admit that this session offered to them their only "healthy good-bye" experience, since other good-byes may have been said in haste, in rage, or never said at all.

These directives are far from exhaustive, but offer a starting point for intervention in short-term therapy for families in crises. Their flexible nature offers much room for expansion and adaptation for the creative therapist.

Summary

Because of the inherent brevity of recovery programs like Haven House, adjunctive art therapy is focused on helping the family cope with the transition of moving from a battering and abusive household to one with the conspicuous absence of the batterer. Members' experiences and the range of accompanying affects are acknowledged, while they are encouraged to access inner strengths enabling them to cope with their life's changes. The inherent nature of art therapy to concretize and define with clarity issues, which are often elusive and obscure, renders it a potent modality for healing in this population.

References

Ackerman, R. J. (1983). *Children of alcoholics. A guidebook for parents, educators and therapists* (2nd ed.). NY: Simon and Shuster.

Black, C. (1981). *It will never happen to me. (children of alcoholics as youngsters, adolescents, adults).* Denver: M.A.C. Publications.

Blos, P. (1962) *On adolescence.* NY: Free Press Div. of MacMillan.

Callaghan, G. M. (1992). *Art therapy with alcoholic families.* Art Therapy with Families in Crisis: Overcoming Resistance through Non-Verbal Expression. D. Linesch, ed. NY: Brunner/Mazel.

Callaghan, G. M. (1989). *Roles in alcoholic families as seen through the art therapy modality.* Master's thesis. Los Angeles: Loyola Marymount University.

El-Guebaly, N., and Offord, D. R. (1977). *The offspring of alcoholics: A critical review.* American Journal of Psychiatry, 134(4), 356-365.

Engel, B. (1990). *The emotionally abused woman.* Woman to Woman. Los Angeles: Lowell.

Ford, F. R. (1983). *Rules: the invisible family.* Family Process. 22 (2), 135-145.

Hanson, G., Liber G. (1989). *A moral for treatment of the adolescent child of an alcoholic.* Alcoholism Treatment Quarterly, 6 (2), 53-69.

Jacob, T., Favorini, A., Meisel, S., and Anderson, C. (1978). *The alcoholic's spouse, children and family interactions.* Journal of Studies on Alcohol, 39 (7), 1231-1251.

Landgarten, H. (1987). *Family art psychotherapy.* NY: Brunner/ Mazel.

Linesch, D. (1988). *Adolescent art therapy.* NY: Brunner/Mazel.

Phillips, A. M., Martin, and D., Martin, M. (1987). *Counseling families with an alcoholic parent.* Family Therapy, 34 (1), 9-16.

Warner, R. H., Rosett, H. L. (1975). *The effects of drinking on offspring.* Journal of Studies on Alcohol, 36 (11), 1395-1420.

Wegsheider, Sharon (1979, May/June). *Children of alcoholics caught in a family trap.* Focus on Alcohol and Drug Issues, 2, 8.

Wilson, C., Orford, J. (1978). *Children of alcoholics* (Report of a preliminary study and comments on the literature). Journal of Studies on Alcohol, 39 (1), 121-142.

Youth at Risk/Families in Recovery Multi-Family Group Art Therapy
by Anne Kellogg, M.A., A.T.R.
& Jeannette McEliece, M.A., A.T.R., M.F.C.C.

Anne Kellogg, M.A., A.T.R., a Loyola Marymount graduate, explored "Inner Child" work as Academic Fellow Scholar in Residence at Loyola Marymount University from 1990-1991. Currently she teaches Early Childhood Art at Pasadena City College, and does therapy at Samaritan Center in Claremont, Mt. Baldy School, and Prototypes, a residential treatment program for pregnant substance-abusing women and their children.

Jeannette McEliece, M. A., A.T.R., M.F.C.C., also a Loyola Marymount University graduate, is the Family Recovery Services Educator at the Pasadena Council on Alcohol and other Drugs, the Almansor Early Education Family Therapist in South Pasadena, doing center and in-home treatment of foster and biological families of infants and children at risk for behavior, learning and emotional disabilities in response to in-utero alcohol or other drug exposure and in private practice

Bringing Families Together

Children of alcoholics and drug abusers are at high risk for repeating the addictive behaviors they have witnessed at home. Children who live in families where chemical dependency has been a problem need special help *dealing with fear and anger* and *learning to talk, trust, and feel again.*

Multi-family groups bring together recovering parents and their children for the purpose of addressing common issues and providing support to one another.

Multi-family groups provide a safe place to observe and interact with other families experiencing similar problems in the development of autonomy, social skills, bonding and negotiating emotional hazards constructively.

The family plays a vital role in the general development of children and particularly in children at risk of chemical dependency. Those who have learned and gained strength from their experiences are able to help those who are still struggling. As families go through this process of growth and recovery, they are able to reach their full potential in society as women, men, friends, mothers, fathers, and families. It is only logical that multi-family intervention programs can have an impact on a larger number of families.

Children living in families where chemical dependency has been a problem need special help—*help to deal with the fear and the anger—help to trust and love again—help to balance their daily activities—help to learn how to simply "be a kid."* In this program we create special time for both children and parents in recovery to begin to restructure their lives. Our program helps both children and adults recover from the trauma of chemical abuse in the family.

Helping to Break the Cycle of Abuse

The long term goal of group therapy with families in recovery is the breaking of the cycle of abuse through addressing generational patterns of chemical dependency. The process is committed to early intervention by providing awareness, education and prevention tools.

Restructuring Family Roles and Interactions

Each family member has adapted to chemical dependency, which has a life of its own, by using survival defenses. All of the group sessions are designed to raise awareness about unhealthy roles, rules, and modes of interacting and to learn more positive ways of relating to each other. It is quite common for children to have become parentified or scapegoated to hold the chaotic chemically dependent family together. They also may assume the roles of "lost child" or "clown." As the dependent person and the co-dependent get into recovery programs like AA and NA, they discover that the whole family, parents and children alike, are in need of recovery.

Why Art?

The art experience taps into the creative process, and the creative process is exactly what these families need as they reconstruct their lives together. The variety of art media helps the families use all their senses, auditory, kinesthetic, visual, tactile, gustatory and intuitive. These senses have been numbed by their adaptive defenses and self-medication. However, *when you scratch an addict, you find a creative person.*

The families are amazed at the symbolic quality and dimension of their images. They find their art so revealing of parts of themselves they had lost or had never been in touch with in the first place. Words keep denial in place. The art process breaks through the denial and brings forth unconscious material. In addition, using art materials is a leveling experience—everyone in the family can do it, and they can do it together.

Finally, experiencing the different art materials and projects gets them in touch with their ability to play. Many of the adults have never played in their childhood because they, too, have been caretakers of chemically dependent parents.

General Design of Sessions

As part of a federally funded prevention program for *Youth At Risk*, we designed the sessions to cover specific issues regarding recovery from chemical dependency, with four or five families (with children ages five to eleven) meeting together with us for twelve weeks. Each session started with a body awareness exercise to release tensions and provide centering and balance for the group's work together. The main part of the hour and a half session involved an art therapy experience with a group discussion/sharing following. The group closed with the adults encircling the children in a protective gesture. All sessions were intended to create an environment with defined structures, expectations, and boundaries. We offered ongoing nurturing and support facilitating self-esteem, self-control, expression of feelings and problem-solving.

Session I
Getting Acquainted

Activities

1. Introduction

We introduce ourselves and briefly describe the program. Families introduce themselves and share what brought them to the program.

2. Scribble Exercise

Make a scribble on the paper and turn it into something.

Objective: A scribble is developmentally appropriate for very young children and provides the families an opportunity to get acquainted in a non-threatening playful way. The earliest developmental stage was chosen to permit involvement of all family members.

Materials: 81/2" by 11" paper, felt markers, chalk, crayons, oil pastels, and colored pencils.

3. Non-Verbal Family Drawing

Draw together on large paper, don't talk, use one color per family member, and take turns drawing.

Objective: To assess communication patterns of family structure, interaction and roles.

Materials: Mural paper, drawing paper, felt markers, oil pastels, chalk, crayons, and colored pencils.

4. Group Rules

The group decides together what rules they needed in order to work together in respectful relationship.

Objective: Rules clarify the boundaries and limits of individuals and family groups. Parents are empowered and encouraged to actively reassert themselves as leaders of their family.

Session II
Family Communication

Activities

1. Review Group Rules

Objective: To provide an experience of consistency in setting limits and creating structure. The therapists modeled setting and maintaining appropriate limits, and conflict resolution emphasizing win-win solutions.

2. Kinetic Family Drawing:

Draw separately. Draw your family doing something together. When you are finished, share the drawing with group members.

Objective: To provide an experience for each individual family member to explore perception of the family. It is important that the nonverbal family drawing and these drawings be saved because the exercise is repeated *in the eleventh session* and compared to this one, providing the families with an opportunity to identify any changes which have occurred within the family system.

Materials: 81/2 x 11 paper, felt pens, chalk, oil pastels, crayons, and colored pencils.

3. Draw Together as a Family

Draw your family doing something together. Each family member is to use only one color, talking about what to do together is permitted. When finished you will be asked to share what the process was like.

Objective: To provide an experience for the family members to move from working alone to working together in exploring and changing their perception of the family.

Session III
Why We Are Here
How Chemical Dependency Got Into The Family

Activities

1. The Paper Chain: Families work together with many 1" by 8" strips of colored construction paper.

- Each parent selects one color to represent his/her family.

- Each parent is to trace their family back three generations by writing the name and most remembered characteristic of the family member, such as alcoholism, physical or sexual abuse, eating disorders, compulsive work, criminal activities, domestic violence, on the individual strips of paper.

- The parent directs and assists the child in pasting and looping each strip together, forming a chain. The products are two paper chains, each of a different color.

- When the chains are finished, each parent discusses his family of origin as represented by the different links in the chain.

- The therapist introduces the idea that like the chain, composed of many different links of construction paper, they are composed of the different links of their family patterns.

- The therapist provides construction paper strips of a third color, and offers the parents and children the opportunity of breaking the pattern by changing the color of the chain with which to unite the two families of origin. The therapist reinforces the idea that the pattern presents a high risk of continuing. By changing the color of the uniting strips, their children have a visual choice of continuing the pattern or trying a new way of being.

207

Objective: Help the family identify destructive patterns in their family and create alternative behaviors to stop the cycle.

Materials: 8"x1"different colored construction paper strips, scissors, felt pens, glue.

2. A Genogram to Trace Multigenerational Patterns.

The traditional genogram, as used by Murray Bowen, asks families to trace their families of origin back at least three generations to initiate disclosure of family truths.

With the parents as leaders, the family creates a symbol of the different branches of their family tree to show how chemical dependency got into both families of origin (Fig. 1).

Objective: The genogram is a successful non-threatening family activity to recognize and clarify intergenerational patterns. It breaks through the denial the role of chemical abuse has on family problems.

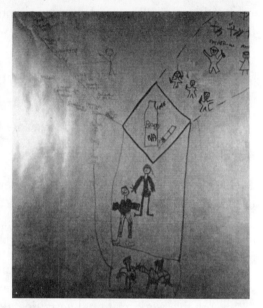

Fig. 1 Family Genogram

Materials: Mural paper, felt markers, oil pastels, collage, chalk, colored pencils.

Group Discussion: Multi-family group shares their tracing of how chemical dependency got into their families.

3. Draw Feelings about Individual Genograms

Each family members draws how it felt to explore and share their findings about their family of origin.

Session IV

Out of Control:

The Effects of Chemical Dependency on the Individual and the Family.

Activities

1. Chemical Abuse Education

The therapists educate the families about physiological damage to the body caused by chemical abuse. They use anatomical pictures such as the poster from the Weekly Reader, *Alcohol, A Drug That Can Harm The Body.*

Objective: To provide education which helps to break through the family denial of the effects of chemical abuse.

2. Show Drug and Alcohol Paraphernalia.

Objective: Develop awareness about variety of harmful substances available.

Materials: Pictures of wine, beer, prescription drugs, cigarettes, syringes, coffee, chocolate, sugar, cocaine, marijuana and hard liquor.

3. Bean Planting

Each family is given two pots in which each family member plants a bean. One pot is fed water, the other alcohol. Each week, the plants are fed as families witness the effect of alcohol on the beans (Fig. 2).

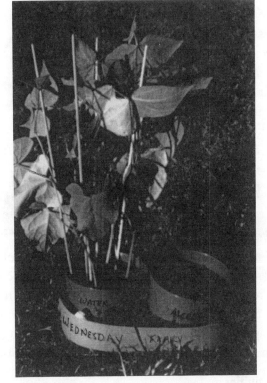

Fig. 2   Effect of alcohol on plants

Objective: Visual proof establishes that alcohol is not healthy for plants and other living things.

Materials: Plastic containers, beans, wine for watering, potting soil.

4. Painting Blindfold

Family members create a painting together taking turns painting blindfolded. The families process this experience together in the multi-family group.

Objective: To experience having a family member behave in an out-of-control manner while offering each family member the experience of enabling and being dependent.

5. Family returns to the original mural and works together to change the painting with the parent as leader.

Objective: Under the leadership of the parent the family is empowered to restructure an "out of control" experience (Fig. 3).

209

6. The therapists teach breathing exercises to emphasize the importance of air as a healthy substance which can be taken into the body.

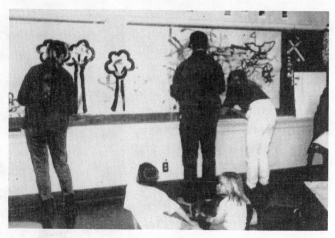

Fig. 3 Restructuring an out-of-control experience

Session V
Rebuilding Trust

Throughout the twelve sessions, therapists give honest feedback and provide models of mutual trust and self awareness. Trust is based on confidence that *parents mean what they say and say what they mean.* Without honesty, there is no trust, and without trust, there is neither communication and cooperation. Because trust has been broken as part of the family disease, there is a strong need to rebuild it. This may be an unfamiliar experience.

Activities

1. Mask making

Families use the following process as they work together building masks. Construction of the mask requires that individual members trust each other in the process. Family members construct masks on each other's faces. If the process is too threatening, they have the option of constructing hands.

Process:
- Cover face or hands with vaseline, making sure all hair is completely covered with vaseline, especially the eyebrows.
- Cut one-inch strips of Plaster of Paris gauze bandage.
- Dip strip in warm water, wipe excess off
- Apply to skin
- Build the mask by covering and layering the face with strips, with the option of covering or leaving uncovered, the eyes and the mouth.
- Two precautions: always leave the nostrils uncovered and do not cover hair with plaster strips.
- Allow time for mask to dry on face (5 to 10 minutes). The mask will pop off with facial movement.

Objective: To provide an experience for the family to rebuild trust. The process shows the degree of trust or mistrust between family members.

Materials: Rolls of plaster of paris gauze bandage, vaseline, paper towels, containers of water. The families should be told in advance to wear old clothing.

2. Group Discussion

Process Family Members' Responses to the Experience.

Objective: To provide an experience where families explore and clarify areas of mistrust that have taken place because of chemical abuse patterns.

Session VI
Coping

Activities

1. What Masks Do You Wear?

Family members adapt to chemical dependency by taking different roles to cope with the inconsistencies and confusion in the family. These defensive roles are like masks worn to hide real feelings which may be too overwhelming to express. The most commonly identified roles are hero, scapegoat, lost child, and mascot or clown.

Offering a variety of media, family members decorate the outside of the masks to show masks worn to cope. (Members who choose to do hands, are given masks of paper and encouraged to decorate both.)

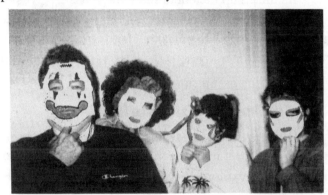

Fig. 4 A clown, pretty woman, person in denial, and good girl

Objective: To explore and clarify the role chosen by each family member to cope with chemical dependency within the family (Fig. 4).

Materials: Tempera paints, brushes, colored tissue paper, liquid starch, glitter, feathers, jewelry, sequins, yarn, stickers, pipe cleaners, glue, scissors, etc.

2. What are Your Feelings Behind the Mask?

Family members decorate the inside of the mask with magazine collage pictures suggesting their true feelings about chemical abuse within the family.

Objectives: To facilitate each family member's ability to get in touch with the effect that chemical abuse has had on their lives. To facilitate communication about defenses and feelings while providing group support.

Materials: Magazine collage pictures, scissors, glue.

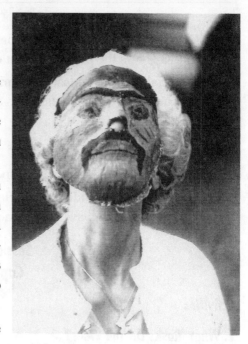

Fig. 5 Mother wears son's mask to provide him an opportunity for self-reflection

3. Group Members Share Their Masks in the Multifamily Group

As the group members share their masks, give permission to disclose or not disclose. In the disclosure, ask the members to place the mask over their faces and share how the mask feels.

Objective: To facilitate communication about defenses and feelings while providing group support.

4. Be a Self Observer by Exchanging Masks

Objective: To provide an experience of self-observation, self-reflection, and self-interpretation for the families to clarify their expressions of love and anger and explore alternative coping behaviors (Fig. 5).

Session VII
Truths and Secrets

If mom or dad is chemically dependent, families feel they have no choice but to hide the truth from friends and even from one another. Families become masters at resistance to disclosure to defend against experiencing shame. Initially we used the word, *secrets*, but found that too threatening. The families withdrew from any discussion until we reframed *secrets* as *truths*.

Activities

1. A Safe Environment

Each family explores the characteristics of what they consider a safe environment in which to share truths before they begin. Then they draw together on mural paper creating a safe environment for telling the truth. When finished, they process the activity in the multi-family group.

Objective: To provide an opportunity for family members to investigate and clarify favorable conditions to tell the truth (share secrets). The experience helps them see the obstacles they create which prevent openness within the family system.

Materials: Mural size paper, pencils, oil pastels, crayons, markers, chalk, paint, boxes, plasticine, etc.

2. Telling the Truth/Drawing Secrets

Each person draws a truth/secret with black crayon on black construction paper. The choice is given either:

• to reveal the secret/tell the truth by painting over the black crayon with water color and sharing it with the group or

• to contain the secret by putting it in an envelope or stapling and taping it shut.

Objective: To provide a safe supportive place to either reveal or contain family secrets.

Materials: Black construction paper, black crayons, water colors, brushes, water, envelopes, staples, glue, tape.

Session VIII
Feelings

Activities

1. Stuffing and Releasing Feelings

Family members are encouraged to write or draw various feelings on sheets of colored tissue paper, and asked to crumple the papers and stuff them inside their clothing. Involve the families in examining themselves. Are they distorted? Does the tissue paper feel irritating? What other feelings are evoked?

Sitting in a circle, invite each family member to unstuff themselves by taking out feelings and either expressing the feeling to the group or simply throwing it away.

Objective: To facilitate *recognition, acceptance,* and *sharing* of stuffed feelings, an experience which is lacking in chemically dependent families

Materials: Colored tissue paper, felt markers.

2. Draw Someone They Trust to Share Their Feelings

Encourage individual family members to talk about their drawings together.

Objective: To explore and identify people in their lives they can trust.

Materials: Felt markers, oil pastels, crayons, chalks, paper.

Session IX
Losses Due to Chemical Dependency

Most family members have incurred some kind of loss as a result of the family disease. These include loss of childhood, loss of authority, loss due to death, divorce, abandonment, loss of health, loss of jobs, homes, and loss of self-esteem.

Activities

1. What Have You Lost?

Magazine Collage or Drawing: Individual family members create a collage or drawing of what he/she has lost as a result of chemical dependency in the family.

2. Share the Experience with the Multi-family Group.

Objective: To provide a forum where each individual family member shares his/her grief about losses with the other families.

Materials: Magazine collage, scissors, glue, paper, pencils, felt pens.

3. Grieving

The family creates some kind of memorial or ceremony to acknowledge and mourn their losses.

Objective: To provide closure and allow the families to let go of their pain.

Materials: Assorted art materials, wood scraps, boxes, construction paper.

Session X
Parents Creating a Healthy Family Environment

In the following exercises the parents are empowered to assume responsibility for running the family and creating a healthy environment.

Activities

1. Problem-Solving Exercise

Parents divide their paper in half. On one side, they draw symbols of what they think their children need, and on the other side, draw how they can provide this. At the same time, the children draw symbols of what they need from their parents.

2. Process the Experience in the Multi-family Group.

Objective: To help the parents clarify their children's needs.

Materials: 11" by 17" paper, markers, crayons, oil pastels, chalk, colored pencils, paper.

3. On Mural Paper Parents Draw a Healthy Environment for the Family

After the parents draw the environment, the children draw and cut out paper dolls representing the family members. Together, the family places the figures in the environment.

Objective: To allow the family the experience of working together to create a healthy environment.

Materials: Markers, crayons, oil pastels, chalk, colored pencils, and mural paper.

Session XI
Change

In this session, we compare and contrast the non-verbal family drawing from the early session with the non-verbal family drawing done in this session.

Activities

1. Nonverbal Family Drawing

Ask each family member to each choose a different colored marker and draw together without talking.

Objective: To provide an opportunity to evaluate changes experienced within their family while encouraging feedback from other group members.

Materials: Mural and drawing paper, felt markers.

2. Compare and Contrast

All the families comment on growth and change as they view their before and after non-verbal drawing, now hung side by side.

215

Objective: To experience self-reflection, with the opportunity to make observations about change and give feedback to one another in a supportive environment.

3. Create Symbols

Ask each family member to create a symbol for him or herself showing how they have changed. Encourage sharing of the symbols within the multi-family group.

Objective: To facilitate another reflective experience which explores self growth and uniqueness of individual family members and clarifies the relationship between individual growth and family growth.

Materials: Plasticene or clay. Wood scraps, if time permits, are also excellent media.

Session XII
Saying Good-Bye

To celebrate our last meeting and our weeks together, we plan a feast, and address the feelings connected with saying good-bye. Our ceremony includes the ritual of eating together, making art, and affirming one another in the process we had gone through.

We talk about how we have created an extended family out of many fragmented families and provided a support system that can continue long after our group has ended.

Activities

1. Pot Luck Dinner

Families are asked to bring a main dish, salad, drink, or dessert to share with the group.

Objective: To encourage families to explore the possibility of creating healthy family rituals particularly around mealtime. To celebrate the

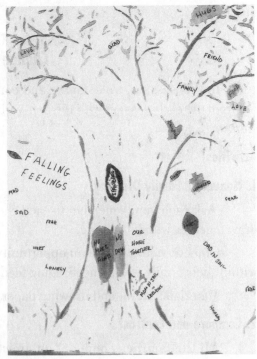

Fig. 6 Mural size 8 foot tree

216

sense of community and support developed during the twelve weeks of working together.

2. A Tree As a Support

Ask parents to work together painting a tree while the children create leaves, fruit, flowers, animals to put on the tree. Ask each family member to write on the leaves words or symbols of things they want to keep in their family and things they don't want. Those things they want to keep can be placed on the limbs of the tree, while those they want to let go of can be placed on the ground beneath the tree (Fig. 6).

Objective: To provide an opportunity for the parents to provide a safe structure which symbolizes a healthy environment for the children and themselves to grow.

Materials: Tempera paint, mural paper, construction and white paper, marking pens, and glue.

3. Family T-Shirts

Family members design T-shirts as mementos of their participation in the group.

Objective: To provide an experience for families to work together creating a *transitional object* to take home symbolic of their potential for change.

Materials: T-shirts can be brought from home and painted with tempera or or fabric paint.

Conclusion

In the beginning of our program, art media works as metaphor for life with at-risk families, focusing on opportunities for self-observation, reflection and change.

In the middle of the program, as the families become more comfortable with the *metaphorical* art process, a sense of competency develops. They become curious about their behavior discovered through sharing group art, providing even greater momentum for learning. The children and the adults develop a sense of autonomy as they begin to take responsibility for their own actions and feelings within the relational system. They *recognize, accept and share* their struggles with each other.

- The use of crayon resist works through the resistance to disclosure of family truths/secrets.

- The tracing of the family genogram gives form to the internal family patterns.

217

• Making and wearing masks is a metaphor for the artificial roles played which covered up the true self.

• Exchanging masks in order to view one's self at a distance creates the opportunity for self-observation, self-reflection, and self-interpretation

• Painting blindfolded symbolizes being out of control.

• Removing their blindfolds empowers the parents to create order out of the chaos.

• Stuffing of tissue paper with feelings written on them helps make them aware of how they stuff feelings.

The process of art becomes the metaphor for processing their issues.

At the end of the program, the family systems become more powerful because they discover, through interaction with the art and media process, deeper self observation and new creative possibilities. Building a network of support allows the many families to move forward as the youth and adult partners meet in dialogue toward positive action even in the midst of difficult circumstances.

This program was funded by the National Office of Substance Abuse Prevention (OSAP).

References

Beattie, M. (1987). *Co-dependent no more.* NY: Harper/Hazelden.

Bowen, M., M.D. (1986). *Family therapy in clinical practice.* NJ: Jason Aronsen

Bradshaw, J. (1988). *Bradshaw on: the family.*FL: Health Communications. Bross, A. (1982) *Family therapy: principles of strategic practice.* NY: Guilford.

de Shazer, S. (1982). *Patterns of brief family therapy: an ecosystem approach.* NY: Guilford

Kramer, E. (1971). *Art as therapy with children.* NY: Schocken.

Lowenfeld, V. (1957) *Creative and mental growth.* NY: MacMillan.

Robbins, A. (1987) *The artist as therapist.* NY: Human Sciences Press.

Stevens, J. O. (1975) *Support and balance, gestalt is—.* Collection of Articles About Gestalt Therapy. UT: Real People Press

Virshup, E. (1979) *Right brain people in a left brain world.* Los Angeles: Guild of Tutors

Wadeson, H. (1980). *Art psychotherapy.* NY: John Wiley & Sons.

Wegscheider, S. (1981). *Another chance.* CA: Science and Behavior.

Whitaker, C. A. (1967). *The growing edge in techniques of family therapy.* Techniques of Family Therapy. J. Haley and L. Hoffman, eds. NY: Basic Books

Establishing a Pediatric Art and Play Therapy Program in a Community Hospital
by Linda Chapman, M.A., A.T.R.

Linda Chapman, M.A., A.T.R., is Director of the Art and Play Therapy Program on the Pediatric Unit at San Francisco General Hospital. A past president of the Northern California Art Therapy Association and board member for twelve years, Ms. Chapman was a 1990 recipient of a NCATA Distinguished Person Award for leadership in the organization and a second award for innovative work in the field of medical art therapy. Currently co-authoring a medical art therapy book, Ms. Chapman lectures and teaches in the area of child art therapy and physical and psychological trauma.

Introduction

Four years ago, at the invitation of Dr. Moses Grossman, Chief of Pediatrics, an Art and Play Therapy Program was created and implemented at San Francisco General Hospital (SFGH) to meet the psychological and psychosocial needs of patients hospitalized on the pediatric unit. This program not only provides preparation for hospitalization and medical procedures, it also employs developmentally appropriate activities and play therapy to assist children and adolescents cope with illness and hospitalization. Most importantly, the Art and Play Therapy Program provides an art therapy assessment and treatment component to address post-traumatic stress disorder (PTSD) symptoms and to treat the psychological reactions to physical trauma.

Physical trauma generates emotional phenomena which consists of a defensive behavioral pattern (Caldwell, 1978), grief reactions (Peterson,

1983) and symptoms of PTSD (Terr, 1991; Eth & Pynoos, 1985; Goodwin, 1985; James, 1989). PTSD symptoms are seen in many of SFGH's hospitalized children as seventy percent of the patients are admitted for traumas including home and school accidents, motor vehicle accidents, burns, physical and sexual abuse, and stab and gunshot wounds. In addition to the trauma of physical injury, patients have often witnessed or experienced violent or catastrophic events prior to hospitalization.

The emotional impact of illness and hospitalization (Prugh, 1953; Robertson, 1958; Freud, 1958; Vernon, 1966; Plank, 1971; Thompson, 1981) on children and adolescents affects the child's developmental process and post-hospitalization psychological and psychosocial adjustment.

The SFGH Art and Play Therapy Program extends the treatment of the effects of illness and hospitalization to include the assessment and psychotherapeutic treatment of the emotional sequelae of physical and psychological trauma. This is essential to address issues which affect trauma recovery including:

• PTSD symptomatology

• recognition of the effects of psychopathology which may predate the injury (Watkins, 1988; Peterson, 1983) and

• effective crisis intervention and family therapy within the context of appropriate cultural norms regarding trauma and hospitalization.

This chapter will describe the components of a therapeutic Art and Play Therapy Program for pediatric patients in a community hospital setting. Issues for consideration while creating and implementing a program which emphasizes the use of art therapy as treatment of choice for physically traumatized children and adolescents will also be discussed. A Graduate Art Therapy Training Program component of the Art and Play Therapy Program is also described.

IN-HOUSE CONSIDERATIONS

Sponsorship

The SFGH Art and Play Therapy Program is jointly sponsored by the Departments of Pediatrics and Psychiatry. *Support by the chiefs of pediatrics and psychiatry provides the essential message to other care providers that assessment and treatment for psychological aspects of trauma, illness and hospitalization are necessary components of pediatric care.*

Fiscal sponsorship would ideally come from hospital operating funds. However, due to limited city and county funds, the SFGH Art and Play Therapy Program has relied on foundation, corporate and individual support since its inception in 1988. The 501(c)3 status required for non-profit organizations must be obtained, and/or a sponsoring non- profit entity associated with the hospital may serve as a fiscal intermediary. At SFGH, both the tax-exempt status and fiscal intermediary functions are provided by *The Volunteers to SFGH*, (SFGH's Volunteer Services department).

Administration & Development

Administrative support is required for fiscal management, correspondence and fund-raising in a foundation-supported Art and Play Therapy Program.

The fiscal management of the SFGH Art and Play Therapy Program is provided by *The Volunteers to SFGH*. In addition to providing the tax-exempt status, this organization is ultimately responsible for management of the Program's financial resources including:

- payment of salary and benefits to the Art and Play Therapy director
- payment of all program expenses
- review of annual program budgets and monthly financial statements
- annual preparation of payroll and tax information for the Federal and State governments
- providing assistance with fund-raising efforts
- recruiting volunteers for the Program's daily activities and special events

The Art and Play Therapy Program Director is responsible for:

- receipt and acknowledgement of all gifts and donations
- maintenance of checking accounts
- purchasing all supplies and equipment
- preparation of monthly and annual financial statements

The Art and Play Therapy Program director position is held by a master-level registered art therapist with ten years experience as a play therapist. Clinical expertise in psychosocial and psychological assessment, and crisis intervention therapy for children, adolescents and families are required. Administrative and program management skills, as well as experience supervising and teaching students is also necessary for successful leadership of an Art and Play Therapy Program.

Writing Grants and Other Fund-Raising Activities

The SFGH program was initiated via a written grant proposal submitted to local foundations and corporations. The proposal expressed the children's and adolescents' needs as identified in previous paragraphs, outlined a program to meet these needs, included the necessary financial and sponsorship documents and proposed a realistic yet adequate budget. Continuation of this grant-supported Art and Play Therapy Program requires ongoing fundraising efforts and contacts as well as a tracking system to follow solicitation guidelines, requests, acknowledgements, track report deadlines, and correspondence.

A correspondence/document file for each donor and an index card system with color coded clips to track the necessary report dates and funding cycles for each foundation provides current information for each donor to the SFGH Art and Play Therapy Program. A simple computerized data base could provide a similar tracking system, if available.

Solicitation of in-kind contributions of toys, art supplies, cameras, film, and other consumable supplies is an ongoing task and essential component of a foundation-funded program. Supplementing existing supply funds with in-kind donations utilizes scarce foundation funds for direct patient services.

Site & Supplies

The setting at SFGH includes a 470-sq.-ft. playroom, furnished office space, and storage space, all located on the Pediatric Unit.

The SFGH Department of Pediatrics provided office furniture, telephone service, office supplies, photocopies, postage, and administrative support when required.

A recent Ronald McDonald Children's Charities grant provided funds to renovate the playroom, with areas designed for art therapy, play therapy and infant play. The playroom accommodates hospital beds (with a four-ft.-wide door), has oxygen outlets, a sink, and a mirrored and matted infant area. Open shelving displays toys and children's books, and locking cabinets contain art supplies, musical instruments, an aquarium display, a tape player and music and story cassettes.

The toys are specifically selected for familiarity, age/developmental appropriateness, creative play, and for use in facilitating expression of issues specific to hospitalization, medical procedures, and trauma resolution.

A variety of art materials, dolls, puppets, animal, superhero and family figures, games, books, and medical supplies and equipment are also available. A moveable cart is stocked with art supplies and toys for use with non-ambulatory patients.

An adjacent teen room is supplied with a computer, small pool-table, television and VCR, games, books, magazines and comic books. The room is furnished with sofas and tables conducive to groups of teenagers relaxing and conversing.

A locked storage room contains dolls, toys, stuffed animals and art supplies. These items are used for replacement of consumable, lost or broken toys, and for gifts for patients.

Patients and The Clinical Team

The SFGH Art and Play Therapy Program serves approximately 1,200 multi-cultural patients annually, ranging in age from four days to eighteen years. Patients' hospitalizations vary from overnight to several months, with an average length of stay of four days.

Patients and their families speak predominantly English, Spanish and Cantonese; however, children from twenty-three countries have been admitted to SFGH during the four years of program operation. Interpreters are essential at times; however, since much of the expression is in metaphor, interpreters are preferred but not essential in every aspect of the therapy. The SFGH Bilingual Services Department employs a cadre of interpreters of fifteen languages (with on-call services for any language) who are available to assist whenever requested.

The children and adolescents at SFGH are admitted for trauma, fractures, surgical procedures, infection, and (sometimes chronic) illness with a variety of medical diagnoses. Patients are also admitted for psychosocial concerns such as abuse, neglect, and substance abuse as well as suicide attempts.

The pediatric clinical team at SFGH includes providers from Pediatrics, Psychiatry, Nursing, Social Work and Art and Play Therapy Departments.

The medical staff includes the Chief of Pediatrics, two pediatric chief residents, residents and interns. Attending and resident physicians from other specialized services, (e.g., Trauma, Plastic Surgery, Orthopedics), as well as medical and pharmacy students, are also part of the medical team.

The psychiatry staff includes a Child Psychiatrist Attending/Consultation Liaison for the clinical team. Under the Director of Nursing at SFGH, nursing team members consist of a head nurse, daily charge nurses, staff nurses, a psychiatric nurse consultant, and nursing students.

Two medical social workers are assigned to the Pediatric Unit. One addresses the needs of children under age twelve, and the other works primarily with adolescents.

The Play Therapy Program staff consists of the director who is a registered art therapist and experienced play therapist, art therapy student interns, psychology and child life students, and volunteers.

Responsibilities of the Art and Play Therapy Program Director

The Art and Play Therapy Program Director must interface with patients and families, other team members and the community. At SFGH, the Program Director attends psychosocial service rounds twice per week, clinical case conferences as scheduled, conducts periodic educational sessions for nursing staff, medical students, residents and attending physicians, and provides specialized consultation services as requested. On occasion, the Program Director is required to testify as an Expert Witness in cases of abuse and neglect. The Program Director receives weekly clinical supervision and periodic case consultation from the Child Psychiatrist, and is responsible for providing supervision to Art and Play Therapy Program Intern Trainees and volunteers.

The Art and Play Therapy Program staff provides information regarding psychological and psychosocial issues to the clinical team which assists in the development of effective treatment plans and case management. It is imperative for the clinical team to work in collaboration as each member provides different, yet essential components of comprehensive pediatric care.

The clinical aspects of the SFGH Art and Play Therapy Program include assessment, crisis-intervention and ongoing treatment for the physical, psychological and social components of pediatric care. SFGH emphasizes the use of art therapy for trauma resolution, based on the effectiveness of non-verbal crisis-intervention-oriented therapy for treatment. In addition, art, play and verbal therapies are utilized to address issues related to illness and hospitalization.

It is critical for the Art and Play therapist and other team members to communicate concerns and findings to the primary medical providers in order to a) support and enhance the primary relationship between physician and patient/family, and b) to inform the physician and other team members of underlying problems which may not have surfaced during the history, physical exam(s) or treatment(s). Physician support and participation in communicating concerns and patient issues with family members maintain a strong team approach, reduce resistance, and eliminate staff or family splitting which may result from an independent team member's action.

Physical Assessment, Intervention and Therapy:

Although the physical care is primarily provided by the medical and nursing staff, the Art and Play therapist must obtain and review information about the patient's medical diagnosis, pain status, drug therapy, medical procedures and prognosis before proceeding to assess the need for psychological intervention.

Assessing the physical condition of hospitalized children and adolescents is primarily focused on physical and motor development, pain status, and physical condition as it relates to development and current level of functioning.

Specific pain control and pain reduction techniques using guided imagery and art therapy assist patients in coping with pain, painful procedures, and for relaxation.

Psychological Assessment, Intervention and Therapy:

The psychological assessment consists of using art therapy techniques to identify emotional and social issues of concern, neurological impairments, affective state, cognitive functioning, ego disturbance, conflict and anxiety, thought content and reality orientation, PTSD symptomatology, and the child's current psychological stage of trauma.

An accurate assessment of the child's perception of the illness and his/her coping strategy for the illness/injury and hospitalization is essential for successful treatment/resolution of possible PTSD psychological sequelae.

The Child Psychiatrist formally assesses all suicidal and substance abuse admissions to determine whether subsequent psychiatric hospitalization is necessary.

Trauma is experienced in the body; therefore treatment must impact the child physically and psychologically (James, 1989). Specific art therapy techniques have been designed and implemented at SFGH to treat the psychological sequelae of trauma by carefully eliciting and facilitating the expression and management of feelings and sensations experienced while recalling the event. Recalling traumatic events is typically a visual, auditory or sensory experience, most commonly visual or "in pictures" (Terr, 1991). Art therapy is an excellent tool for concrete expression of the event from inner to outer existence as it is drawn on the paper. Art productions are used to properly sequence events, for reassociation (or retelling) of the event, for affective discharge, education, and for documentation of progression and change.

Children, often in a regressed state, experience numerous fears and anxieties associated with hospitalization, including fear of dying, fear of bodily change or damage (e.g, castration or amputation), fear of abandonment, anxiety, helplessness, embarrassment, guilt, and depressive symptoms. Therapeutic interventions to address these issues include art and play therapy, role play, puppet play, medical play, verbal therapy and family therapy.

Psychosocial Assessment, Intervention and Therapy

Medical Social Work staff members provide case management and address the clinical team's social concerns for the patients.

Psychosocial issues of the hospitalized child or adolescent include isolation, apathy, separation from parents, siblings, caregivers, friends, school and some semblance of the child's "normal daily routine," invasion of privacy, excessive stimulation to the senses and forced passivity.

Psychosocial interventions offered by the SFGH Art and Play Therapy Program include individual and group therapy, activity therapy, and special events at holidays or other occasions.

The activity therapy component of the SFGH program includes a volunteer program wherein individuals in the community spend time with the hospitalized children providing play, stories, art activities and games. The San Francisco Public Library "Book Buddy" volunteers read stories to the hospitalized children on a weekly basis, and the San Francisco SPCA Assisted Pet Therapy Program volunteers bring animals for visits twice per month. A local musician also provides weekly guitar and singing sessions for the hospitalized children.

Graduate Art Therapy Training Program

The Graduate Art Therapy Training Program is a vital component of the Pediatric Art and Play Therapy Program as it provides patient services in exchange for education, training and supervision.

The SFGH Art Therapy Training Program provides the interns with an in-depth clinical experience as an art therapist-in-training. Practical experience in the assessment and treatment of traumatized and ill children who are hospitalized is augmented with training in child development, child sexual abuse, crisis-intervention-oriented art and play therapy, cross-cultural psychology, family therapy, and case management.

Interns are encouraged to apply in early spring for the SFGH positions which commence the following autumn. Applicants must submit a resume, course schedule identifying completed courses and a letter describing their interest in the SFGH Pediatric Art and Play Therapy Program. Interviews are held during May, and selection and written notification are completed in early June for September placements. Applicants are selected on the basis of education in the fields of art therapy and psychology, interest in the medical setting and traumatized children, and professional characteristics.

Interns complete the admission process for the SFGH Training Program, including a required medical screening, completion of university/hospital contracts and necessary documentation prior to beginning the nine-month placement.

A liaison with the Child and Adolescent Sexual Abuse Resource Center (C.A.S.A.R.C.) at San Francisco General Hospital provides the interns with an opportunity to provide 15 weeks of ongoing child therapy for a child referred for assessment and treatment of sexual abuse. The interns are supervised by an assigned C.A.S.A.R.C. therapist and receive bi-monthly joint supervision from the Art and Play Therapy Program Director (art therapist) and C.A.S.A.R.C. therapist.

Weekly, interns complete 16 hours of placement, receive one hour of clinical supervision from the art therapist, attend psycho-social service rounds, and participate in individual and group art and play therapy assessment and treatment sessions. Interns also attend and participate in clinical case conferences as requested.

Interns are required to submit written process notes for all C.A.S.A.R.C. sessions and a minimum of two sessions per week from the Pediatric Unit. Required readings are assigned, and a final case presentation and art therapy in-service presentation to other professionals must be completed by the end of the internship.

Verbal and written evaluations are completed by the Art and Play Therapy Director in the middle and end of the internship period. Students are evaluated on professional characteristics, communication skills, assessment skills, treatment planning, therapeutic interaction, art therapy skills, and acceptance and use of supervision.

Summary

A commitment to excellence in pediatric trauma medicine must include a psychotherapeutic assessment and treatment component of the hospital care. Current Joint Commission on Accreditation of Healthcare Organizations (JCAHO) and California Title 22 mandates include limited psychosocial services for pediatric patients. However, the recent advances in the knowledge regarding the psychological effects of trauma indicate a need for psychological interventions for traumatic injuries and resultant psychological trauma. Immediate intervention is essential for complete care of the pediatric patient.

A comprehensive clinical assessment and treatment program for an urban community hospital serving low-income and disadvantaged children and adolescents is highly cost effective. Preliminary assessment for learning disabilities, difficulties in expressive and receptive language, sensory-motor, cognitive and social development, as well as physical and sexual abuse provides the opportunity for early intervention. Providing in-patient psychological services for traumatized children, adolescents and families prevents the development of PTSD by assisting in the resolution of trauma and the development of appropriate coping mechanisms for adjustment during and following hospitalization. In addition, treatment for families is essential in reducing anxiety, fear and denial, adjusting to changes that have occurred, mobilizing support, and accepting further rehabilitation or psychological treatment if necessary.

References
Medical Art And Play Therapy

Achtenberg, J. (1985). *Imagery & healing.* Shambala: New Science Library.

Achtenberg, J. & Lawlis, F. (1980). *Bridges of the bodymind.* IL.: Institute for Personality and Ability Testing.

Aguilera, D., & Messick, J. (1982). *Crisis intervention: theory and methodology.* St. Louis: Mosby.

Appleton, V. (1989). *Transition from trauma: art therapy with adolescent and young adult burn patients.* Ann Arbor: University Microfilms, Int'l. Publication No. 9027812.

Burnstein, S. and Meichenbaum (1979). *The work of worrying in children undergoing surgery.* Journal of Abnormal Child Psychology, 7 (2), 121-132.

Caldwell, E. (1978). *The psychological impact of trauma.* Nursing Clinics of North America. 13 (2), 247-54.

Cotton, M. A. (1985). *Creative art expression from a leukemic child.* Journal of the American Art Therapy Association. 2, 55-65.

Crowl, M. (1980). *Case study: the basic process of art therapy as demonstrated by efforts to allay a child's fear of surgery.* American Journal of Art Therapy. 19, 49-51.

D'Antonio, I. J. (1984). *Therapeutic use of play in hospitals.* Nursing Clinics of North America. 19 (2), 351-59.

Eth, S. and Pynoos, R. S. (1985). *Post-traumatic stress disorder in children.* Washington, D.C.: American Psychiatric Press.

Gabriels, R. K. (1988). *Art therapy assessment of coping styles in severe asthmatics.* Journal of the American Art Therapy Association, July, 59-68.

Geraghty, B. (1985). *Case study: art therapy with a native Alaskan girl on a pediatric ward.* American Journal of Art Therapy. 23, 26-128.

Gibbs, J. and Larke, N. (1989). *Psychological interventions with minority youth.* San Francisco: Jossey Bass.

Gil, E. and Edwards, D. (Ed.). *Breaking the cycle: assessment and treatment of abuse and neglect.* Cambridge, MA: Cambridge Graduate School of Psychology Manual for Professionals.

Goldberger, J., Gaynard, L. and Wolfer, J. (1990). *Helping children cope with health-care procedures.* Contemporary Pediatrics. March,141-160.

Green, A. (1978). *Psychiatric treatment of abused children.* Journal of the Academy of Child Psychiatry. 17, 356-71.
————(1983). *Dimensions of psychological trauma in abused children.* Journal of the Academy of Child Psychiatry.. 22, 231-37.

Horowitz, M.J. and Kaltreider, N. (1980). *Brief treatment of post-traumatic stress disorders.* New Directions for Mental Health Services. 6, 67-79.

James, B. (1989). *Treating traumatized children.* MA: Lexington.

Jospe, M. (1978). *The placebo effect in healing.* MA: Lexington.

Kiely, A. (1992). *Volunteers in child health: management, selection, training and supervision.* Bethesda, MD: Association for the Care of Children's Health.

Kivnick, H.Q. and Erickson, J.M., (1983). *The arts as healing.* American Journal of Orthopsychiatry. Vol. 53:602-17.

Kleinman, A. (1980). *Patients and healers in the context of culture.* Berkeley: University of California Press.

Kremberg, M. R. (1982). *The doctor as toy-fixer: a combination of art and play therapy.* American Journal of Art Therapy. 21, 87-91.

Kubler-Ross, E. (1969). *On children and death.* NY: Macmillan.

Landgarten, H. B. (1981). *Clinical art therapy, a comprehensive guide.* NY: Brunner/Mazel.

Lee, J. M., (1970). *Emotional reactions to trauma.* Nursing Clinics of North America. 5 (4), 577-87.

Levine, S. (1987). *Healing into life and death.* NY: Anchor Press/Doubleday.

Lusebrink, V. (1990). *Imagery and visual expression in therapy.* NY: Plenum.

Mehl, L. (1986). *Mind and matter: healing approaches to chronic disease.* San Francisco: Mindbody/Health Resources Press.

Mehl, L. and Peterson, G. (1988). *Hypnosis, healing and physical illness.* NY: Irvington.

Moore, A.C. (1989). *Crisis intervention: a care plan for families of hospitalized children.* Pediatric Nursing. 15 (3), 234-36.

Nagera, H. (1981). *Children's reactions to hospitalization and illness.* The Developmental Approach to Childhood Psychopathology. NY: Jason Aronson.

Olsen, E.H. (1970). *The impact of serious illness on the family system.* Principles of Preventive Psychiatry. NY: Basic Books.

Peterson, L. (1983). *The psychological impact of trauma: recognition and treatment.* American Journal of Emergency Medicine. 1, 102-106.

Plank, E. (1962). *Working with children in hospitals.* OH: Western Reserve University Press.

Pribram, K.H. (1971). *Languages of the brain: experimental paradoxes and principles in neurophysiology.* Englewood Cliffs, NJ: Prentice-Hall.

Queen, S., Habenstein, R., and Sobel, Q. J. (1985). *The family in various cultures.* NY: Harper and Row.

Rae, W. A. (1991). *Analyzing drawings of children who are physically ill and hospitalized, using the ipsative method.* Journal of the Association for the Care of Children's Health. 20 (4).

Romero, J. T. (1982). *Hispanic supports systems, health and mental health promotion strategies.* Chapt. 11, Hispanic Natural Supports Systems, Valle and Vega, eds.

Schaefer, C. E. (1991). *Play diagnosis and assessment.* NY: John Wiley.

Schaefer, C. E. and O'Connor, K. J. (1983). *Handbook of play therapy.* NY: John Wiley.

Serinus, J. (ed.), (1986). *Psychoimmunity and the healing process, a holistic approach to immunity and AIDS.* Berkeley, CA: Celestial Arts.

Sgroi, S. M. (1982). *Handbook of clinical intervention in child sexual abuse.* Lexington, MA: Lexington Books.

Solnit, A. J. (1975). *Psychological reactions to facial and hand burns in young men.* Psychoanalytic Study of the Child. 30, 549-66.

Sue, D. W. and Sue, D. (1990). *Counseling the culturally different—theory and practice.* NY: Wiley-Interscience.

Terr, L. (1991). *Childhood traumas: an outline and overview.* American Journal of Psychiatry, January 148, 1.
————(1991). *Psychiatric consequences of child abuse: conceptual models.* American Academy of Child and Adolescent Psychiatry 38th Annual Meeting. San Francisco.

Terr, L. (1990). *Too scared to cry.* NY: Harper and Row.
————(1988). *What happens to the memories of early childhood trauma?* Journal of the Academy of Child and Adolescent Psychiatry. 27, 96-104.

Thompson, R. H., and Sanford, G. (1981). *Child life in hospitals.* Springfield, IL: C. C. Thomas.

van der Kolk, B. A. (1984). *Post traumatic stress disorder: a psychological and biological sequelae.* Washington, D.C.: American Psychiatric Press.

Watkins, P. (1988). *Psychological stages in adaptation following burn injury: a method of facilitating psychological recovery of burn victims.* Journal of Burn Care and Rehabilitation. 9 (4), 376-84.

Webb, N. B. (ed.), (1991). *Play therapy with children in crisis.* NY: Guilford Press.

The Development of Camarillo State Hospital's Art Therapy/Fine Arts Discovery Studio
by Jack Cheney, M.A.

Jack Cheney is the founder and director of the Art Therapy/Fine Arts Discovery Program at Camarillo State Hospital and Developmental Center for the past 6 years. Recipient of the 1993 AMGEN Teacher of Excellence $10,000 Award, he graduated cum laude as an art major from University of California, Santa Barbara and did his graduate work in the art therapy program at California State University, Los Angeles. Committed to community arts outreach as illustrated by years of involvement as a multi-media artist, musician, performer and teacher in the Ojai-Ventura County region, Mr. Cheney firmly believes that art is a primary language which makes available means by which we may dissolve the artificial boundaries dividing us.

California's Camarillo State Hospital and Developmental Center, nestled in seclusion among arid coastal foothills adjacent to the rich farmland of Ventura County in Southern California, serves a diverse population of approximately 1200 individuals. This unique facility is divided into two main bodies: the State Hospital treating about 600 individuals with severe mental and emotional disorders, and the Developmental Center serving the needs of approximately 600 developmentally challenged individuals. The 37 living units house a diverse population who are challenged by just about every acute and chronic mental, emotional and developmental dysfunction imaginable.

When I began work in the winter of 1987, I was asked to develop a program which would, operating through Central Program Services, serve as many programs and address as wide a range of disabilities as possible with group and individual art therapy. The resulting program has been and continues to be a work in progress. I have assessed the needs of my many clients, the state of communications, creativity, and relations in general within the institutional environment, as well as the status of understanding and support within the greater community. At considerable stretching of my own capabilities and the utilization of all available resources, including the goodwill of like-minded colleagues and community volunteers, I have worked to create a program which provides optimal avenues of communications, expression, and relatedness within the microcosm of the art therapy studio and the macrocosm of the institution and the community. In this way we have created a supportive and flexible environment, rich in artistic media and creative choice, in which my clients can blaze their own unique paths from confining limits to new realms of personal integration, self-discovery and development.

This chapter will concern itself with the fundamentals of this multi-level multi-media approach and the effect it has had on our clients, staff and community. Finally, I will present a few case histories to illustrate some of the unique paths individuals have taken toward more complete and fulfilling states of being, focusing specifically on children and adolescents with histories of sexual and/or physical abuse, and a woman with whom I worked individually who suffers from Multiple Personality Disorder. My final case study will present work in progress with a group of adolescents who display the symptoms of Post Traumatic Stress Disorder. These youths, the blocked and enraged by-products of inner-city physical and social disintegration, are some of the most treatment-refractory and dangerous individuals with whom I have attempted to evolve intervention strategies. We must place a high priority on helping the many children in our culture who are born and grow up in the depressing cauldrons of our smoldering cities. The ranks of the disenfranchised in our society are growing. In terms of the continued viability of our culture, the problems presented by our informally maintained system of apartheid represent our biggest challenge.

The Microcosm—The Art Therapy/Fine Arts Discovery Studio

Considering the challenge of serving the needs of such a spectrum of individuals, I resolved to develop a flexible modality, rich in creative outlets, positive regard, therapeutic dialogue, and expressive freedom. Drawing on my own long-standing involvement in two- and three-dimensional arts, music, drama, and poetry, I have developed an approach which is varied and adaptable to a very wide range of functioning levels and therapeutic needs. Each individual has his or her unique way of learning. Creating an environment rich in constructive and expressive choices allows each individual increased opportunities to gravitate toward those forms of expression which are appropriate for the point of learning and development at which the individual is poised and with which each feels most capable and comfortable. I have found that such an environment and approach facilitates a relaxed therapeutic atmosphere and reduces depression and aggressiveness, while increasing self concept, positive self-regard, conflict awareness, and empathy between participants. In addition, convinced that the development of creativity is a powerful adjunct to personal integration, I have considered it a primary goal to also facilitate and reward artistic development.

The Studio

The art studio is a somewhat intimate space, being only 15 feet by 25 feet wall to wall. It has a large bank of north-facing windows which provides indirect light throughout the day. Inside the studio I keep it much like the art rooms I have seen on many college campuses. There are several easels, a clay-throwing wheel and several work tables. A large round table sits in the middle of the room around which as many as twelve people can sit to share their art, concerns, insights and issues.

When one first walks into the studio, one is struck by the contrast between the art therapy studio environment and the otherwise predictably neat, orderly and somewhat sterile offices and other rooms common to the rest of the hospital and developmental center. One is struck by a riot of colors, compositions and forms of student artwork celebrating their existence from every surface of the room including the ceiling. There are musical instruments of every description, drums created by students and tables full of art materials and supplies. Everything in the environment seems to reach out to the visitor, stimulating a natural creative response in almost everyone who enters. Countless times, students and staff have said that to come into the art studio is, in a very real sense, like leaving the hospital altogether. There are colors and media everywhere. Participants are reminded not to wear their favorite clothes because the emphasis here is on expressive choice and freedom, rather than the otherwise strict norms of sanitation.

Active Participation of Staff

In addition, I insist on the active participation of the other staff members and volunteers who visit the art studio. There is no room for dispassionate clinicians to sit aside aloof from the creative and expressive activities. To do so contributes to an artificial and impeding sense of isolation among residents who are, in general, struggling with a profound sense of rejection

233

and abandonment from society. With staff singing and making music and art alongside residents, there exists a spirit of discovery in which the creative and therapeutic processes are afforded much respect. In a very real sense, this accepting, stimulating, involving and media-rich environment does much of the work on its own to reduce client anxiety and facilitate openness to therapeutic and developmental work.

The General Structure of Group Activities

Almost without exception I begin each group, after a simple, spontaneous welcoming, with a shared period of music. I bring a lifetime of love of and involvement in music to this aspect of the program. In general I will play the guitar or harp and lead the group in several songs. Most of my students are not adept musicians, but all of them have voices and can play the many rhythm instruments that I make available. No matter what the functioning level of the participants, I find that music at the beginning of a session facilitates group relaxation, cohesion and communication. Depending on the current needs of the group, we proceed with songs I may choose, songs chosen by members of the group, pure rhythm exercises, and/or directive songs which require input from each of the participants on a particular theme to complete each verse of the song. In this way we work deep emotions and issues closer to the conscious surface of our awareness where they more easily are accessed and processed in the art therapy exercises which follow.

Art Therapy

Stimulated by the art studio environment and the shared music experience, group members are now invited to participate in a focused art therapy exercise. The themes of these exercises vary depending on the functioning level of the participants and the general issues being addressed by the group. This part of the visit to the art therapy studio is usually accomplished around the round table. I put soft music on the stereo. Participants usually work on paper using pastels, acrylic paints or watercolors or clay. Directives generally focus on family issues, other important relationships, color/feeling compositions, personal strengths/weaknesses, long and short term goals, early memories, etc. I take great pains to instruct everyone to view these works as means toward therapeutic ends and not as reflections of the person's artistic abilities. I intervene at any attempt by group members to negatively criticize another's art. At times, I offer no directives and allow individuals to create whatever they wish or work with abstract media such as string and ink techniques.

Whether the activity is directive or non-directive we reach a point where the members of the group have completed their expressions. We then share our work and discuss the meanings and issues which emerge. It is here that much important work is accomplished. At this time students reveal their complex and often fragile inner worlds. Combining their own insights, the shared experiences of their peers, and the therapist's interaction, their participants receive support for their strengths and sensibilities. They break through barriers of isolation and rejection and evolve skills for dealing with their traumas. They gain a sense of being one of a support group which gains strength from the others and asks for support and understanding in return.

Sovereignty over Meaning

I am not, in general, an overtly interpretive therapist. I have found that being interpretive and confrontational with chronic patients increases their resistance. Ultimately I prefer to allow my students sovereignty over the meaning of their own art work. In this way they are encouraged to reveal themselves to themselves. To the patient, insights seem to come much more from within, and permanent change is more likely to take place in the developing personality. In this way, also, trust between the patient and the therapist is preserved, and the individual is not as likely to become skeptical about his or her own creative impulses.

The Studio is a Creative Sanctuary

Following the formal session of art therapy, the participants are rewarded with a free period of fine arts discovery. During the time that is left, usually 45 minutes to an hour, the art studio becomes a creative sanctuary, a laboratory of free will. Participants choose from a vast array of expressive options, painting at the easels, throwing clay on the wheel or creating a clay sculpture. One chooses to decorate articles of clothing with paints or tie-dye. One chooses bead work, writes a poem, works on the latest dance steps or receives instruction on one of the many musical instruments available in the studio.

In art there are no wrong answers, only expressions which help one establish identity and develop ability. During this period, life in the art studio can become challenging for the therapist. With work proceeding on many different levels in many different media, it can be difficult at times to keep up with the requests for instruction and material help. This is where the support of other therapists who accompany the groups is critical. With their help, and the assistance of the many fine community volunteers which this program has attracted, the creative growth of these students can and does proceed uninterrupted during the free art period.

235

The Macrocosm—The Institution and The Community

I have found that cultural events at the facility, developing creative and expressive roles for staff, and educating and involving the community all help predispose clients to benefit from their work in the art studio. Therapy cannot be isolated from the general life of the hospital and developmental center. Cultural celebrations, art shows, and other special events provide creative and expressive opportunities that stimulate growth, as each person explores his or her relationship to others in new and different ways.

My program functions as a catalyst of communication, relatedness and imagination, creating a climate in which the community as a whole is united in the healing process. This principle has been well-recognized for ages by countless civilizations. If our goal is to create the unique circumstances by which chronically challenged individuals may progress therapeutically and developmentally, then we must open and develop avenues of community involvement, cultural expression and education.

Developing Staff Talent

So many people enjoy and appreciate the many talent shows, plays, art shows, dances, and day-long celebrations that the Art Therapy/Fine Arts Discovery Program is perceived as an entity which actively cares about the quality of daily life. Co-therapists discover and pursue their own personal and artistic realms through their involvement in the art studio. Staff members use talents not in their job description to entertain, coordinate parades and booths, or create their own art work to display in our Regional Mental Health and Developmental Community Art Shows. Through resident art which is often on public display, community members have their prejudices challenged and discover the creativity and humanity of our residents.

Our residents, in return, receive enthusiastically positive feedback from the community from which they have been isolated. Community members have spent thousands of dollars purchasing the fine art of the residents. Spending cash in their hands is the type of reinforcer our emerging artists really understand and appreciate. In addition, our residents have won by their creative endeavors hundreds of ribbons at the Ventura County Fair over the last five years. All of the area's local newspapers have devoted much space to lauding the artistic triumphs of our residents. Many community members have become aware of the innovative activities taking place at the hospital and have become volunteers seeking to involve themselves in the unique dynamics of the art studio in service to our clients.

The resulting good will of all these things goes a long way toward helping our residents feel that they are welcomed, encouraged and appreciated by the the surrounding community. In the art studio this sense translates into reduced client resistance, and the enthusiastic participation and support of fellow colleagues.

I view my program as a turning point in space which provides a vast array of safe paths along which participants may discover their potentials and evolve toward more complete states of conflict resolution, personal integration and creative development. In the case studies which follow I will try to illustrate how some individuals have taken advantage of the choices offered to arrive at milestones of personal growth.

An Early Group of Four Emotionally Challenged Boys, 9 to 11 Years of Age

One of the first groups I established was with four young boys, ages nine to eleven, from Unit 75 of the Children's Treatment Program. The transformation of the dynamics of this group from a state characterized by distrust and low impulse control to one of trust, communication and cooperation serves to illustrate how *clients play crucial roles in determining the best media and context for therapeutic arts interventions.*

These four boys, Alex and Jerry, age nine, and James and George, age eleven, had all been referred to the art therapy program by the Unit 75 clinical team headed by Dr. Calvin for treatment of their affective disorders, particularly deficits in the areas of socialization and impulse control, including assaultiveness. It was hoped that through this modality each young person could better understand himself and learn to appropriately and freely communicate his thoughts and feelings with others. All four boys had similar backgrounds marked by extended episodes of physical and/or sexual abuse. As is the case with most of the people we treat, all four had been moved to and from several residential treatment facilities before coming to Unit 75. All had been removed from their family at a very early age. Only in Jerry's case did the long term plan include preparations to reunify with the dysfunctional family of origin.

In mid-March, 1987, two months after beginning my program, I brought these four lads up to the art therapy studio for the first time. I was supported in my efforts by one of my first volunteers, a professional artist, Carrie Hunt. This group entered the art studio for the first time like a cadre of hyper-kinetic commandos. Though we tried to exert some control, it was clear by their behavior that they were determined to test the limits of my patience. Once inside the studio they fanned out in all directions. In the following ten minutes it took us to persuade them to sit down around the round table, they had managed to open and explore every unlocked door and drawer in the place. In fact, through some form of psycho-motor diffusion every nook and cranny of this strange new environment had been touched by at least one of them.

When we were all seated together, I began by trying to explain the goals of our group; how we use our art to better understand ourselves, etc. I then introduced them to the string and ink exercise. I demonstrated how lovely abstract patterns could be created by dragging an ink-soaked piece of cotton string across a piece of white paper. I proudly displayed my pattern and invited the group to identify forms which they might see hidden in the abstract design. I explained that these forms could be developed further using the pastels which I had in the center of the round table. I then let each member take his turn with the string and ink to see what unique art he might create.

Moments later, all of the group members had stopped using the string to apply the jet-black ink, and, with their hands immersed in the ink, each member was trying to outdo the other to see who could put the most ink on the small, saturated, dripping piece of white paper. The ink mess was getting all over, and I was beginning to wonder what therapeutic needs were being addressed.

Building Blocks

After a cursory period of cleanup I decided to try a shared wooden block exercise. I asked the boys to work in pairs to accomplish a building block project which I hoped would give us a vehicle by which we might address issues of socialization. Alex and George decided that they wanted to work together. That left Jerry and James to be the other team. From the beginning, Jerry showed no interest in the project. James willingly took over the project and Jerry was reduced to a bystander. Alex and George disputed one another's design and implementation ideas from the start. At the height of the conflict, George threatened Alex when Alex tried to rearrange a section which had been completed to George's satisfaction. Alex was about to thrust an angry foot through the entire construction when I intervened. Alex then isolated himself in a far corner of the room, a heap of rage and frustration.

It seemed that we were not making great progress.

As we prepared to leave the studio that afternoon, Jerry decided to crawl into a large packing box which was lying on the floor next to the door. When I finally noticed him, he had become completely immersed in play, pretending that the simple, plain cardboard box was a car. Preceding this moment, Jerry had show all the signs of being the most withdrawn and overtly depressed of the group. At this moment, however, his eyes were shining, and he was having a wonderful time making the noises of the racing motor and the screeching tires as he leaned back and forth to counteract the imagined centrifugal force one would experience racing around hairpin turns. I was reminded of a classic holiday scene of a room full of new toys with the children too busy playing in the packing crates to notice their new expensive gifts. Half-jokingly I suggested to the group that rather than the type of activities we had attempted that week, I should instead next week bring in a bunch of large boxes that we could all play in. Their response was an immediate, unanimous, and enthusiastic yes.

The Box as Fortress

The next week, I brought in four large refrigerator boxes, duct tape, string and markers. With obvious delight the boys took their boxes each to a site well separated from the others. For the rest of the period they were absolutely consumed with developing boxes into defensible fortresses. Reflecting their shared distrust of everyone, each one of them had me cut narrow slits in the walls of the boxes so that each inhabitant could see out but no one else could see in. Each created cardboard weapons which fit through the slits to thwart any threat or would-be invader. They did not invite one another, me or Carrie within their fortress. All parties worked with a seriousness and resolve. There were no fights that session, no inappropriate behavior or language.

At the end of the session I began an informal discussion on the vulnerability they might feel in the world. They were much more willing to talk. Jerry stated that when he was in his fort he felt safer. "I just like to sit in there because it helps me to relax," he said. George offered some insight about the feelings he had about his fortress. "It feels good to have your own place," he said. It was clear that these boxes gave them a means to ameliorate their emotional turmoil; a place, womb-like, to feel safe and get away from everyone. I realized that working on and in these boxes, these children had found a means to feel safe and in control.

In the six weeks that followed, I brought in more boxes which each member integrated into his particular fortress. Unique aspects of each habitation began to emerge which reflected the processes and personality of each creator. Alex built his fortress deep with a closet at the west end of the studio. His box arrangement, which had the form of a war bunker, was the least accessible of them all. In his interactions with other group members he displayed the highest level of hostility and suspicion. On his outermost box he mounted a turret gun with which, he was proud to say he would "blow everyone away."

George, who displayed the most ability in social interactions, created his domicile closer to the center of the studio than anyone else. His fortress was more casual and informal. He was the first to give up the cardboard weaponry and ask to have the narrow slits on the sides of his boxes enlarged to the size of normal windows. He was also the first to invite others into his "home."

Jerry was more preoccupied with the aesthetics of his arrangement than any of the other boys. His arrangement soon sported a round entryway and became methodically arranged inside and out. In his main room he hung round wooden rings and carefully placed white hospital towels on them.

James maintained the most consistent interest in the building process itself. He seemed to enjoy reworking the boxes each time he came in. He also was the most easily annoyed when the random movements of the other group members interrupted his work or threatened his structures.

At the end of each session I led a simple discussion centered around the feelings each was having at the time. Resistance to processing personal feelings was beginning to evaporate, and the individual members of the group began develop a constructive rapport with one another, and with their two adult facilitators. By our fourth session the boys were willing to engage in a short art therapy exercise before they were free to pursue their box work.

As often happens in a facility like Camarillo, by the sixth meeting the makeup of the group was changed by one member. Alex was released to another residential treatment facility, and, after conferring with the treatment team, a ten-year-old boy named Bob was recommended and included in the group. I worried at first that the change might impair the progress of the group. This, however, was not to be the case. As I have witnessed many times since that point, once a group has overcome initial resistance and become embarked on a mutually satisfying creative course, new members readily assimilate the atmosphere of security and discovery.

The Box as a Community

On the ninth week, something remarkable took place in the box work. Instead of working on their houses independently, as had been their usual pattern, they began to fasten their boxes to one another using George's box as a nucleus. In this way they found themselves cooperating in ways that would have been unthinkable nine weeks before. By the tenth week, half of the studio was filled with an elaborate labyrinth of cardboard box work. Box over box taped next to box stretched floor to ceiling. Among the boys, a complex system of pretend social relations had begun to emerge. George was "the boss" and the other boys answered to him as he instructed them to do this or that construction work for customers who called on his flexible tube "phone."

After a few more meetings of the group the boys began to show interest in using the other materials in the studio. By this time we began each group with some music and an art therapy exercise. The boys now displayed a willingness to talk about some of their hopes and painful memories. With their box work the boys had overcome the initial chaos and conflict which had first characterized the group. In the months which followed each individual created artwork which helped them get in touch with some of the roots of their primary conflicts.

A skull created by Jerry (Fig. 1) demonstrates this. I had a clay sculpture I had been working on. Jerry was fascinated by the process of building a hollow form and asked me to help him with a creation of his own. When asked what sort of form he would like to pursue, without hesitation he said a skull. Jerry had done several drawings of skulls during art therapy exercises. I helped him wrap the paper armature and showed him how to slab the clay and wrap it around the form. Jerry took the process from there.

Symbols of Abuse

Working with the focus and intensity of a pint-sized Rodin, he created a very accomplished, if somewhat ghoulish, form. The next week after it had dried, he removed a section of the top of the skull which had begun to crack. "This is where he got hit over the head. It killed him! See!" I asked him if it reminded him of the many times when he had endured severe physical abuse. Jerry became very quiet. The form before him had become a symbol of his own suffering. He stayed close to me. The tears in his eyes were all the answer to this question I needed. After the skull had been fired Jerry glazed most of the skull bone white. The cracked portion where the "injury" had been he glazed blood red. After the glaze firing Jerry shared his creation with the rest of the group. He was proud of the technical and artistic job he had done. In the next breath he shared some of the trauma which he had endured which he found that this skull so well embodied. Everyone supported Jerry for his artistic abilities and the courage he showed in sharing such personal and painful memories.

Several members of the group shared similar stories from their tortuous past. The group had come a long way and was surely moving together with understanding and purpose.

This group, like many others, was able to avail itself of other advantages offered by the program. At one point, with the help of several community volunteers, the boys joined the rest of their unit in constructing a bamboo club house on the grounds outside their residence. Using bamboo from a nearby river bottom, saws and twine they were able to participate in the realization of most kids' childhood fantasy in building this structure. Such a project worked to enhance the spirit of constructive socialization and cooperation among all the members of the unit.

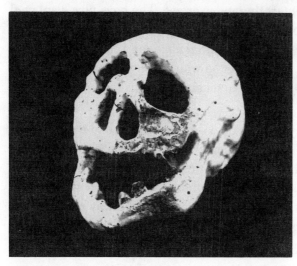

Fig. 1: This skull, created by Jerry, helped him identify, externalize, and process the rage he experienced enduring severe physical abuse.

Annual Art Shows

In addition, the members were able to enter and sell their artwork in the first annual art show we sponsored on the grounds of the facility. All work was carefully prepared and carefully presented. The boys' self esteem was enhanced both by how good their work looked when presented in custom mats, and by the fact that people from the community were willing to pay good money to them for the works of their imaginations.

The boys also evolved a very constructive and special relationship with our volunteer, Carrie, during the time they were in the program. Among countless other things, Carrie did wonders for their self image by painting portraits of each child, one at a time in the studio as the opportunities presented themselves.

A California Arts Council Grant

Two of the boys, James and Bob, were still on their unit when, through the Department of Mental Health and the California Arts Council grant I wrote, we produced with the children of several units a full-length presentation of Lionel Bart's *Oliver!* James and Bob proved a lot to themselves as well as to peers and staff as they stuck with the tedious rehearsals to finally triumph on stage in front of two very live audiences.

This was one of the first groups to participate in the multi-dimensional expressive arts of the Art Therapy/Fine Arts Discovery Program.

MARY'S STORY
Art Therapy With an Individual Suffering From Multiple Personality Disorder

Mary, a young adult woman, was admitted to the Developmental Center in March, 1989. She was admitted under an assumed name through Regional Center network. She exhibited symptoms of severe developmental disability and cerebral palsy. She was treated for some time in the physical therapy program for this physical disorder. A couple of months after admission, one of Mary's administrative personalities surfaced and the story of her true history and diagnosis began to unfold. Upon some careful research, it was discovered that Mary had assumed the name of and had obtained the social security number of an individual residing in the mid-west, Mary's region of origin. Further, it became obvious that her symptoms of cerebral palsy were a mock aspect of one of the many personalities Mary had evolved over the years to cope with a horrific childhood of sexual and physical abuse and neglect. It was theorized that Mary evolved the developmentally challenged personalities in order to obtain necessary services available to such individuals, as compared to the decreasing services which are available to those who are mentally ill. A thorough check of Mary's history of hospitalizations uncovered at least 100 separate instances of admission to psychiatric and developmental facilities.

From that point of accurate diagnosis, Mary was provided the weekly services of two primary analysts as well as several occasional interns. She was also enrolled in a program of job training and vocational development. The treatment team, understanding the importance of symbolic representation as a means of treating individuals suffering from multiple personality disorder, referred Mary to the Art Therapy/Fine Arts Discovery Program for weekly Tuesday afternoon drop-in periods. At that time, I operated two drop-in periods per week to allow residents with free time and campus access to come and create art, play instruments or merely hang out and enjoy the stimulating ambiance. This is the closest thing to Adler's Therapeutic Social Club that I employ.

When Mary was first escorted to the art studio, she entered under the name of Jennifer. "Jennifer" was strict and disapproving of the untidy state of the environment in the art studio. She seemed rigid and emotionally fragile. I provided her with paper and pastels and a place to work and went back to dividing my time between the other artists and my own creative pursuits. After a few minutes, I noticed that "Jennifer" had nothing on her page. Her face was full of anxiety. "I don't know what to do!" she cried. "Isn't someone going to help me?" Seeing that she badly needed to loosen up and relax, I suggested that she try an abstract design with the string and ink. As we worked together to create that first high-contrast abstract form on white paper, change came over her. The anxiety lifted from her countenance and the pure joy of creative discovery took its place. She completed several designs, then turned to me and smiled. "Oh, by the way, my name is Mary."

From that point on, Mary thoroughly enjoyed the rest of her visit. She reacted with appropriate laughter to the many scenes of creativity and humor which surrounded her in the studio. She explored the clay, paints and other media that were about. She derived some deep sweet pleasure from the few songs which I was asked by others to sing. When her escort returned for her at the end of the two hours she almost pleaded, "You will bring me back next week, won't you?"

Mary returned every week like clockwork. She worked on several projects with multiple faces in them and was becoming more aware of the monumental task of reintegration which faced her. One day, Mary was escorted to the studio and entered under the name of "Sunny." "Sunny's" disposition was too joyous for this world. With constant giggles and ooohs and aaahs reminiscent of childhood abandon, she came into the environment as if it was the first time she had been there. I asked her what she would like to do. "Paint!" was her immediate and enthusiastic response. When I asked her what color, she responded immediately again "Sunny" likes yellow." I provided her with paint, paper and brushes. When we got the gallons of paint out of the closet, she requested red as well. Having set up her activity, I turned my attention elsewhere. Every minute or so I would look over to "Sunny" and watch her collect vast quantities of yellow on her brush and drip the semi-fluid mass with great tactile satisfaction thickly on the paper, easel, and floor. I turned my head away for another minute and when I looked back over "Sunny," her face full of regressive abandon, had her hands thrust into the bucket of yellow paint. By the time I got to her, she had thrust both hands into the gallon of red paint. To look in her eyes, it seemed that she was deep within herself.

As I wiped the paint from her arms, she collapsed on the floor and began to make sing-song sounds of a little child. I called the unit for assistance. When I returned, Mary was in a fetal position, looking as much like a new born as is possible for a grown woman. She was looking for things on the floor and was trying to put the things she found (pencil, paper scraps, etc.) to her lips. I lay there on the floor with her underneath one of the worktables and gently kept her from putting objects in her mouth. After a while a little bit older personality surfaced and Mary was able to sit up. By the time the escorts from the unit arrived Mary was again in the mode of "Sunny." She happily greeted them. As she left the studio she said to her escorts, "This place is fun, and (gesturing to me) he's nice."

I shared the events of that afternoon with Linda Terry, Mary's social worker, who in turn revealed them to Mary's other therapists. This became an important pattern in Mary's treatment. Deep personalities and issues stimulated by symbolic art would rise to the surface, and the information would be relayed to other primary therapists who would use the information to help Mary further reveal and process through the implied issues.

After several more months of visits to the art studio during drop-in period, I received a request from the treatment team for me to work with Mary, as a primary one-to-one therapist. The therapeutic team requested that I work with Mary to reveal as much as possible the dynamics of the sexual and physical torture Mary had endured as a child.

Mary took well to the increased intensity of our inquiry. Being an excellent illustrator, she produced graphic representations of the closet in which she had been locked as a child. She revealed her great fear of doors, because it was through her bedroom door at night that her father would enter to engage Mary in countless forms of sexually aberrant activity. Her mother was portrayed as a severe woman who colluded in the abuse and even occasionally took part. Commonly during this period, Mary discussed some aspect of the torture which caused her personality to fracture out of adaptive necessity (Fig. 2).

Then we discussed the failed marriage she had left before her hospitalization. This union, as often happens, was with a man who, according to Mary, suffered a similar childhood and diagnoses. Next, Mary drew pictures of her five children, and expressed great feelings of loss at being separated from them. She was especially anxious about her oldest daughter who still lives in the custody of her abusive parents. She is certain that her daughter is enduring the same sort of childhood that she did.

At the end of these sessions Mary would insist that I sing to her. She most often chose songs about going home (*Country Roads*, etc.) or spiritual songs which supported the reemergence of her Christian Faith. As I sang to her, I felt I was filling a need for nurturing spirit and security that one feels when singing to a newborn. The music seemed to assuage the pain of her nightmarish past.

In the Spring of 1991, another primary influence entered Mary's life in the person of a new chaplain who began an active outreach program to all of the programs at the facility. He invited Mary to attend services and visited

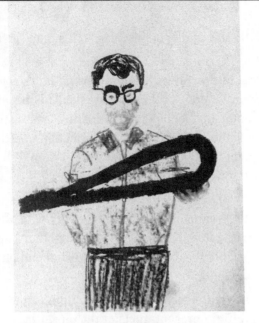

Fig. 2: Mary depicts her father as the overbearing abuser, emphasizing the leather belt with which he used to beat her as a child.

Mary on a weekly basis. During the Easter Services, we were privileged to hear a talented and accomplished soloist. The week after these services, Mary entered the studio absolutely lifted by the gift of inspiration she had received at the Easter Service in general, and by the singing, in particular. Raised as part of a religious community, Mary had some memory of what was good and nourishing within the Christian tradition. This religious experience gave her an opportunity to reestablish one portion of her childhood self which she felt was worth salvaging. An important step in her healing, it provided her a nucleus around which to reestablish a core value system. Religious themes emerged more frequently in her spontaneous art, as she continued the tedious work of integration (Fig 3).

In the time which followed until her release to a well-supervised group home in April of 1992, Mary worked diligently in the art studio and, with her other analysts, reconstructed the fractured pieces of her being. She worked simultaneously to forge meaningful relationships within the context of the hospital community, seeking out the emotional support and appreciation necessary to any person's mental health.

In her art, she journeyed from compositions showing twisting black and purple mazes full of blind corners and dead ends to luminous outward spirals done in pinks, light blues and greens. Early landscapes which Mary created showed half-dead forests full of trees with severed limbs, with anxious eyes peering out from knotholes and from behind rocks and shattered tree trunks. Later landscapes were inhabited by lush flora, healthy trees and green grass (Fig. 4). The recoiling eyes had become rabbits and mice and owls, more in plain view, though still slightly hidden in the undergrowth. It was apparent through her symbolic images that Mary counteracted the destructive attitudes she had internalized along with the abuse she had endured.

A Directive for Two Drawings

One such symbolic image evolved from a directive to make two drawings; one to represent the destructive lessons, attitudes and values which she had internalized from her parents; the second representing those things which she gained from her childhood which she wanted to preserve.

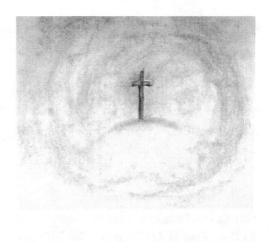

Fig. 3: Christian values are the focal point of this drawing, done by Mary, after Easter services

After Mary completed the project, we discussed the familiar issues which each drawing represented. I then instructed her to take the drawing based on the destructive material and physically purge herself by destroying the paper and throwing the pieces in the trash can where it belonged. She completed this aspect of the assignment with much enthusiasm, ripping, crumbling and stomping on the offensive drawings. With the other paper I instructed her to embrace herself while thinking of those aspects of her roots which she truly held dear. She did this with so much tenderness that it was obvious that she found this exercise to be quite meaningful and transforming.

In similar activities Mary worked diligently and with great interest, apparently determined to capture as much important self-awareness information as possible.

The last meetings before her discharge were rather informal and unconventional. Mary had recently begun to pay much more attention to her appearance. She was careful that her outfits matched and that her hair looked clean and well cared for. In short, she simply seemed more present than ever before. We talked about the three years we worked together. By this time we had become something more than client and clinician. She spoke with great interest and enthusiasm about the arts program, the art shows of which she has been a part, the carnivals and other special events she has attended. She reminded me of the sense of relief and joy she experienced when she first entered this non-institutional creative haven, and I realized that we had paved, in our time together, a two-way street of mutual support. During some of the sessions she did some ar,t but for the most part we would just visit. Invariably she would ask me to play and sing for her a song or two. She talked about the new apartment she was getting and about the roommates and staff with whom she would be staying. She discussed the job training and coaching she was receiving, her hopes and dreams for her future and the future of her children.

Mary has left the institution and is currently residing in a small group home. She still has many challenges ahead of her as the maturation and integration of her personality progresses. I cannot help but think of the many ways we have gained from knowing and working with her. Those with whom she has struggled to find herself have discovered hidden aspects of their own selves in return.

Chronic Emotionally Challenged Adolescents—
An Overview of Art Therapy/Fine Arts Discovery Intervention Techniques

At any one time at Camarillo State Hospital there are in treatment approximately 100 youths between the ages of 13 and 18 divided into five separate living units. The majority of these children were born into the world with the potential of any normal child. What happens to turn them into youths who must be considered either threats to the safety of themselves or others is found in the environments and most often the dysfunctional family networks in which they are raised. By the time most of these young people are admitted to our facility they have been removed from their family of origin and have

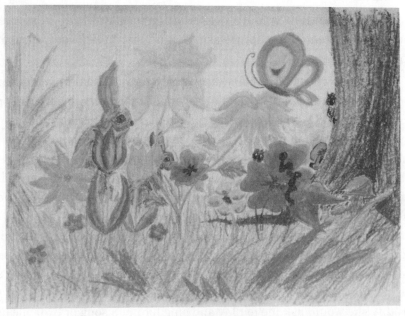

Fig. 4: Mary's later landscapes become much more grounded in reality.

248

resided in more than a few less-restrictive foster home and psychiatric treatment facilities.

In general, only the most chronic individuals end up at Camarillo. These children have endured holocausts of sexual and physical abuse—neglect and abandonment so severe that it is hard to imagine that they have been raised in a civilized culture. These adolescents can be wild, impulsive, assaultive and self-destructive. By and large they enter our facility haunted by suspicion and fear, unable to trust anyone, especially themselves.

Following are artwork and poems which illustrate the sense of devastation, abandonment and betrayal experienced by these teenagers.

Life Experiences by Jane, age 16

> *My life is flying by/Memories of places I've lived/Thoughts of people I've met/Changing sizes of clothes/Learning new things every day/Meeting new people every day/My life is flying by.*
>
> *Looking through dark windows/touching in cold places/Remembering my first love/Remembering my first hate/Painful thoughts cluttering my mind/Losing the friends I make/Being too afraid to make new ones/My life is flying by.*
>
> *Sharing my love with someone/Getting my love broken in two/Getting hurt and nowhere to turn to/ Getting hurt more and more/ Crying for help but nobody listens/What should I do now?/Please listen to my crying/My life is flying by.*

Skip by Helene, age 16

Once, on a yellow sheet of paper he wrote a poem...He called it "Skip," because that was the name of his dog and that's what it was all about. His teacher gave him an "A" and a gold star and his mother put it on the kitchen door to show to all his

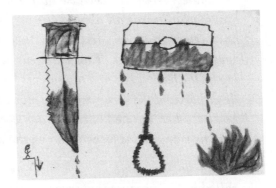

Fig. 5: Jane exhibits several means by which she has contemplated taking her life

aunts. That was the year his sister was born and his parents kissed all the time. And the little girl around the corner laughed when he

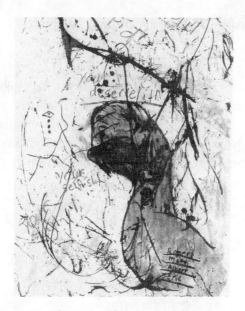

Fig. 6: Jane discovers a threatening clenched fist in this abstract string and ink pattern. Using pastels she darkened the perceived arm and fist. Surrounded by a sea of hurtful and disparaging remarks, she depicts herself weeping at the repetitive abuse.

fell down with his bike. And his father tucked him into bed every night.

Then, on white paper he wrote another poem... He called it "Autumn," because that was the season, and that's what it was all about. His teacher gave him a hard searching look and told him to write more clearly. His mother told him not to hang on the kitchen door because it has just been painted. That was the year that his sister got glasses and his parents didn't kiss any more. And the little girl around the corner sent him a postcard signed with rows of Xs. And his father didn't tuck him into bed at night.

On white paper with a typewriter he typed another poem...He called it "Absolutely Nothing" because that is what he thought he was. And that is what it was all about. His professor gave him an "A" and a hard searching look. His mother never said anything because he never showed it to her. That's the year he caught his little sister necking on the back porch and his parents fought all the time. And the little girl around the corner wore too much makeup, so he laughed when he kissed her, but he kissed her anyway. And he stayed up until 3 a.m. listening to his father snore in the next room.

On the back of a matchbook cover he scribbled his last poem. He called it "?," because that was his main concern and that's what it's all about. He gave himself an "A" and a slash on each wrist. And he hung it on the bathroom door because he couldn't make it to the kitchen.

Intervention Strategies

To evolve arts inter-
vention strategies for this
group has been one of the
most profound challenges I
have faced in my tenure at
this facility. It is a profound
tribute to the resiliency of the
human spirit that these kids
allow themselves to be
reached at all.

Several factors help in
reducing suspicion and en-
listing constructive responses
from our adolescent participants.

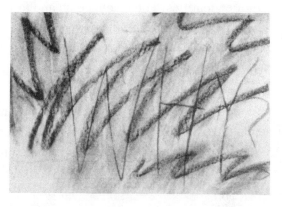

Fig. 7: Helene, in a composition of feverishly
slashed lines and lightning bolt forms, asks why
she was born into a family where sexual crimes
against her were perpetuated and tolerated.

• First of all, the studio environment, with its flexible and accepting
non-institutional atmosphere, tends to set our chronic youths at ease. In general, chronically disturbed adolescents mistrust the rigid conformity found
in the rest of the facility. In the art studio they find an environment which is

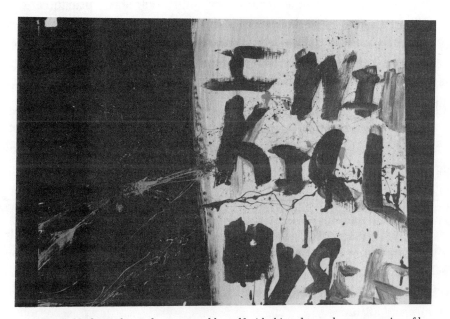

Fig. 8: Marla confronts the group and herself with this splattered representation of her
suicidal thoughts.

colorful, stimulating and non-rigid, that they can identify with, where personal expression is welcomed. These adolescents are struggling to forge unique identities. The many media and forms of expression open to them give each the opportunity to make choices and pursue artforms unique to themselves, thus facilitating constructive differentiation.

• In addition to all of the two and three-dimensional media, we encourage *music, dance, poetry, and creative writing*. If there is one expressive medium with which almost all adolescents identify, it is *music*. All the adolescents have their own favorite groups, and most own audiotapes (if not always stereos on which to play them). Music is one thing we have plenty of in the art studio; many instruments, most of which are simple to play on some level, are scattered throughout the room. Included are guitars, harp, mountain dulcimer, piano, autoharp, conch shell, recorder, as well as a vast array of rhythm instruments.

• At the beginning of each session, it takes no coaxing to involve everyone in a "get down" period of music. Sometimes it is good old rock and roll; sometimes it is plaintive ballads like *"The Rose."* Somewhere between *"La Bamba"* and our own improvised *"The Camarillo Blues"* a tribal-like bond is forged, and the group becomes ready for the next shared art therapy exercise.

Whether the exercise is directive or non-directive, we provide ample materials with which to work. While sitting around the table for this shared activity time, participants are allowed to use paint, pastels, watercolor or charcoal. Again, freedom of choice facilitates expression, expression facilitates sharing, and sharing paves the way for processing, insight and intervention.

It is during this shared time that important issues surface in the art. Themes of suicide, depression, betrayal, rage, abandonment—the emotional baggage of victimization—are all brought before the group whose members recognize and discuss similar experiences, offer coping strategies, vent hurt and rage, and reach out for love and support.

To access the feelings which are at the root of these adolescents' maladaptive behaviors is one of the major goals of the program. We now use knowledge of the feelings and memories which have risen to the surface to help the individual reassess the resulting self-destructive and maladaptive behaviors and attitudes.

Illustrations of the progressive movement of adolescents toward self-aware-ness and integration.

Walk With Me by Helene, age 16

> *I may not be the greatest passion/But lower flames burn longer/And I may not overwhelm your soul/But gentle strength is stronger/I may not be the most beautiful/But with time all beauties fade/And I may not be your sunshine/But when you rest you choose the shade/I may not fill your heart with laughter/But there is joy in just a smile/And I could be anything you ever wanted/ Come walk with me awhile.*

I Finally Found My Best Friend by Dawn, age 17

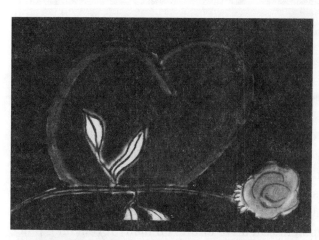

I finally found my best friend/She is someone I know better than anyone else/I know her deepest, darkest secrets, and to me that means a lot.

Although there are conflicts between us, we are still close/If you haven't guessed who that best friend is by now/take a wild guess/for that best friend is me.

Fig. 9: In a rose and vine composition, Helene placed a large purple heart, acknowledging the atmosphere of love which has allowed her to come to terms with herself and her troubled past.

"Free Art Period"

After this period of intense and revealing work, my groups are ready to use the remaining time to explore the creative media of their choosing. This "free art period" serves a spectrum of needs. After an emotionally intense period of group introspection, this time functions as a release valve, allowing a time for the participants to sublimate in spontaneous expressions the intense impulses which have risen to the surface. It is a time to allow the insights of the group work to sink in; a way for each individual to find his or her own unique way to relax and decompress.

It is during this period that some of the most intense and accomplished art is created. Some feel the need to connect with the earth and so gravitate

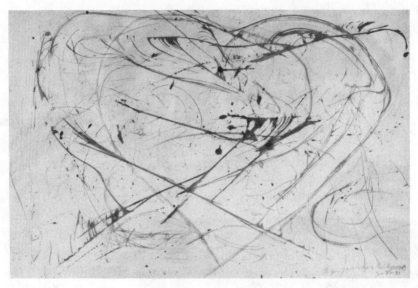

Fig. 10: Jennifer finds and develops this colorful and generous heart in the midst of a string and ink abstract pattern.

toward ceramic sculpture or the clay wheel. Others crave the visual and tactile stimulation of large scale painting. Some do body prints using paint that they readily apply to their hands and arms. Some put on their favorite music tape and work on the latest dance moves or sing along with the lyrics. Some play the piano or the drums in the adjacent room. The studio becomes a laboratory of identity development. Creative efforts on many levels take place simultaneously. Though it seems chaotic to the casual observer, it reminds me more of so many stars assuming their own direction and relatedness in an expanding universe.

Auxiliary Aspects of the Art Therapy/Fine Arts Discovery Program: The Reparenting Dynamic

For most residents of the hospital, cultural offerings and the direct involvement of community members provide fulfillment which is important to the emotional growth, social development and integration of these young people. For the previous years of their young lives they have lived in impoverished social environments. Before their court-mandated separation from their families, they had been surrounded by abusive, dysfunctional relationships where their needs for support were virtually ignored. The cultural events which we produce for their benefit have the effect of providing special environments and circumstances by which these young people can explore their unique identities as well as their social identities.

Each individual finds his or her own way of participating. Among the chronic adolescent patients, a number of individuals take pleasure in helping attend to the organizational aspects of such activities. Either by painting posters for the dances, organizing parade entries, helping set up and maintain booths for the cultural festivals, or matting and organizing artwork and setting up displays for our yearly art shows, these youths are able to practice active relatedness and citizenship. They are gratified to see that by contributing their energies to produce events they create opportunities for many people to derive personal growth and meaningful social pleasure. While working on these activities, sharing with others a common sense of mission, they experience what it is like to participate in a larger social fabric

They also learn how to have fun at the dances, carnivals or art shows. Within the context of these shared efforts and celebrations the symptoms of their consuming emotional disabilities decrease noticeably. New attitudes and constructive alliances find their way back to the therapeutic context and progress is quickened along the continuum of personal reclamation and social integration. These necessary social principles are at work within the context of any normal junior high and high school environment. Providing these experiences within the psychiatric hospital setting pays countless dividends for our chronic adolescents.

Bonding

We have discovered another transforming principle at work in our program. Through the years, many individuals from the community have been drawn into service at the art studio. Attracted by the opportunity for personal growth and the desire to help others less fortunate, many highly-educated, creative and dedicated volunteers have joined us in the studio. Many commit time on a weekly basis to the same group. Both men and women have dedicated countless hours directly serving the adolescents who consider the art studio their special haven. As time passes and the children adjust to the presence of the other adults, a unique and gratifying form of identification and bonding occurs. Time and again, group members begin to identify the community volunteers as a surrogate "mothers," and "fathers." There are many reasons that I see for the emergence of this dynamic, and why it works to facilitate therapeutic progress.

Customarily, soon after a volunteer has begun work with a group, he or she begins to identify with the suffering and needs of the individuals who frequent the therapeutic environment and attempts are made to address those needs with what I call the "cornucopia response." Great bowls of fruit find their way onto the art therapy table at the beginning of each session. Cakes, candles, and balloons are brought in to celebrate birthdays and other special events. Requests for special resources are granted if within the means of the volunteer. All these responses are appreciated by group members as demonstrations of real caring: true mothering and fathering.

The volunteer, though not usually a professionally trained clinician, can and does offer sensitivity. Clients in crises who feel a special affinity or "chemistry" with the volunteer, sometimes choose to disclose important feelings and issues to a trusted volunteer instead of to me or another paid staff member. Volunteers are apprised of the complex nature of our clients' disabilities and are counseled not to conduct interventions on their own. Instead, the volunteer is encouraged to be an active listener with whom the client can trust his or her innermost feelings. By having such an individual in the therapeutic environment, young people enjoy increased safe opportunities for therapeutic relations and exchanges. They experience the increased support of having someone who takes time out of their regular life "on the outside" to come to the hospital and be there just for them.

Volunteers each come ready to share their special talents and abilities. Most who are attracted to the program have an interest in art and have special artistic skills which they are happy to share with the kids during the "free art period."

For all these reasons, young people identify with the art studio as a "home" where their true natures can be explored and developed. This haven atmosphere allows them to seek out primary, archetypal relationships to fill the void left by the disappointing dysfunctional and abusive relationships of their childhood. They come to identify me and other men as father figures and women volunteers as mother figures, often spontaneously referring to us as "Dad" and "Mom." They often take any extra time available during free periods to be in the studio to gain as much as they can from this reparenting. They seem to bathe in the aura of our constructive relatedness and role modeling. During these drop-in periods they will not be there as much to create art per se as to be with their "adopted parents."

The reparenting dynamic which I have seen at work is not exclusive to community volunteers. It also exists in relation to co-therapists who escort groups to the art studio. That the community volunteer is not paid, however, seems to make a difference to the clients. No conflict of interest is perceived by the clients. The volunteer is seen as one who is there out of the goodness of her heart, compelled by genuine love and concern for them.

Adolescents from Inner-City Environments:
Post Traumatic Stress Syndrome and Intervention Resistance

In recent years we have been receiving for treatment many youths from inner-city environments. They are generally admitted with diagnoses of low impulse control and conduct disorders, especially acute assaultiveness. These young people have histories of confinement in what is usually a series of psychiatric and foster care placements. In general, they are the most dangerous subgroup of youths to house on the units. They are prone to violent outbursts, gang-like affiliations, serious assault and A.W.O.L conspiracies. Sadly, most youths with this personality profile are housed within our criminal justice system, either in juvenile halls or by the California Youth Authority where the emphasis is on control and punishment rather than treatment.

These youths present our mental health system as well as the society as a whole completely different challenges than do youths that come to us from dysfunctional families but otherwise functioning communities. They may have endured sexual and physical abuse to compound their problems ,but having the added daily stress of growing up under constant threats from their community environments has had a profound effect on these young people.

Like youths growing up within the context of constant civil unrest such as children growing up in Northern Ireland, these kids exhibit the classic symptoms of Post Traumatic Stress Syndrome. Growing up in inner-city "war zones" in one-parent family units that are chronically over-stressed and under-supported, these kids evolve adaptations to their environment reminiscent of William Golding's *Lord of the Flies*. Denied support by their families and communities, these youths turn to one another and their "code of the street" for relationships, meaning, and structure.

In the past we have treated youths with this psychological profile along with others with more usual maladies. The more I work with these kids, however, the more I am convinced that their needs are unique and require interventions specially designed for their origins. I have found that they are refractory to the usual approaches which work with survivors of "mere" sexual and physical abuse.

Following are some of the dynamics I have seen operating with PTSD children who are the members of other therapy groups. I am developing plans for a treatment modality which may more effectively deal with their unique problems.

The most obvious behavior exhibited by these inner-city youths is their propensity to group together *away from the general population* in any

257

given situation. Whether or not they are from the same neighborhoods, these kids gravitate toward one another and sit together in groups if allowed. Contrary to abuse survivors who generally tend to isolate, these kids are constantly seeking one another's input and approval in group-sharing situations. Their relationships with one another are marked by open mutual abuse, sarcasm, and antagonism. *When confronted by external confrontations or stress, however, they band together against a common enemy.*

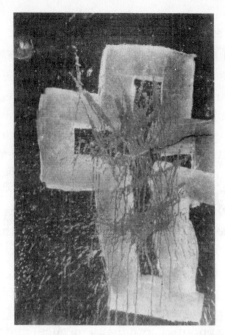

Fig. 11: Shawna created this large painting in memory of her grandfather who was killed in a drive-by shooting as she watched.

One of the most difficult things to do with these kids is to get them to reveal any feelings. When first asked to create therapeutic art, they most generally work in pure black and white or in colors reminiscent of the gang colors of their neighborhoods. Tending toward the familiar, they will create art along an established line of respected graffiti. When asked to talk about any feelings which may be contained in their work, they will generally decline with broad generalizations, saying, "It's nothing" or "I don't know. I just did it."

One girl, when asked to create a "self" box (a shoe box or other cardboard box collaged inside and out with pictures and symbolic "things") found the smallest box possible, decorated it within the span of five minutes and glued it shut. When it came time to share the meaning of her creation with the rest of the group, she stated "Here I am. I did it quick, and I don't have anything on the inside." These youths have had to stuff so many feelings for so many years they really don't have any idea of what they feel.

A directive I asked a group of young adolescent boys to accomplish illustrates this aspect of their syndrome.

I asked the group to think back upon the earliest memory each had as a child. After some coaxing, they, along with the other members of the group complied. *In each case with the inner-city kids, they remembered being threatened with great bodily harm.* One remembered being knocked unconscious at the age of four by a much larger club-wielding youth (Fig.12).

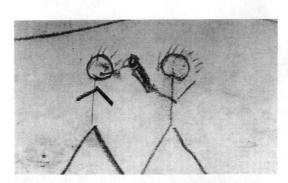

Fig. 12: Raphael, in this simple drawing, relates that his earliest childhood memory was of having to fight for his life "with sticks, rocks and bottles."

Another child remembers being threatened by another child at the age of seven (Fig.13). His response was to "knock the living shit!" out of this kid. "I've been fighting for my life ever since," he concluded. The other PTSD kid in this group reported that at the age of five he was threatened by a street gang that wanted to "lean on" his big brother. Under a deluge of dangerous circumstances it is no wonder to me that one's inner world and life of feelings have little space in which to develop.

The other kids in the group, from suburban neighborhoods, discussed domestic uncertainties; the threat of abuse from an alcoholic parent, the joy in adoption at the age of five. It was much easier for these kids to generalize about their current emotional states in relation to these early experiences than it was for the PTSD kids.

The inner-city kids seemed to accept their childhood experiences as the way of the cruel world, a world they intended to rejoin and subdue. The abuse survivors seemed to view their unhappy childhoods as unreasonable aberrations which saddled them with many conflicts they didn't entirely deserve.

Here is where the dynamics of the combined group process began to unravel. As we started to relate in depth to work through substantive issues which our childhoods left us with, the three inner-city kids started to relate on a level disconnected from the total group process. With non-verbal looks, hand signs and mumbles, they worked one another toward

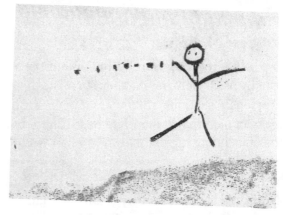

Fig. 13: Hunter depicts his earliest childhood memory: "Having rock fights with the other kids from my neighborhood. I got a bloody head a lot at first, but then I learned how to beat up anybody."

259

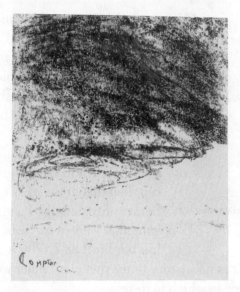

Fig. 14: Don typically filled the skies above his "home turf" of Compton with the darkness of fear, foreboding and pollution.

a frenzy of antagonism, disrupting the constructive work from which the other two members were profiting, while completely losing sight of and being consumed by their own dysfunctions.

I now, as much a possible, work with these PTSD youths in homogeneous groups. There are a number of art media and expression forms to which they gladly gravitate. I have noticed, for example, that inner-city kids love to *work with clay* which, I feel, gives them a chance to connect with the earth from which their wretched environments have kept them estranged. When encouraged and allowed, they greatly enjoy the *regressive tactile sensations of finger painting, and splatter painting.* In general, they love the *grounded sense of repetitive drumbeats* and keep up this activity longer than any group of kids with whom I have worked.

As the Los Angeles riots of 1992 illustrate, there is much rage within the hearts of the disenfranchised of the inner city. These kids are products of this rage and of a society who has effectively ceased to care.

String and Ink as Whips

In a recent group, I brought out the string and ink materials which I usually use to help my students stimulate their creative imaginations. They had previously seen me and others use the string and ink to create compelling abstract patterns on the white page. These boys used the materials to express the consuming rage of their own inner world. Rather than carefully drag the ink-soaked string across the page, they began to forcefully whip and whip and whip the page with the string (Fig. 15). Working together and taking turns, adding red to the black they created one large page after another of violent whip marks, which when viewed in the perspective of their lives, assumed the symbol of the uncontrolled flame of rage which consumes their young lives and the lives of those who are sentenced to live in despair in their communities.

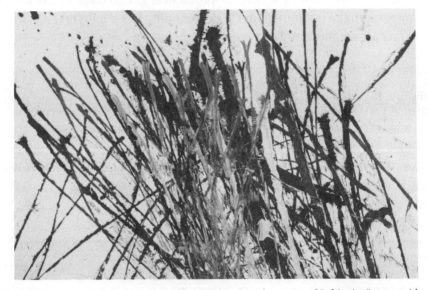

Fig. 15: Like so many flames leaping to the sky, this shared exercise of "whipping" paper with black, red, and yellow paint-soaked string allowed the group of inner-city PTSD youths to work together to identify and vent some rage.

I have established, with the Children's Treatment Program, one weekly group with adolescents age 13 to 15 who represent the PTSD profile I am determined to address.

My first goal is to take whatever steps are necessary to establish a sense of safety which the members can feel and enjoy. I intend to allow as much expression in clay, rhythm, and tactile media as possible. From this point, I hope to help them define and understand a range of feelings through their art. If we accomplish work along these lines, I feel that they may begin to avail themselves of the advantages that other adolescents have enjoyed within the scope of the Art Therapy/Fine Arts Discovery Program. From there, they may be ready to look beyond the communities which contain them and entertain notions of a future much different and much richer than any they have experienced in their past.

If we reach these goals, we have come half-way. If these youths, reclaimed and harboring some fragile hope, are released back into communities still reeling from unemployment, environmental decay, and social disintegration, they will most likely revert to old familiar patterns of self-preser-vation. There is no health, mental or otherwise, in a society which ignores the needs of vast sections of its population. We cannot build enough prisons to make these problems disappear. We must all become concerned agents of caring and transformation. He who ignores these problems contributes to every act of destruction by which the problem is gauged. If there is anything that my work in the institution and the community has taught me, it is that the fates of us all are inexorably intertwined.

References

Ansbacher, H.L., & Ansbacher, R.R. (Eds.) (1964). Alfred Adler: *Superiority and social interest.* A Collection of Later Writings. Evanston, IL: Northwestern University Press.

Capacchione, L. (1991). *Recovery of your inner child.* NY: Simon and Schuster.

Edwards, B. (1979). *Drawing on the right side of the brain.* Los Angeles: J.P. Tarcher

Gardner, H. (1983). *Frames of mind: the theory of multiple intelligences.* NY: Basic Books.

Green, H. (1964). *I never nromised nou a rose garden.* NY: Signet Press.

Kramer, E. (1971). *Art as therapy with children.* NY: Schocken.

Jung, C.G. (1964). *Man and his symbols.* NY: Doubleday.

Naumberg, M. (1966). *Dynamically oriented art therapy: its principles and practice.* NY: Grune and Stratton.

Oaklander, V. (1978). *Windows to our children.* Utah: Real People Press.

Rubin, J.A. (1987). *Approaches to art therapy.* NY: Brunner/Mazel.

Rubin, J.A. (1978). *Child art therapy: understanding and helping children grow through art.* NY: Van Nostrand Reinhold.

Rogers, C. (1961). *On becoming a person.* NY: Doubleday.

Virshup, E. (1979). *Right brain people in a left brain world.* Los Angeles: Guild of Tudors Press.

Wadeson, H. (1980). *Art psychotherapy.* NY: John Wiley and Sons.

A New Age Art Therapist
in a Psychiatric Nursing Unit
by Marissa Rubin, M.A., ATR

Marissa Rubin has worked on the adolescent unit at the Neuropsychi-atric Institute/Hospital at the University of California, Los Angeles for the past ten years. A graduate of California State University, Los Angeles' art therapy program, she combines her interest in far eastern thought and the art therapy process by blending the expressive arts, including dance and poetry, and far eastern concepts of yoga and acupressure in her work.

Eyes closed below dark sunglasses, I sit relaxed, walkman headset piping in 'Sounds of the Healing Waters' by Erik Berglund, harp music to help me disengage from the array of movement and clatter of bus travel. It's 12:45 p.m. I arrive in Westwood Village from Venice, forty minutes away. The time has been used to prepare my inner ground for the shift just ahead, as a member of the evening nursing team on A-West, an in-patient unit for developmentally disabled adolescents at the Neuropsychiatric Institute/Hospital, University of California, Los Angeles. At Westwood Blvd. and Le Conte, I enter a bookstore to look for an I Ching-like message of guidance from any book that attracts, to kindle an idea for an Art Group—a line, a word, a pattern.

"Please allow us to assist you in making your stay both a comfortable and memorable one," I glean from a bed and breakfast catalogue.

What comforts can I offer patients other than a consistency of scheduling, some predictability, attitudes of caring in the face of his and her stories of rejection, abandonment, violation, either environmentally or biologically inflicted? The task, however, has been articulated. Crossing Le Conte, on Westwood Blvd., towards NPI, rows of ancient Eucalyptus trees above a rich carpet of grass yield, on this July day, a harvest of bright slender leaves in their red-orange-yellow leave taking stage. I select a few, scoop up several dozen, then walk to my next mecca, the tropical fish tank on the B-Floor. I resonate with that fluid, effortless flow of movement for awhile.

As I approach the glass entry window of A West, I take note of the AWOL alert and begin the process of keying in on our locked ward. I walk to the staff room, unlock that door and join the evening team. Tonight it consists of three R.N.'s, the team leader, one psychiatric technician, one nursing assistant and myself, a senior Mental Health Practitioner. The usual air of alert attention is heightened by recent days of decompensation by tall and physically strong Jenny, who has been diagnosed schizophrenic. Her behavior has also seemed borderline in that with certain people, particularly male staff, she has not displayed the blank look that usually means voices are directing her to harm herself or others. This condition was first recognized two years ago when Jenny began to act out internal commands on herself and her mother. Then began the hospitalization of this intelligent, pleasant young woman. "Marissa, I like your Birkenstocks, I'm buying a pair for myself when my folks come to visit. Then I'll be a hippie, like you." We laugh, as I protest.

The team schedule is formulated, assignments made, and the report from the day shift is heard to help with our planning. My art group will include: Jenny with her one-to-one staff, Mitchell, diagnosed OCD, Obsessive Compulsive Disorder, an observant orthodox Jew who is being scapegoated by James, ADHD (attention deficit hyperactive disorder), of the same faith, but rebellious against it and all authority figures and quick to become enraged as well as Eric, also ADHD, who sponges up peer pressure, and Jonas, a moderately high functioning autistic (not a "classic" autistic in that he seems always to tolerate a stimulating milieu and can express affection and feelings appropriately), who in our community has not displayed the physical aggression experienced by his mother, and Tomaso, Hispanic/Afro American, 14 years old with a seizure disorder and a tumor growing in his brain. He is not targeted for scapegoating as he is not perceived as a threat. He laughs, draws figures and houses in primitive ways with stick arms and hands. The beauty of his soul was recently expressed by one of his stick figures with arms stretching out at forty-five degree angles from the head (location of the tumor) and touching the perimeter of a huge sun that completely surrounds the smiling figure.

Art group will be held in the dayroom, instead of the dining room where Treatment Planning is taking place, or the den, where the reinforcement of

T.V. or Nintendo may be earned by patients who comply with their contracts. The den will be occupied by Ted, a 21-year-old autistic who looks as if he has been working out at Gold's Gym—a local Venice institution for body builders. Just prior to arriving here, Ted had broken thirty windows in thirty two days. Our record is a dramatic improvement, only one breakage in the two weeks he's been with us. Nonetheless, we treat him with kid gloves. At ten minutes of 4:00 p.m., I gather art materials, music tapes, vials of peppermint and lavender essential oils, several white hospital sheets and squares of intensely colored origami paper. We will not do origami, but I've been experimenting with creating a functional and intentional mandala in the center of our round art table. It is composed of colored pencils, marker pens, oil pastels and chalk pastels. I also utilize particularly expressive or texturally exciting pieces of potential collage material to compose this constantly changing and compelling center piece. I hope to break through the ennui, to overcome some of the resistance expressed in such statements as "Art group sucks" and arrive at a more harmonious response which also frequently comes through as "I love art group." I sprinkle drops of essential oil on the white cloth (peppermint has a tonic freshening effect, lavender is calming), then place our 11x14 sheets of drawing paper around the table, arranging chairs to correspond with each paper. Music will be turned on after I've described the task. This is the preliminary ritual. Each group member will be a spoke of the wheel. At times I'm at the rudder.

The group that assembles now knows that they will be earning points for participation and behavior. Jenny sits down to my right, quiet and appearing interested in drawing, as usual. Jonas hasn't arrived and I choose to begin without him as the collective attention span is limited and I can more easily fill the late comer in than risk early disintegration. As the materials have been arranged like treasures, hands are starting to dart out and gather them, appropriating arsenals of color.

Throughout the hour, along with relaxation music in the background, I will be liberally providing verbal suggestions in a soft voice tone:

Begin to relax all parts of yourself; feel your body resting comfortably with the force of gravity; let go of all your cares during this special time; feel your writing hand relax on the paper as you draw your picture; notice your breath; soften any tension in your face (shoulders, etc.), in an on-going way, interspersed with spontaneous conversation.

The end of this group produces some divestment of defensive armor and a few welcome yawns.

A Few Journal Notes

1/30—Redefining a good art group…it begins with me at center and using the healing components joyfully—the sound (music), essence oils (now, lemon & lavender), color and materials for art and my own peaceful grounded presence. Note: In art group, with the direction of "Be still and listen to your heart beat" {I gave this direction to the group}, I had a general sense of lightness, better functioning — due of course, to Yoga, meditation centering techniques. After, "listen to your heart beat," I gave the direction to draw (within a circle) the "contents of your heart."

2/4—I did a Yoga relaxation group for three girls at work, it felt good doing it with good results for them.

2/19—A super busy day, perhaps too much so—prior to and mainly at work. An ambitious attempt at pre-art group relaxation for an unruly group of thirteen. And needing to rush to T.J. Cinnamon's for rolls (for Ben's discharge party) and to vending for Mike's treats. Running, racing (and to pick up the video machine) and run it and do a story for the girls. — Too much—I am tired but not tense, will sleep well. I'll try for a more relaxing Wednesday

2/20—Good planning for art group on the (outdoor) deck including other staff, specifying in advance, the expectation of the kids, etc.

2/24/91—Art group got out of hand due to a misguided attempt at patients' "coolness" through argument and put downs by a male patient. Generally outrageous social manners. I should try a tea party! It gave me a pain the neck, literally which I worked out during my dinner break via yoga and relaxation.

3/4—The quality of the day at work and beyond reflected the inner-work.

3/11—Major nursing inter-shift meeting about the stress of working on A West, trauma, aggression and how should we deal with it?

4/12—A challenging shift, with two art groups. One at 4:00 p.m. and one at 7:00 p.m. — we made large body outlines to fill in.

5/17/92—Working with a borderline on a drawing to help her learn and give her ego strength. Dr.Andrea Moskowitz described and demonstrated her method of working with explosive borderlines:

a) keep your voice soft.

b) appeal to their thinking, not feeling.

c) responding in reverse terms, i.e. "You guys lock us up, hate us," with "We care about you."

To Have and Have Not—A Mini-Oasis of Art Therapy

Ten years of working at UCLA NPI/H, hired as a mental health practitioner and member of the psychiatric nursing team, evening shift, have accrued to date. Here, art therapy does not constitute a separate discipline, as do occupational therapy or recreational therapy. So, I have the rather unique position of being an ATR, practicing art therapy and having the privilege of a nursing perspective. I perform a multitude of psychiatric nursing functions but instead of dispensing medications which I'm not licensed to do, I dispense colors, art materials, as healing media. And although I'm well utilized on A-West, I'm the only art therapist on any of the psychiatric units.

The following explanation about the practice of art therapy on A-West appeared on a large collage of patient artwork that I prepared. It was mounted in a glass case outside of the Nursing Office during the months of April and May, 1992. Full of color, affect, and intensity, it attracted the notice of doctors and others in the hospital who had previously been unaware that this activity was taking place.

Philosophy

Art Therapy Group is a non-judgmental, non-competitive experience. All work produced is valued as expressing an essential part of the individual with the purpose of communicating in the moment.

Nursing and Clinical Use of Drawings— Tangible drawings produced during art group provide a lens to our patients' inner world, about which most are not capable of verbally articulating. Drawings reflect moods, attitudes, values. Contents frequently feature on-going events and struggles in relation to family, to self-image, etc. Unconscious contents reveal the dark side of past trauma. *Drawings also anticipate aggressive acting out behavior,* that may first have begun to emerge symbolically via a spiraling volcano which enlarges as it ascends. Shared during treatment p 0lanning meetings, the (frozen) form metaphorically seems like a slice of the patient's psyche made available by his/her own effort. The record formed by art work produced during hospitalization can be seen to parallel various stages of treatment. Vicissitudes of mood, responses to medication, strong or weak defenses, integration or lack thereof, appear through changes in content, form, color, technique and the kinetics of material use.

Drawing is done in a therapeutic ambiance that includes the use of music and aroma and is process-oriented. Writing poetry or narrative responses to drawings or simply giving titles or word/feeling equivalents for color, shape and form are encouraged. This is combined with the structure of our behavioral and psychodynamically based program.

267

The utmost flexibility is required to meet the needs of our diverse population. Organic disorders intensify the unpredictability of behavior and group dynamics. ADHD (attention deficit hyperactive disorder), autistic and schizophrenic patients may simultaneously be a part of the same group. I.Q. disparity may be as high as 100. Therefore, in addition to single group tasks and themes, individual tasks, goals and teaching are essential.

Patient Benefits from Art Therapy:
Self Esteem

The all-embracing philosophy of art group rewards the most seemingly meager efforts. Many pieces are framed and displayed on the unit. Favorite drawings are taped on bulletin boards in patients' rooms. Occasionally patient portraits are sketched by this writer as a positive reflection of one's image back to them.

Empowerment

Creating a part of one's own environment within the hospital setting has involved using drawings—both large and small scale to decorate bedroom bulletin boards. Patients can choose to give gifts of their drawings to peers, family, friends and staff members.

Community

A recent project involved small scale constructions of poster board houses that were individually designed by patients within an eclectic town or village. Seasonal miniature Halloween trappings were added in October.

Another on-going group project is the shared creation of "Good-bye" posters for peers about to be discharged—one of our rituals dealing with the issue of separation.

Addendum—Economic Crisis

Recently, the hospital has reeled under the impact both of the larger U.S. and California economy and its own budget difficulties. Tightening up at NPI/H has threatened to involve layoffs of a few of the most recently hired nursing staff and extremely limited use of per diem or registry personnel. It feels as if we are walking in a cloud, not knowing where this is taking us, but hoping for the survival of our jobs and the very institution that has presented the wonderful programs that have evolved over the years.

Strategies, Themes & Techniques
Anger

The attempt is to facilitate the safe expression of anger and uncomfortable contents. I frequently work on a one-to-one basis with patients who would otherwise have landed in our seclusion room for aggressive acting out of their anger. One method I prefer is a combination of bodywork and art therapy where stretching, tensing and relaxing body parts and moving towards a full breath is followed by drawing, to capture, as much as possible, the rage that is released. This is then discussed in a caring, supportive way. Affect is expressed through, for example, the dense, pressured application of color and at times the puncturing of one's paper with pencils. Once, to prevent the need of two male patients to actually come to blows, I had them do battle on a shared paper. They became contenders in a symbolic boxing ring.

Catalysts

For visual stimulation, either at the beginning or during group, if interest declines, I may use the following:

• Laser Discs—They spin on a flat surface, color and design change with the rate of speed. It is also a centering device—in that one is focusing on a mandala.

• Kaleidoscopes—Focus on the surroundings that feed through the multi-faceted glass surface.

• Magnifying glasses (the plastic variety, for safety)—to closely examine the unseen texture in one's own drawing and other visual material.

• Cut 1" square in white board to slide over surface of drawing and examine slowly, meditatively.

De-Escalation

• Periods of total silence during group while drawing. The amount of time is based on individual tolerance, (five to ten minutes in most cases and with a reinforcer of a small gift from our community store). I have been thanked in private afterwards by several patients for helping them slow down.

• Direction to draw for awhile, then *"Freeze"* one's position and be silent, for 30-60 seconds. Relaxation messages are dispensed, and we continue working and stopping intermittently in a game-like atmosphere, where gifts may be earned at the end.

• Usually utilized after very chaotic contents have been released in the art therapy process. The direction to form a large sphere (or any other shape) and fill it in slowly with a selected color. This seems to have a calming effect to help bind the painful release.

Family

Drawing of oneself with family members, in family settings of home, outings, etc. is used regularly.

269

Feelings

The most basic and essential directive is "Draw your feelings."

Gangs/Violence/Sex

These themes are initiated by patients. If sexually explicit, sometimes the drawing and the patient are removed, in a group situation. A method I have used in dealing with violent (sometimes Heavy Metal) themes is to respond to the aesthetics of the drawing and not the shock value. I work with expanding drawing skills and help enlarge his/her scope beyond the limitations of the identity they have formed within the context of gangs or violence-dispensing Heavy Metal groups. I also discuss shocking or inappropriate contents with individuals privately, outside of group.

Goals

Extremely therapeutic at almost any stage of hospitalization. Short term and long term goals may be visualized and drawn. A question like "What do you want in your life?" may be asked. This positive framework can be an immediate antidote to drawings that express hopelessness.

Integration of Opposites

Either on a single paper divided in half or a circle divided, or two separate pieces of paper, the following are examples I have used to attempt to bring extreme opposites into a framework of awareness. I sometimes ask for another drawing of how the contrasting elements can relate (or enhance one another).

- draw what you don't like—what you do like
- chaos, confusion, anger—peace, harmony, happiness
- darkness—light
- self-as you feel you are—self-as you'd like to be
- sharp, hard edges—soft, muted, delicate.

Journals

Useful for fairly high functioning patients for processing feelings during time alone. They may choose to share contents with staff or keep the journal private.

Maps

These may feature the treasure of one's choice at the end, or relate to past, present or future (imagined) circumstances. If past or present, they can be re-charged with more positive aspects (or ideas) than actually were experienced. Any obstacles may be drawn and over-come symbolically. Map-mak-

270

ing always feels like an adventure. Maps of emotional terrain, trails and pathways, may take any form—circular, linear and so on. Draw a map of your life with the memories you're in touch with at this moment.

Multicultural

A large group collage combining people of different races, cultures, ages and gender, forms a backdrop for addressing multi-cultural issues. Guided discussion targets personal experiences, ideas and attitudes of patients.

Orientation

To time, place, season, weather, etc.

• On a hot summer day, the group task was a drawing of a large (6' high x 3' wide) waterfall in blues and greens. The butcher paper was mounted on the wall and patients took turns adding to the development of the waterfall. The music background was "Oh the Water" by Holly Near and environmental tapes of water.

• Travel—I offer pictures from travel magazines and calendars of a wide range of vacation agendas to jump-start drawings of chosen vacation sites.

• Themes may also be developed around holidays and times of day.

Problem Solving

• Use of cartoon framework. Creation of a wise person (or object) who is able to provide helpful input or a solution to a particular problem. Written dialogue is placed in the cartoon bubbles. In a variation, sometimes I will use guided imagery to evoke the wise person who may be anyone from a book, movie or sports hero to a relative or teacher.

• Draw the obstacle. How do you get around it? How do you deal with it symbolically?

Reclaiming Disowned Parts of Personality

• Masks—Create one out of a simple brown paper bag. Embellish with color, glitter, as desired. Wear it and dialogue with a peer. Switch masks and dialogue from the perspective of a different persona.

• Puppets—Shadow puppets, constructed of light weight cardboard faced with black construction paper and tied at joints with string, are mounted on two sticks held by the puppeteer (patient) who perches on his/her knees behind a white sheet. A flashlight provides illumination around the puppets. They represent good, evil, etc. in the character of a witch, a princess, a cat and so on. Hidden from view, hidden parts of oneself can vent, unself consciously.

Resistance

• Use a copying machine to magnify an observed skill; to build self-esteem. For example, I photocopied and enlarged three cartoon characters a patient had done alone in his room. He had refused to join our group, saying that he preferred to work alone. I cleared it with him before allowing peers to color copies of his work. Peers were impressed, complimented him. Before long he decided to join the group and share directly.

• Reducing the time period in which art group occurs is sometimes advantageous if it is followed by a preferred activity, e.g., outdoor physical activities (especially useful for ADHD patients).

• Providing simple white frames along with a nice plastic cover often entices the resistant group member to participate. This instant sense of completion helps to encourage work in subsequent groups as well. Pictures are displayed in community spaces or in the patient's own room.

Self Image/Identity

• Draw yourself as a baby—may use magazine photos to draw from.

• Design your own T-shirt, record album.

• Full Body Outline—filled in with features, clothing, collage.

• Design a greeting card *for yourself*, producing positive, esteem-building messages.

Song Themes

• Choose from song titles on a list provided for the group or your own title and draw a picture of what the song suggests to you.

• Design a record album cover for your favorite music.

Still Life

• Draw pre-arranged composition of fruit, objects and drapery.

• Arrange your own miniature combination of small objects and draw them.

• Take turns within the group to add objects to a still life composition or within a group making a collage.

Video

Use a nature film for pictorial inspiration without sound (may use environmental music tape instead.

Summary

Art therapy invites creativity. Art is produced from the fabric of oneself, like a spider spinning webs out of the materials of its own being. Single drawings frequently encompass large areas of experience in a rapid telescopic disclosure of the patient's psyche.

On the unit, I am keenly aware of positive and negative aspects of external stimuli. During art groups, I manipulate the environment, reducing superfluous clutter to create a compelling void or emptiness to attract its opposite. I also seek to awaken the senses via the use of aroma and music.

Over the years, I have done many art therapy in-services for staff members. The pleasant ambiance of the art group spills beyond its walls attracting staff participation. Nurses and doctors often join the patients during these groups, observing their patients as well as participating in the art process. An educational art therapy display representative of our patients and program has been on view for some time in the hospital.

The unit psychologist and chief psychiatrist are both knowledgeable and responsive to the on-going outpouring of art. Drawings move through treatment planning meetings and are informally shared with nursing staff on a regular basis, as well as with interns and fellows who pass through on time-limited educational tours. Most value the depth of clinical information these drawings provide, as well as the humor, helping the staff deal with the seriousness and difficulty of diagnosing and planning treatment.

Beyond scheduled formal art groups, my 10-hour days allow for many art therapy-related experiences. My position as "keeper of the pastels and markers" permits me to respond immediately to patient requests for materials as ideas arise, for example, for large scale posters or journals that are hand-crafted. On weekends, some patients prefer to be involved in art activities while peers watch videos or play on our outdoor deck. Recently a high-functioning female patient with Post Traumatic Stress Disorder and I worked one-to-one on a large mural after her peers had gone to bed, a special experience allowing for good personal contact.

I feel it's an advantage to be seen in contexts other than art groups. I may take a patient to radiology, distribute snacks or help settle someone with a bedtime story. The children feel more comfortable with me as one of the family of staff members, when they see me in and out of group therapy settings.

What we are capable of imagining and drawing, I believe, may be seen as a contemporary sampling of where we've been, where we are and where we're heading. To be able to take one's own measure, that is, to increase awareness of who we are while at the same time searching and drawing out our inner imagery leads us to more choices and greater consciousness.

References

Arguelles, J and M. (1972). *Mandala.* Berkeley: Shambala Publications.

Brena, S. F. (1973). *Yoga & Medicine.* Baltimore: Pelican Books.

Chan, W. T. (1963). *A Source Book in Chinese Philosophy.* Princeton: Princeton University Press.

Keyes, M. F. (1974). *The Inward Journey.* California: Celestial Arts.

Lavabre, M. F. (1990). *Aromatherapy Workbook.* Vermont: Healing Arts

Muktananda, S. (1978). *Play of Consciousness.* NY: SYDA Foundation.

Neruda, P. (1971). *A New Decade. Poems 1958-1967.* NY: Grove Press.

Art Psychotherapy and Eye Movement Desensitization Reprocessing (EMD/R) Method, an Integrated Approach
by Linda Cohn, M.S., M.F.C.C., A.T.R.

Linda Cohn, M.S., M.F.C.C., A.T.R., has been a registered art therapist for 20 years. Formerly director of graduate art therapy at Antioch University and assistant professor of Art Education at the University of Illinois in Chicago, she also served as president of both the Illinois and Northern California Art Therapy Associations and has designed three graduate programs in art therapy. She has conducted many national and regional seminars in art therapy, art education, and the creative process. Currently, she teaches art therapy at the University of California, Berkeley Extension and at San Francisco State University and has a private practice in San Francisco and Marin counties.

> *The irrational fullness of life has taught me never to discard anything, even when it goes against all our theories or otherwise admits of no immediate explanation. It is of course disquieting, and one is not certain whether the compass is pointing true or not; but security, certitude and peace do not lead to discoveries.*
>
> C. G. Jung

New modes of therapy, before they are completely tried and defined, challenge the professional status quo as well as our individual skills and preconceptions. Eye Movement Desensitization Reprocessing (EMD/R) presents just such a challenge. The method, barely three years old, has shown excellent results in the treatment of post-traumatic stress disorder (PTSD), but is as yet incompletely documented, and the reasons for its success remain open to speculation (Shapiro, 1989). Even so, only by continually exploring new methods can art therapists integrate advances in mental health care.

Three current trends encourage exploration of EMD/R: first, the tendency among insurance companies toward covering only short-term therapy; second, the pressing need to develop effective treatments for long-term PTSD and abuse-related problems; and finally, the increasing evidence, based on both empirical studies and clinical observation, validating the importance of imagery for healing the mind and body. (In this paper, I use the term "imagery" to mean client-generated images, whether internally experienced, verbally expressed, or visually represented using art media.)

I maintain that in treatment of limited duration, art therapists can address blocked memories and emotions more fully through a combination of methods used in art psychotherapy with those of EMD/R. We must remember that any method, whether old or new, is only that: a tool chosen by the therapist to organize the various aspects of treatment. No method used in isolation can supplant the full dimension of the therapeutic process.

Individually, both art psychotherapy and EMD/R use imagery in different ways to help clients release blocked emotions connected with painful memories, conflicts, and symptoms more rapidly than in traditional, verbal therapies. By combining these methods, one can work simultaneously on all client systems—which is to say, one can integrate the client's cognitive, perceptual, affective, and sensate processes on multiple levels, verbal and nonverbal, active and passive, conscious and unconscious. Integration of all human systems leads to personal development, balance, and health (Lusebrink, 1990; Wolpe, 1991; Shapiro, 1989).

To clarify how I have combined art psychotherapy and EMD/R in an integrated therapeutic approach, I will define the two methods, discuss their individual and complementary qualities, and present case examples from my own private practice as an art therapist.

Definitions

EMD/R

EMD/R was developed in 1987 by psychologist Francine Shapiro, Ph.D., a research associate at The Mental Research Institute in Palo Alto, California. Her original research supported the value of EMD/R as a rapid treatment for anxiety and traumatic memories (Shapiro, 1989).

Shapiro discovered EMD/R procedures by accident. She reports experiencing recurring, disturbing thoughts. She found that whenever the thoughts arose, she spontaneously began certain repeated, rhythmic eye movements, after which the unpleasant thoughts lost much of their power. Further repetition of the eye movements completely eliminated the thoughts, which if deliberately retrieved, were no longer upsetting. To explore this maneuver's therapeutic possibilities and evolve a standardized procedure, Dr. Shapiro induced these eye movements in a wide range of volunteers. The promising results of these preliminary clinical experiments led to a controlled investigation of the procedure. The results demonstrated fast and effective treatment of PTSD-related symptoms and traumatic memories.

Dr. Shapiro continues to refine the procedure based on clinical data and feedback from extensive trial applications of EMD/R to a variety of clinical issues and populations. A number of follow-up investigations of EMD/R are in progress around the United States. Although complete empirical data are not yet ready, a few studies (Marquis, 1991; Puk, 1991; Wolpe, 1991) and many reports by licensed clinicians imply that EMD/R facilitates: 1) reduction of past emotional charges and somatic complaints; 2) cessation of flashbacks, intrusive thoughts, and sleep disturbances; 3) development of insights and self-esteem; 4) installation of new beliefs and thoughts that prepare subjects to develop previously limited skills, abilities, and attitudes; and 5) rapid implementation of behavioral change that otherwise might require much longer in conventional therapy.

In EMD/R the therapist's emphasis is on the interplay of cognitive thoughts, emotions, and body sensations, and on relieving undesirable thoughts and feelings associated with past conflicts or trauma. Rhythmic eye movements help bring buried thoughts and feelings to consciousness, thus relieving stress on a somatic level. Shifts among client systems characterize the unfolding of therapeutic material; e.g., a memory may be experienced perceptually, as a mental image, then somatically, as a physical sensation, before shifting to the cognitive level, as a new idea. Any affect that is disassociated from memory is reintegrated via imagery and converted into coping mechanisms.

In this paper, I give only a general description of EMD/R procedures. These may seem simple, but require specialized training because they involve multiple patterns and responses which require specific choices and reactions on the part of the therapist. To insure therapist competency and client well-being, Dr. Shapiro will teach EMD/R only to licensed clinicians.

Initially, the client and therapist discuss the presenting problem, and then, after a thorough history, formulate a working hypothesis about the client's current experience and goals in therapy. Through these initial discussions, the therapist should be able to conduct EMD/R sessions with a thorough understanding of the client's symptoms, their duration as well as the initial causes, how the client is presently affected, and parallels with or connections to past or present memories or behavior.

After history-taking is complete, clients are asked to create a mental image representing the problem from which they wish relief. After establishing this visualization, they add to the mental image the negative belief or self-assessment connected with the problem. For example, a client who had been raped might hold the picture of the rape scene in her mind along with negative belief statements such as "It was my fault," or "I am helpless."

As clients continue to concentrate on their original mental picture, including the words of the belief statement, they are also directed to identify the emotion they are experiencing. Next, using Wolpe's scale of Subjective Units of Disturbance (SUDs), they assign to this emotion a score from 0 (neutral) to 10 (worst possible) (Wolpe, 1982). They also identify where the emotion is located in their bodies. For example, the rape victim might feel anxiety that is a 9 on the SUDs scale and presently located in the chest area.

Next, clients are asked to provide a positive belief statement reflecting how they would prefer to feel. (For the rape victim, perhaps "I did the best I could," or "I'm in control now.") They then rate the statement according to the Shapiro's Validity Cognitive Scale based on how true the new message feels to them now, from 1 (not true) through 7 (very true) (Shapiro, 1989).

As the clients continue to hold the mental image, negative belief statement, and the localized physical sensation in their minds, they are asked to track the therapist's finger with their eyes as it sweeps rapidly from side to side across their full line of vision. After this back-and-forth movement is repeated 12–36 times, the client is asked to give feedback as to what is happening on a visual, auditory, somatic, or cognitive level. Once the therapist has the client's free association, the eye movements are repeated. This process of eye movement and client feedback is continued until the SUDs level is neutralized (0 or 1). Then, the client is asked to hold the positive cognition in mind. The eye movements are performed again, followed by further client feedback; this process is repeated until the validity of the positive cognition is increased to very true (7). By accepting the new, positive belief on an experiential level, the client accepts a new organizing principle throughout the various systems, making the belief more accessible.

The reprocessing dynamic is a critical component of the method. Clinical experience indicates that besides desensitization of trauma and shifting of cognitive beliefs, reprocessing of information is accelerated as well. This reprocessing is not limited to the original symptom, but also reprocesses layers of the client's emotions (e.g., anger, shame, guilt, sorrow) as they unfold

278

during the process. Clinical feedback has also indicated that a single session of EMD/R can reprocess some traumas, while others require multiple sessions as the reprocessing may proceed more slowly. These clients are informed to expect further memories, insights, and associations to arise between sessions and are advised to keep a log of such material so that it can be reprocessed in the next session (Shapiro, 1991).

Art Psychotherapy

Art psychotherapy emphasizes using the artistic process for therapeutic purposes, working toward insight rather than completion of an artistic product. Images are created spontaneously and often may be fragmented or incomplete. The artwork is viewed as symbolic speech, and there is verbal free-association with the images created. Then a more phenomenological approach is used to discuss the artwork with the client. The client views the image as a total gestalt, which Betensky (1973a) defines as a "psychological occurrence," which simultaneously reinforces the physical, emotional, and rational. In this way the art facilitates communication between the client's inner and outer realms: the client cognitively explores the relationship of the subjective experience of feelings and thoughts with objective reality. The movement to and from the perceptual, emotional, subjective realm and detached, neutral objectivity is therapeutically valuable for the client. Limiting consciousness to either objective or subjective experience keeps the client "stuck" (Betensky, 1977); a major goal of art therapists is to help clients increase flexibility in utilizing both spheres.

EMD/R and Art Psychotherapy as Complementary Processes

EMD/R and art psychotherapy share quite a bit of theoretical common ground. First, both involve internal and external imagery. According to Lusebrink (1990), inner experiences of imagery and their external representation influence one another; at the same time, they differ because of the manner in which they are expressed. The internal image is based on sensory, affective, perceptual, and cognitive processes. The image is then externalized through verbal descriptions or through manipulation of art media. Encouraging clients to externalize their internal images through drawing or by describing their perceptions of the image enhances image formation, helping clients bring to consciousness more specific details from memory. This imagery stimulation also encourages ideation, fluency, and cognitive flexibility, including generation of novel information, which may contribute to novel solutions (Lusebrink, 1990).

279

Second, repeatedly drawing or discussing images facilitates interaction of visual and verbal processing of information by the right and left hemispheres of the brain, respectively. This interaction, in turn, helps to integrate sensory and kinesthetic experience with verbal, cognitive, and symbolic processes, imparting new perceptions to the client and increasing the possibilities of creative solutions (Ornstein, 1972).

Third, the visual tracking in EMD/R and the creation of drawings in art psychotherapy use the same systems to bring information to consciousness quickly and interfere with the same systems to reduce the emotional response—both work through eye movements. Both processes have been said to be like "dreaming awake," inviting comparison with the processing of memory as dreams in Rapid Eye Movement (REM) sleep.

In order to be saved, memories are removed from short-term memory banks, broken into fragments, and stored in long-term memory circuits. When one of these circuits is stimulated in REM sleep, the entire memory and related memories flood into dreams. While the brain is activated during REM sleep, neural circuits that had been active during the day are aroused, along with related circuits, including those for unresolved problems, worries, or emotional issues (Reiser, 1992). According to this theory, images in a dream carry meaning related to current and unresolved life problems.

Likewise, "dream" visions are brought into conscious awareness through finger-tracking in EMD/R and drawing in art psychotherapy. EMD/R eye movements in particular seem to stimulate some neural process that interferes with the connection between a stimulus and its emotional response. Possibly, the currents generated by the eye movements block the pathways connecting the frontal lobes with hypothalamus and the hippocampus, thus weakening the connection between stimulus and response (Shapiro, 1989).

The fourth major similarity between EMD/R and art therapy is that both reduce the time spent in therapy, by 1) reducing transference, and 2) bringing up unconscious material more quickly. Art therapy is often considered to uncover unconscious material more quickly than verbal therapy. Even so, EMD/R involves more direct, intensive manipulation of eye movement than occurs through drawing in art therapy, and therefore fosters even faster uncovering of information and desensitization. In combination, the two methods facilitate the therapeutic process in flexible, multidimensional ways. Their use together provides a source of "the random," which Erikson (1965) believes helps ensure that clients discover answers for themselves rather than blindly following a therapist's lead, and thus become more active participants in their own therapy.

280

In addition to these similarities, major differences distinguish art psychotherapy from EMD/R, differences that highlight the added dimension art therapy techniques bring to the EMD/R process. The most evident is art psychotherapy's rendering of images in concrete form. Unlike mental images, drawings become a tangible, permanent record not subject to transformation in memory recall. Drawings can be reviewed with clients at any point, enabling them literally to see their progress. This visual record also can be a diagnostic tool for the therapist to determine multiple factors, e.g., ego states, defenses, and regression. The expression of symbolic images is often a prerequisite for verbal association, insight, and behavior—sometimes expression of an idea in a drawing precedes verbal expression by weeks.

Unlike the linear, verbal processing of EMD/R, drawings provide a spatial matrix. The design elements of line, form, color, texture, and page placement are used to magnify the relationship of one image to another. As Wadeson (1980) states, "in a picture I can portray it all at once. I can show closeness and distance, bonds and divisions, similarities and differences, feelings, particular attributes, context of family life, ad infinitum." This magnification provides a tremendous amount of information to be processed through therapy in future EMD/R sessions.

The built-in properties of different art materials—the hardness of pencils, fluidity of paints, elasticity of clay, etc.—serve specific functions and operate on multiple levels (Kagin and Lusebrink, 1978). Thus, the client's choice of media assumes therapeutic significance.

The uses of art media could be coordinated with EMD/R methods in any number of individual formulas, in order to foster a particular system. This is a promising area for future research. However, for the purpose of my own preliminary integration of the two methods, art materials available to the client were limited to pencils, markers, oil pastels, chalk, and 18 x 24 inch paper. In general these art materials were chosen because they emphasize eye/motor coordination and they are resistive, simple, and structured, i.e., the built-in properties of the materials favor control over expression; few mental operations are required to use these particular media; and the art experience is directed by the therapist (Kagin & Lusebrink, 1978).

By definition, art psychotherapy proceeds through creative acts. The art media may be used symbolically to create boundaries and set limits, as well as in acts of symbolic risk-taking. Robbins (1987) sees making art as creating a "mirroring container that organizes an array of different impressions coming from levels of awareness." Creative expression assists the client in sublimation, the replacement of instinctual behavior by socially acceptable behavior. Thus, the visual expressions created become the basic agent for change in therapy (Landgarten, 1981).

As my case histories will show, methods originally developed in art psychotherapy practice and in early trials of EMD/R complement one another effectively in treatment situations, providing rapid and permanent relief of trauma in both children and adults. I believe from my own practice that the eye movements speed the process of uncovering information, while the art therapy solidifies the uncovered information in a tangible form, thus addressing all systems to increase awareness and learning.

In the following two cases, expression with art media, when used in conjunction with EMD/R, is in response to specific topic assignments, e.g., draw the emotion, physical sensation, symptom, conflict, or issue. The client's drawings are used in two ways: as in case 1, by interweaving them with EMD/R to define and direct more attention to a specific system, thereby enhancing client focus, or as in case 2, by analyzing them with the client before or after EMD/R, helping the client to gain objectivity.

Case Histories
Case 1

G., a 7½ year-old boy, was brought into treatment by his aunt. He had come from his parents' home in Ohio, leaving home for the first time to come visit his aunt in California; the visit was scheduled to last nine days. G. had been excited about his visit and had no trouble separating from his parents at the airport or flying on the airplane alone. However, upon arrival on the first day, he began crying and was unable to sleep at night, saying he wanted his mother and wanted to go home. Talking with his parents on the telephone did not help to alleviate his behavior. When G.'s distress continued on the third day of his visit, his aunt contacted me to see whether G. could be helped with art therapy. We arranged an appointment for that afternoon.

G. entered the session easily, exploring the different art materials on the table. When using EMD/R with children, one must convey the process in age-appropriate language; therefore, I explained to G. that he would get to draw, then play an "eye game" in which he would follow my fingers with his eyes. After that, he would have time to make more pictures.

G. was asked to draw a picture of what made him feel so sad (Fig. 1). For this initial drawing, G. used only a black marker, with no added color. He said, "That's me crying, and that's my house in Ohio. I wish I was home. I miss my Mommy." Then G. began to cry. I asked him to watch my fingers. After one set of 24 eye movements he had stopped crying, but stated that his stomach hurt, indicating a change in body sensation. He was told to hold his stomach (to focus his concentration on the body sensation) and to watch my fingers for another set of eye movements. After this set, G. spontaneously looked up and smiled, saying "My stomach ache is gone." After another eye-movement set, G. asked to draw a picture (Fig. 2).

Fig. 1 G.'s drawing of his sad feelings

"That's me in a chair. I feel better," he said. The relative sizes of the two figures indicate increased self-esteem, just as the addition of color in the second drawing (the pants are blue, the bow red, and the hair brown) indicates a more positive affect.

After this statement, I initiated a fourth eye-movement set, after which G. was asked to draw a picture of his family doing something (Fig. 3). G. seemed comfortable, humming as he drew the jump-rope, symbolically connecting himself with his mother. One final set of eye movements was completed, after which G. excitedly told me about the members of his family in Ohio as well as what he and his aunt were going to do after the session.

The next day, G.'s aunt reported that G. had changed his mind: he wanted to stay in California and go to Golden Gate Park. He completed his visit, slept through the nights, and never mentioned a desire to go home early. Two months later,

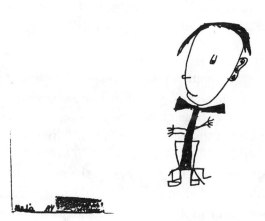

Fig. 2 "That's me in the chair. I feel better"

G.'s mother told his aunt she felt G. had matured on his trip. He no longer "clung" to her around the house and was much more active with his friends.

With G., the use of drawings interwoven with EMD/R procedures was helpful in several ways. First, they helped him to clarify the emotion or thought that was to be the stimulus for the EMD/R procedure. For example, after he drew the picture of himself and his distant home (Fig.1), I instructed him to look at his drawing and focus on it during the EMD/R method.

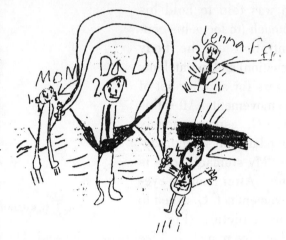

Fig. 3 G. draws his connection with his mother

The drawings were also used in between applications of the EMD/R method to reinforce his experience of personal changes; G. himself could see the change in his own drawings, which represented change in himself. According to Tower, children encode information largely in visual terms. Therefore, the use of imagery in therapy with children contributes to cognition by increasing attention and concentration and by providing for quicker processing of the information. Imagery has further effective benefits to children, contributing to increased resources in handling stress and strengthening self-identity and self-control (Tower, 1983).

Finally, using drawings as a substitute for words facilitated the application of EMD/R with a child, who may have less sophisticated verbal skills or ability to abstract than an adult.

Case 2

S., an attractive, 34 year–old, pregnant mother of one child, came into therapy to work on a "shift" in her sexual relationship with her husband. The change began before her first pregnancy and had since "gotten worse." S. explained that she began to feel "dirty and disgusted" at the initiation of sexual foreplay. She felt she didn't want to be touched vaginally and would start "drifting off." Eventually, she would pull away, feeling anger toward her husband and shame over her behavior. Although at one point she had feared her growing aversion to sexual contact would end the relationship, S. felt that, otherwise, she had a good marriage with a man she loved. She had discussed her feelings with her husband, and they decided to enter therapy separately to work on specific issues in their past that they thought might be affecting the present relationship. Before her marriage, S. had been involved in hypnotherapy, psychodynamic therapy, and group therapy for about two years.

Background

S., the eighth of 13 children, described her parents as heavy drinkers who were not emotionally equipped to raise so many children. She felt her mother was always depressed and was the controller of the family. "Mom set the punishment, and she would tell Dad to carry it out. Then he would strap us." S. said she knew her father loved her, but couldn't say the same for her mother. She felt she couldn't possibly depend on either parent for emotional support.

When S. was 10 years old, she was molested by a group of boys. Her sister had convinced her to have sex with them for money. She could not remember the details and felt disoriented when thinking about the incident.

Throughout her adolescence, she recalled, her parents rebuked her constantly for wearing miniskirts and spending time with boys. Her father would tell her that she looked "disgusting," and her mother once called her a "slut" in front of her friends.

Between ages 18 and 28, S. had four abortions and was hospitalized once for a urinary infection. At age 22 she became emotionally involved with a man in a relationship that lasted four years. After that, she had several short-term relationships until she met her husband at age 30. They had been married two years at the time she began therapy with me. Both her parents were alive and, according to S., still incapable of handling their own problems without using their children as scapegoats.

Treatment

S. wanted to be in therapy only for five months, ending just before the birth of her second child. For this reason, a combination of EMD/R and art psychotherapy was chosen for treatment. Many pictures were drawn throughout the five months; four representative examples are shown here.

After the initial history-taking sessions, S. began a session by remembering the first time she experienced the symptoms for which she now sought treatment; this had occurred during her four-year relationship, one night when she and her boyfriend were lying on the couch. She was asked to hold that picture in her mind and draw the sensation she had in her body. She drew "Fear" (Fig. 4) and ranked it at level 9 on the SUDs scale. She described the picture as herself—a very small pink dot directly in the center of the picture—surrounded and overwhelmed by sadness and fear—the black swirls encircling the dot.

During the ensuing eye-movement sequences, she realized that her fear was related to not feeling in control of her life. Therefore, she allowed others to control her, especially sexually, feeling angry but never voicing her own needs. She realized she gave all her energy to pleasing men, feeling sad and inadequate when she was alone. She felt that she had no idea of who she was or what she wanted.

As her fear, anger, and shame were desensitized through EMD/R, S.'s mental image changed. She was no longer lying on the couch, but rather standing separate from her boyfriend, telling him what she didn't like. Her positive thought, "I can claim my energy and control my life," went to level 7 on the Validity Cognitive Scale. When asked to draw a picture of how she was feeling, she drew "Clarity" (Fig. 5), describing it as a feeling of "movement—like my fear was opening up." For the first time, she said, "I felt as if I could begin to take control of my life".

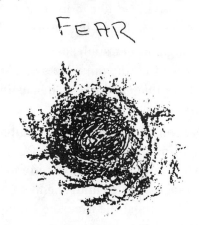

Fig. 4 S.'s symbol of fear

In the following months, continuing to do drawings and EMD/R in each weekly session, S. remembered her childhood molestation in detail and realized it caused her to feel angry, helpless, and mistrustful in the presence of men. She also became aware of her extreme anger at her parents for their emotional neglect and rejection when she voiced her feelings, concerns, or ideas while growing up. She realized she had felt unable to tell anyone in her family of her pain from the molestation because she "had to be the good girl who pleased everyone by being seen and not heard."

At the same time, S. began to notice changes in her behavior. She spoke out to her husband, neighbors, and friends expressing her desires as well as things that bothered her, directing anger appropriately without feeling guilty. She was able to establish boundaries between herself and family members and to distance herself from involvement in her parents' problems. Overall she felt more confident.

Once S. desensitized and reprocessed memories and beliefs about her molestation and certain parental memories, she wanted to address her remaining fear about her sexuality. When asked to show where the fear was located in her body, she drew "Stagnant Fear" (Fig. 6). Next she was asked to carry on a conversation with the fear. By drawing the picture, she located the fear in her pelvic region; through the conversation, she realized it was connected to her negative sense of self related to her previous abortions.

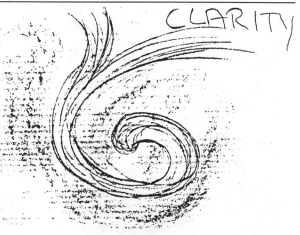

Fig. 5 S.'s symbol of clarity

EMD/R was used to desensitize the traumatic memories and negative beliefs she held about herself. In the following sessions she rated her fear, anxiety, and guilt at SUDs level 10. The negative cognitions she held were "I'm stupid and careless like a child," "My sexuality will get me into trouble," and "I shouldn't enjoy sex." Through the EMD/R process she came to understand how she carried these messages into her sexual relations with her husband. She discovered that she didn't always want sex, but "like a child I couldn't say no because I would be reprimanded—that's probably why I did what my sister and those boys wanted." As S. shifted her negative cognitions to positive ones ("I'm an adult now," "I have choices," "It is OK for me to be a sexual human being," and "I can enjoy sex"), she reported a change in her sexual relationship, which became more comfortable, playful, and satisfying. She no longer thought of sex as an obligation, but rather as a desired choice.

In her final session, S. used EMD/R to diminish her anxiety about childbirth. Her first pregnancy had been extremely difficult. She had planned on having a home birth, but complications forced her to go to the hospital to deliver the baby. She felt she had physically prevented the baby from emerging because she didn't feel capable of completing labor; thus, she failed at home birth. The negative cognitions she used for EMD/R were "I'm not capable," and "I'm a failure." She wanted to reprocess this belief to "I am capable and trust my own process." S. scored her anxiety beyond "10" and located it once again in her pelvic area. She was asked to draw what that anxiety looked like (Fig. 7); this drawing, "Churning" reflected S.'s emotional state in more detail than her statements. As she drew, she pressed the oil pastels hard against the page, using orange hues of great visual intensity. The spiral in the drawing twists from inside outward, mirroring her increasing anxiety.

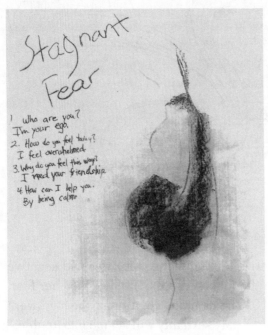

Stagnant
Fear

1 Who are you?
I'm your ego.
2. How do you feel today?
I feel overwhelmed.
3. Why do you feel this way?
I need your friendship.
4 How can I help you.
By being calm.

Fig. 6 Where S.'s fear was located in her body

She held both her drawing and the negative belief in her mind. After five sets of EMD/R, her SUDs level decreased to 5. She had processed her first pregnancy, releasing her pain and fear of the unknown. As her SUDs level decreased and her positive cognition increased, S. saw the anxiety and fear flowing out of her vagina, and warm, blue calm coming in to fill her body.

Once the validity of her positive cognition had increased to "7" and her anxiety had decreased to SUDs level "0," S. said "I have a feeling of completion and trust. I feel grounded and connected with being pregnant. I know I can do it [i.e., give birth] just fine." Then she was asked to draw some aspect of the EMD/R experience she wanted to keep. She drew "Flowing Calm" (Fig. 8) and said "That's me filled with blue calm." When her drawing from a month before (Fig. 6) was placed next to the new drawing, S. was surprised to see her body positioned in exactly the same place on the page in both. This time, however, she depicted herself as more solid, defined, and without the fear in her body. She said "I gave myself the calm my ego wanted."

After completing therapy, although S. once again had birth complications, she reported having no fear or anxiety before or during the labor, saying "it was an extremely positive experience."

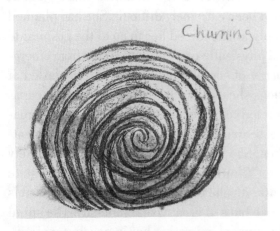

Churning

Fig. 7 A symbol of S.'s anxiety

S. was clear about the specific sexual issues she was confronting when she entered therapy. During the five months of weekly therapy she became remarkably more aware of the underlying dynamics of her sexual dysfunction and fears about the impending delivery of her child. Not only did she gain insight, but simultaneously she was desensitized to many of the underlying fears and anxieties which oppressed her and threatened her marital relationship. Her sense of self-esteem and confidence about

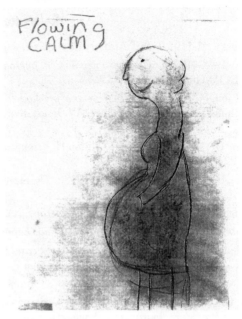

Fig. 8 "That's me filled with blue calm."

her ability to experience sexuality positively increased markedly, as reflected in her drawings.

With S., the connection between art therapy and the EMD/R work was different than was the case with G., although some of the benefits were similar. In this instance, EMD/R and art psychotherapy were essentially parallel therapeutic processes. The application of the EMD/R procedures enhanced the more traditional art-therapy process and precipitated progress.

Conclusion

In the interplay of EMD/R and art psychotherapy methods: 1) the perceptual, somatic, emotional, and cognitive systems are reinforced and integrated more fully; 2) affect is released, desensitized, and distanced, and energy is sublimated; 3) negative beliefs are shifted to new positive beliefs, which the client can "try on and see" in drawings; 4) both the conscious and unconscious work together to create balance; 5) past and present realities are differentiated; 6) less time is needed for client insight and reorganization than in traditional therapy; and 7) clients are more creative in, and have more responsibility for the therapy process.

As Erikson (1948) points out, "not until a person goes through the inner process of reassociating and reorganizing his experiential life can results occur." Combined, EMD/R and art psychotherapy enrich the therapeutic process, each lending support and adding dimension to the other, thereby creating change and a greater whole.

References

Betensky, M. (1973). *Self discovery through self-expression.* Springfield, IL: C. C. Thomas.

——————(1977). *The phenomenological approach to art expression and art psychotherapy.* Art Psychotherapy, 173-179.

Erickson, M. H. (1948/1980). *Hypnotic psychotherapy.* In E. L. Rossi, The collected papers of Milton H. Erickson on hypnosis. IV. Innovative hypnotherapy, 35-48. NY: Irvington.

—————— (1965/1980). *The use of symptoms as an integral part of hypnotherapy.* In E.L. Rossi, The Collected Papers of Milton H. Erickson on Hypnosis. Innovative Hypnotherapy. 212-223. NY: Irvington.

Kagin, S. L., & Lusebrink, V. B. (1978). *The expressive therapies continuum.* Art Psychotherapy, 171-179.

Landgarten, H. B. (1981). *Clinical art therapy.* NY: Brunner/Mazel.

Lusebrink, V. B. (1990). *Imagery and Visual Expression in Therapy.* NY: Plenum Press.

Marquis, J. (1991). *A report on seventy eight cases treated by eye movement desensitization.* Journal of Behavior Therapy and Experimental Psychiatry. 22, 187-191.

Ornstein, R. (1972). *The psychology of consciousness.* San Francisco: W. H. Freeman.

Puk, G. (1991). *Treating Traumatic Memories: A Case Report on The Eye Movement Desensitization Procedure.* Journal of Behavior Therapy and Experimental Psychiatry. 22, 149-151.

Reiser, M. F. (1990). *Memory in mind and brain: what dream imagery reveals.* NY: Basic Books.

Robbins, A. (1987). *The artist as therapist.* NY: Human Sciences Press.

Shapiro, F. (1989). *Eye movement desensitization : a new treatment for post-traumatic stress disorder.* Journal of Behavior Therapy and Experimental Psychiatry. 20, 211-217.

Shapiro, F. (1991). *Eye movement desensitization and reprocessing procedure.* Behavior Therapist. 14, 133-135.

Tower, R. B. (1983). *Imagery: Its role in development.* In A. A. Skeikh, Imagery: Current theory, research and application. 222-251, NY: Wiley.

Wadeson, H. (1982). *Art psychotherapy.* NY: Wiley.

Wolpe, J. (1982). *The practice of behavior therapy.* NY: Pergamon Press.

Wolpe, J. & Abrams, J. (1991). *Post traumatic stress disorder overcome by eye movement desensitization: a case report.* Journal of Behavior Therapy and Experimental Psychiatry, 22, 39-43.

Learning to Love:
How Art Therapy and Authentic Movement
Transform Being
by Suzanne Lovell, Ph.D., A.T.R.

Suzanne Lovell, Ph.D., A.T.R., has worked in both public and private agencies for 14 years. Currently she teaches in the Psychology Department at Sonoma State University in Northern California, advises students in the External Degree Masters Program in the Creative Arts Therapist, and shares in a clinical practice with Wolf-Corey, Inc., in Napa. She also teaches privately and teaches and presents nationally. Her video, "Symbolic Healing: a Personal Story," demonstrates how imagery through art and movement affected her experience with cancer. A book and video are in progress on how symbolic healing works.

> *"To transform, you need to go down into the body—Otherwise nothing will ever change, it will remain the same—I seek my way downward—The way I am seeking is always descending, descending—It's never going up, it's always descending.*   The Mother/Satprem, 1981, p. 60

> *"At this time in the Western world, in response to our deepening need for authentic spiritual experience, all we can do is to return to our physical selves."*   Adler, 1991, p. 14

The day before surgery for uterine cancer, I went to an Authentic Movement session. As soon as we began, I felt the impulse to close my eyes, move into the middle of the circle of women, and open up to what needed to happen. In the center of the room there is a tall pole with a rope wrapped around it. At some point in my movement, I discovered the rope and began to tug and pull on it. An inner voice said, "I have to get hold of this! My healing depends on this snake's energy!" I felt under extreme tension and pressure. I felt a fear of darkness enveloping me, of being trampled if I failed or let go. I cried and fought—And then something changed. As my arms rose slowly upward to my head, I experienced antlers growing: my inner healer appeared as Deer woman—At home later, I spent hours drawing and honoring the loving image which appeared through me. Lovell, 1990, p. 25

History and Definition

For a number of years Mary Whitehouse explored the question of the authentic self with the eyes and heart of a dancer and lay Jungian analyst. For over 20 years Janet Adler, my teacher and one of Mary's students, has explored the question of the authentic self with the eyes and heart of a movement therapist and mystic. For 20 years I have been exploring this question with the eyes and heart of an art therapist and wounded healer; the last 5 years have been through learning and teaching the integration of art therapy and Authentic Movement.

Conceptually, Authentic Movement has roots in developmental, ego, and Jungian psychologies. The premise is that through the reflecting eyes of an other we come into conscious being, we grow a self. For an infant to grow in a healthy way, s/he must be "witnessed" by a loving or good-enough other. Developmental gaps occur in those places where insufficiently or inadequately "seen," a child remains a mystery to him or herself; an emptiness or hollowness persists. Developmental wounds occur when an interaction diminishes, ignores or negates the infant's very real experience. These unwitnessed gaps or wounds form the emotional and somatic issues which we seek to address later in our lives through therapy and life experiences. The ability and the willingness to be the "witness" for a client in therapy is understood as essential for the client in healing those gaps and (re)creating a healthy self.

Other roots of Authentic Movement—as well as art therapy—derive from deeper sources fed by our innate abilities to seek healing through direct experiences in imagery and by our longing for union with the Divine, the Whole. Imagery is understood as the language of all of our senses, visual, auditory, olfactory, kinetic, and tactile. As transpersonal experience, art therapy and Authentic Movement can lead the Mover through personal unconscious terrain onward into collective unconscious experiences, into the imaginal world, into direct experiences of knowing healing and Oneness with all of life. Psychological theory that includes the transpersonal comes to its edge here. "Here" is where the mystic, the shaman, the wounded healer are called to journey. This "here" is a little understood, certainly under-valued and rarely acceptable form of experience in our Western society. But it is "here" that we can recover "at-onement" with ourself and the Other; it is here that we learn or remember our wholeness and "speak" our common human language, the language of imagery.

The shaman, the wounded healer, the mystic—these names are both personal and archetypal embodiments of the energy which carries images between the invisible or spirit world and our ordinary material-seeming world. Art and movement are contemporary forms which can make this imaginal energy visible. Meditational art-making through color, form, and body-aware-ness in combination with Authentic Movement offers the opportunity to attend inward to personal needs and transpersonal longings.

By allowing our art and movement to answer the personal questions or issues that arise, we learn to integrate consciousness with the unconscious; we act in a manner both oppositional and balancing to our culture's teachings about conscious mind.

The Forms

The form of Authentic Movement involves a *Mover* who closes her eyes, "listens" and expresses the impulses, sensations or feelings within, and a *Witness* who "holds" the safety of the space and practices seeing truthfully. When the Mover finishes moving, she is free to share anything about her experience. The task of the Witness is, with permission of the Mover, to share her own felt responses to those parts of the movement which the Mover has spoken about.

• Having been taught in our society to discriminate and to judge, Authentic Movement reminds us to *simply witness.*

• Having been taught to practice and take apart, this form reminds us *to hold the whole experience together.*

• Having been taught to project our own world onto the world of oth-ers, this practice teaches us *to own our own world and to receptively hold and respect the world of the other.*

A question in the Mover might be: how am I responding in this moment?

A question in the Witness might be: how can I be present for another without judgment, analysis or interpretation? A goal is the practice of loving compassion as both Mover and Witness in the experience shared together in the moment; and to learn to take this compassion out into the world around us.

The form of meditational or focused art-making—what I consider an

293

organic cross-cultural root of contemporary art therapy—involves opening our eyes inward, learning to make visible the sensations, feelings, impulses or images that arise within without judging, censoring or interpreting. This form of art-making is a bridge.

It helps us move through the worlds in several important ways. It navigates between the heavy seas of traumatic experience locked in our bodies to the distant shore where hope rests and conscious words offer ground to stand on.

It offers an inviting or compelling window inward when our minds are still racing around with "outer" demands.

It offers a visible memory of our journey, and it carries truth about our experience which can continue to inform us long after the movement has stopped.

Finally, it gives us edges and a container, first closeness and then distance so that we rest in right relationship to the emerging material. Art making and Authentic Movement together form a strong bridge between seemingly parallel worlds—internal/external, personal/transpersonal, matter/spirit, mind/body.

Authentic movement and art therapy, while being contemporary therapeutic forms, simultaneously touch into deep universal human truths. While each form is taught separately by qualified teachers in the San Francisco Bay area, I have chosen to combine them in a nine-month training option for mature non-students and art therapy students in the External Degree Master's Program at Sonoma State University. This experience, called *Symbolic Healing Through Art Therapy and Authentic Movement*, as you will read below, involves four hours once a week between September and May. As a nine-month commitment, it allows equally for the development of an art-based, experientially-based theory of human healing as well as for the birthing of significant personal change and the evolution of transpersonal group dynamics.

While the form welcomes both genders, it is relatively recent that more men are expressing interest; one recent group, for example, had four men and eight women. In introductory weekend classes through Extended Education, which have limited enrollment but are open to the general public, one might expect twenty women and four men. Regardless of gender, students come wanting an opportunity to listen and look inward in order to become more intimate and competent as parents, lovers, workers: to be in the world with compassion and awareness. Given the humanistic-transpersonal focus of the Art Therapy Option at Sonoma State, this experience provides also a strong container for those students wanting to know directly the perennial ways of the Wounded Healer's journey.

The Experience

The wood stove has been lit since 7 am. The smoke swirls out of the stove pipe and mixes with the morning fog, rendering the nearby vineyard a place of peace and mystery. I drive up the short driveway and park, gather the flowers from the car and enter the studio. When the sitting mats are set out in a circle, when the art materials are set out in their pale straw baskets, when the flowers are set and the candle is lit, I am ready to begin.

Students arrive, greet each other, quietly move toward the art materials and choose. We begin in silence by evoking the images inside us, honoring them by making them visible, reaffirming our commitment to trust process by practicing it. Sometimes the image comes from a dream, sometimes it is a precise continuation of some theme a student is wrestling with; through the months it becomes more clearly an extension of body expressing itself on paper, the impulse for color or shape coming out of the hand with little reference to conscious mind.

Sometimes there is a need for verbal sharing; other times we move directly into Authentic Movement.

I sit as "Witness"—honing my own commitment to practice seeing without judging, projecting or interpreting; my task is to hold the "container" so that what is true for each "Mover" can be expressed in safety.

The students find a spot within this container, close their eyes and as they go inward, invite their bodies to inform their minds through both stillness and movement. During this time, the only sounds are the Mover-initiated sounds. One might hear foot stomping, laughing, crying, cursing, cacophony or chorus, hands drumming, clapping, thumping, giggles, sighs or stillness. One might see enormous movements as a mover runs around the perimeter of the circle, battles with something fearsome, or leaps with joy and abandon. One might see small movements like a newborn child's hand finding its face, or sacred, timeless movements that might occur in a temple or a field or at a hearth. One might witness an extraordinary, small micromovement of one finger or no movement at all, simply stillness, a deeply moving and penetrating stillness. When the time is up (and it is a precise time agreed upon, 30 or 45 minutes), I say, "It is time to bring your experience to a close."

Students slowly return to the ordinary world of room, windows, sunlight, oak trees with birds or wind sounds. While early on, students describe their experiences verbally and I respond as a witness with *how their movement moved me*, as they deepen their experience, they turn more and more to seeking silence in order to do more art, to write in their journals. Their internal witness is growing—this internal experience of a self compassionately witnessing self, not being critical or negative, but simply present.

Then it is art time. Progressively I see it as the movement continuing albeit through a different form. I continue to witness. Students gravitate to materials which are congruent with, or in response to, their experiences so far. Sometimes it is clay, with eyes closing once more, to allow the fingers to seek and draw out the invisible form waiting. Sometimes it is clay to catch and hold a moment from earlier movement or to move the movement further or to bring it as a whole into closure. It may be watercolors to continue the flow of imagery or watercolors to make visible feelings or sensations that continue beneath the surface. There is a stillness and a depth to the art process which is as moving to this witness as the previous movement.

When it is time to bring this experience to a close, we reform our circle; there is the option to verbally share any part of the previous time.

In response as witness I share my experience, *how I felt or was moved by* what I witnessed. I honor the person and his/her work by not judging, interpreting or analyzing it. As on-going witness I am privileged to follow the imagery that unfolds—to see how the movement on paper shifts over time—to mark how impeccable the psyche is in unfolding the healing story of the Mover.

In the spirit of the Authentic Movement form which Janet Adler teaches, discussion about anyone's artwork is discouraged. Unlike group therapy, this is not a time for everyone to work on their issues through interaction. Students may speak about how an art piece moves them, on a feeling level, or how it helps them gain insight about something personal to the speaker. *It is a time to practice witnessing*, to listen inwardly to discern between what is compassionate witnessing and what is old mind-telling stories about ourselves in the guise of someone else's imagery.

Throughout the nine months of the class, there is a slow progression in the length of the time periods, how the time periods are used and what happens during them. Each session begins with art: art as transition from the outside world to the one within. And often we end with art. The interweaving of the two forms remains organic as group consensus for art or movement or talking generally sets the timing of each session.

In the fall, I am the only witness; all students close their eyes and wait for their own internal imagery to arise as source of their movement. By spring, students are also practicing witnessing, working in dyads or triads, taking turns moving and being witnessed, learning to witness and to move deeper.

By spring, also, many students have experiences of no longer moving themselves but rather feel the distinct sensation of *being moved* by their body without conscious interference (a phenomenon first described by Mary Whitehouse). Mind becomes witness in these events; an "internal witness" is growing stronger. Through the will to experience their truth directly and through the surrender to the internal wisdom in their bodies, each one discovers idiosyncratically—in an individual way in response to individual timing—what is true and what is not true.

One common discovery may be that in emptying their mind of ordinary thought processes through body experience, mind itself becomes a curious and interested participant as witness in the unfolding process. The shifts in the art imagery mark the unfolding stories of trauma healing, lost self-parts being retrieved, discoveries about the co-existence of pain and joy in the healer's journey.

These words are simple but the process is not; it may take several years to develop the trust in self necessary to allow the self to *fully* witness self. Put in other words, learning to love begins at the beginning, but it may take a while to know that that is what is happening. It certainly takes time to trust that all is process and the self is not separate from that one whole process. All this time, however, is leading toward more conscious loving. When a personal issue has been addressed, another may arise to take its place. Interestingly, development comes to be experienced not as linear so much as "spiral."

In the repetition of certain gestures, for example, a Mover becomes aware of the gesture's existence first, and then its meaning. Eventually specific movements may recede because their meaning has been integrated into the Mover's life or because they are not to be recognized at this time. Additionally, Movers begin to experience how personal and transpersonal moments are often woven together with a synchronicity or orderliness that is surprising. The art-making shifts between being faithful companion to a movement experience or guide opening a door to a new movement exploration.

From fall through spring, the body speaks through art and movement. Giving time and attention to letting the body speak is going to the door of the unknown, the unconscious, surrendering to what the body needs to say, learning the courage and the way to be still, to listen and to see. This then is the intention: to learn to listen, to learn to see, to learn to feel, and to learn to know directly what is true for ourselves, so that we may become more truthful in our relationships with others.

297

This practice is what I know as learning to love. For me, experiencing these forms as sacred human expression, meaning (w)holy and deserving of reverence and respect, I feel a lively gratitude for the role I play and the growing I continue to do. Teacher and student alike practice this honing of learning to love.

Evidences

Excerpts from three stories that unfolded through the Authentic Movement-art therapy process may help to demonstrate the effect of this approach. They bridge the worlds from intensely personal to midlife situational trauma to the gift of a transpersonal experience with death.

Becoming Visible

During a period of one and one-half years, a young woman, Annie, age twenty-four, attended two course offerings in the creative arts therapies at Sonoma State, "Symbolic Healing Through Art Therapy And Authentic Movement" (twelve months) and "Introduction to Art Therapy" (four months). She focused on coming to terms with the wounds of growing up in a seriously dysfunctional family. Her dilemmas included: splitting (dissociating from painful truths and memories); rage and grief with authority figures; fear connected with issues of abandonment; a delusional system (false beliefs about reality); and the development of a false self to compensate for the lack of development of a congruent authentic self.

Annie's despair at rarely having her childhood emotional needs met and the lack of early modeling of healthy self-care behaviors combined to make her young adult life a fast roller coaster ride with emotional peaks and valleys. Annie was often either reacting against the world or attempting to exert control over it. While she had achieved highest honors academically and was intellectually capable of pursuing any vocational path of interest, the disparity between her facade and her internal self-concepts seriously compromised her best efforts. Through the symbolic healing process she found a light to help her along her path.

Annie demonstrated remarkable courage and persistence in facing her unconscious through movement and art. Through "being seen" by an external witness while experiencing the pain of returning to her childhood-self—the rage and grief of being invisible, unseen and abandoned—she began to develop an internal witness for herself. With this new experience Annie began to heal her past and to create a possible life of her own.

One evening, we reviewed approximately sixty paintings from her collection. The quotes from twenty pieces are in chronological order; they are her own words to what most "moved" her. The word "Image" [I] refers to a picture she made; the words "Authentic Movement and Art" [AM&A] condense both body and visual imagery during a four-hour session. Following a thematic approach will hold the power of her experiences for the reader.

Experiences of Pain, Rage and Splitting

Image: "A knife cutting away at all the people who told me that I shouldn't feel. The knife rides on the energy of anger and pain."

I: "A sad little girl going crazy, her eyes turn inward: there is a girl inside a girl, crying endless tears."

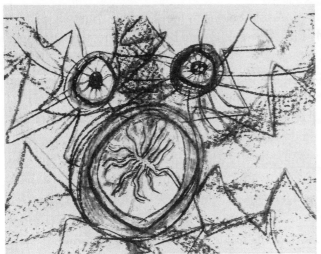

I: "I split into fours to try to stabilize myself; my emotions split up and with the confusion I can't figure out what's happening."

I: "Everything is dying, upside down flowers. One flower, nipped in the bud, the last of its kind, its breed, is slowly dying,

Fig. 1 An early picture of Annie's rage.

slowly joining the pull of the dead old-fashioned flowers. It's a question what the new flower looks like: it's not here yet."

I: "I feel I'll never end this pool of grief. I know it [the abuse] happened. I'm crying alone in my room, forever alone in my badness."

Authentic Movement & Art: Annie begins pounding the walls and discovers that she is both beating and feels like she is being beaten. "Fuck you!" she shouts and cries over and over. Black and red paint and oil pastels fill pages of paper.

I: "To be me I have to fade away or I have to be so angry."

AM&A: "Rage hurts, I hurt. Expressing my rage consumes my energy. I feel like one huge ball of pain. It's so overwhelming I'll get lost in it. All I am is fear, pain, rage, sorrow. Where am I going with it? It's so hard when it's my only experience of myself.

Experiences of a Door Opening

AM&A: "If I allow myself to fully enter into those feelings, on the other side comes some compassion for myself."

I: A shark with large teeth. "It's humorous, sharp. I feel powerful, 'I can get you!' I used to bite people when I was angry."

AM&A (Text of three pictures) 1) "I exist, and I'm afraid to show you who I am. But I am here. I am seen." 2) "Oh the pain, the joy, the light of being, I'm me, I'm here, and I'm beautiful and I'm real." 3) " 'Oh, a rebirth!' I remember dancing, allowing me to be seen."

AM: Alone on the floor, Annie begins to feel her face. She begins crying and later explains, "My face is there!" Annie begins to directly experience herself through her body.

AM&A: Annie writes in big letters, "PROVE IT! Prove that I was so bad as a child!" Annie begins to confront the "authorities" and the effects of the reality of her childhood on her now that she is grown. "Get real. When can I get on with my life? When do I do something?"

I: Annie begins to recognize that when she repeats stressful patterns of her childhood now, by creating a heavy schedule for herself, she evokes intensely painful feelings and feels like "someone is whipping me, I fall down and cry." Only now it is she who is doing it to herself.

I: "Kneeling, no arms, looking away. Scary creatures are around. I feel pushed and compelled to explore my unconscious."

AM&A: After expressing some rage in her movement, Annie paints her hands and then her face. She then returns to more movement and expresses the most rage yet. Smearing paint evoked preverbal body experiences for her.

Experiences of Healing the Self in the Family

Kinetic Family Drawing: "We were only together when we had to be; everyone was always yelling at each other." Sharing this reality, Annie began seeing her family in a new way.

Family Relationships Through Clay and Paint:

"Dad is an awful serpent creature, weak and wimpy. I'm a laughing hyena shaking and howling at the moon. Mom is a bear balancing and then she falls over backwards. T is a snake, wily and laughing; he slips in and out of everything. J is a wolf, strong, but following a narrow path edged in black." As Annie sorted out the relationships within her family she reported surprise to discover her closeness to her father, despite her rage at him for abandoning her.

I: A crying face with volcano coming out of the mouth. "See me, pay attention to me, god damn it!' It's also telling *me* to pay attention to me." With this image, Annie asks, "How can I be my own witness? I am struggling to witness myself and then come to others and say 'I have this need, please help me.' " Instead of demanding: "Take care of me, fulfill my needs!" Annie expresses more awareness of her rights and needs, and that there is a healthier way to take care of herself.

I: A shaman-bird and a heart being cut open. "The sexual abuse question is hard for me to separate out because of my mother's sexual abuse: what is hers, what is mine? And because of the taboo of even discussing sex in my family. There was no place for me to share my pain."

AM&A: "I was running around looking for care, finally got some from R. Feels like I'm striking out, but it isn't overwhelming rage, it's more me wanting attention." After several months of moving "alone" and being focused on expressing her rage in corners or against walls, Annie begins to move in the circle with others and tentatively to seek what she needs.

I: Making a "sad center" on a page, she then wrote: "It's hard to remember to take care of myself, to love myself first. Annie, I love you, and you are not responsible for anyone else's feelings. I love you and forgive you. I'm strong, I can stand up, I can act sexually appropriate, I can ask for nurturing and affection when I want it."

In her self-reflections, Annie said, "This stuff isn't fun and games. It's about making choices, saying no to people and yes and I'm scared by that. I've gone from an amorphic and amoebic form to being maybe ten years old. I've learned a whole new vocabulary and possible way of working with these things. When I choose to practice, I'm mighty good at expressing these feelings."

Putting her foot down

A mature woman, Juliana had been experiencing pain in her marriage of 20 years. In her words,

> At this time, I had a dream of a five-year old boy sitting: his hands were up and they had no bones; they had been removed. The reason was: punishment. During the Authentic Movement, the next week, one of the symbols that came up was the boy with the hands. I remember moving my hands and putting them to my face, to nurture myself, to feel nurtured. [Then] I began to stomp my feet; that was so empowering for me, to just be able to put my foot down.

Juliana retrieved her memories of how unacceptable it had been for her to be assertive like her brothers; her desires to express her "little boy" self were put down and taunted and made fun of. Putting her foot down, "felt like the first time that I had ever stood up for myself, and said, 'It's too painful! I can't go on with this label [wife] that's been on me for twenty years. Life isn't worth it. I really need to look and see what I need to do about this.' "

Which she did. Moving from her Authentic Movement and dream experiences through a series of images with various media, Juliana succeeded in accepting divorce, working through her own responsibilities and empowering herself to begin a new career more congruent with her belief system.

The Sacrifice of the Deer

The following is from the transcript of a field research project carried

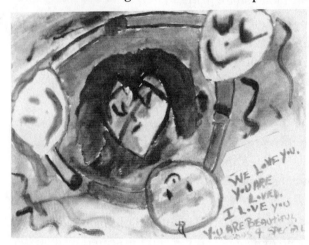

out during a 10-week period of Symbolic Healing. Karen, who left an business executive position in order to become an Art Therapy student, speaks about a transformative experience she had while moving. She began her movement by walking slowly in a large circle around the room.

Fig. 2 An example of Annie's later art

It was right before I was to visit my younger brother who's dying. He's 34 and has cancer. Within a few minutes of the time that I closed my eyes, I had what I call a waking dream—but this time it was different. I saw a scene where a baby deer was sick, and I had to kill it to put it out of its pain, and then we were to eat this deer. And so I had to dress the deer. And I didn't want to—it was so young and innocent and fragile and seemed so incredibly sad. But it was something that had to be done. What I was doing was going around the room in a circle, this interior scene kept changing.

I went through a process of agreeing that yes, it was time: I had to kill it, eat it, and then I honored it. (Karen stops moving, kneels down and experiences the killing, the eating and the sewing movements.) I used the leather for different things, including a pair of baby moccasins.

302

After that happened, eating it and making these beaded moccasins with its leather, I was walking and I had a sensation of seeing this intense, intense green, which for me is a very healing color. And my sense of the whole experience for me personally was accepting my younger brother's impending death. There was a personal message of "Yes, you have to accept this, let it go," and in doing that, there was healing.

Death could be healing. It is a natural part of this cycle. It didn't have to be tragic. Yes, there is sadness and mourning, but there is an honoring. And as it turned out, when I met with him a few days later, we had an incredible time together—I could also see transpersonal dimensions in this experience, that what I was doing was very ritual-like. And it was (also) part of a group experience, that death and change are such constant patterns in our lives, but it doesn't have to be tragic. I've had other experiences in Authentic Movement that had a similar quality to that, a universal and mythic kind of quality to it.

Conclusion

There is an invisible bond of power between the wounded healer and the healee. The bond is the essence of the work of the healer. All else—all ritual, gadgets, medical maneuverings of the body and manipulations of the mind—are merely reminders of the divine process. The shamans know this full well and strengthen the bond with ritual. Some call this bond love. It comes forth from the desire to make and be made well or whole.   Achterberg, in Doore, 1988, p. 122.

The implications for our lives as therapists are broad and far reaching. Beyond the problem-solving which we may do as therapists, helping our clients with ordinary reality issues, there are two other realities worthy of our commitment: a personal one and a transpersonal or collective one.

On the personal level, there is a deeper calling to "witness" clients, to be a compassionate *other* who sees and accepts their wounds and losses. This calling we can answer only to the degree to which we see and accept our own wounds and losses and live in a balanced relationship with them. As Naomi Remen and Rollo May express it,

The archetype of the Wounded Healer asserts that there is no difference between the two people engaged in a healing relationship. Indeed both are wounded and both are healers. It is the woundedness of the healer which enables him or her to understand the patient and which informs the wise and healing action. The healer within the patient is evoked by the wound itself and also in the response to the woundedness of the heal-

303

*er. It is the synthesis between the healer within the patient and the heal-
er within the (healer) which maximizes the healing of the patient's
wound. Healing is a mutual process. We cannot heal unless we acknowledge our woundedness and we cannot heal without being healed ourselves. (1985, p. 85)*

There is an aliveness—an at-onement—in our work in those true and
deep moments when we encounter our own wounds. Those healing moments
come as a surprise; we can't plan them. In the work described above, they
happen visibly in the Mover's body and in his/her art-making and in the witnessing itself. As Witness, I am moved again and again by the strength and
courage which we human beings possess to face adversity and transform it,
and in the process, to transform our being. We arrive at where we were in our
beginnings, open and vulnerable; now we know and embody our being in our
lives.

On the transpersonal or collective level, as we witness the uniqueness
and commonality of all humans, there is a calling to contribute to the well-
being of the whole. Through our practice of the creative arts therapies for
healing and learning to love, we develop the wisdom we need—to know what
we each can do to be of service. And when our path gets unclear or difficult,
we can descend again, return to our body wisdom and the images forming to
learn how to proceed. In this way, we remain in loving connection with ourselves and the whole.

Learning to love is a practice. Just the way a child learns to walk, we too
heal and grow our ability to love. Slowly we extend this practice of moving,
art-making and witnessing with compassion out into the world.

References
Imagery & Healing

Achterberg, J. (1985). *Imagery in healing: Shamanism and modern medicine.* NY: Shambala.

Eliade, M. (1972). *Shamanism: Archaic techniques of ecstasy.* Princeton: Princeton University Press.

———— (1988). *Symbolism, the sacred, & the arts.* D. Apostolos-Cappadona, ed.). NY:
Crossroads.

Halifax, J. (1982). *Shaman: The wounded healer.* NY: Crossroads.

Kalweit, H. (1988). *Dreamtime and inner space: The world of the shaman.* Boston: Shambala.

Krippner, S. and Granger, D. (ed.) (1985). *Art, creativity, and consciousness.* Saybrook
Review. Fall/Winter, 5 (2).

Remen, N. (Ed.). (1985). *Dimensions of healing,* Saybrook Review, Summer/Fall, 5 (1).

Samuels, M. and Samuels, N. (1990). *Healing with the mind's eye.* NY: Simon and Schuster.

Sandner, D. (1979). *Navaho Symbols of Healing.* NY: Harcourt Brace Jovanovich.

Art Therapy

Arguelles, J. (1975). *The Transformative vision: Reflections on the nature and history of human expression.* Boston: Shambala.

London, P.. (1989). *No more secondhand art: Awakening the artist within.* Boston: Shambala.

McNiff, S. (1981). *The arts and psychotherapy.* Springfield, IL: C.C. Thomas.

———— (1988) *Fundamentals of art therapy.* Springfield, IL: C. C.Thomas.

———— (1989) *Depth psychology of art.* Springfield, IL: C. C. Thomas.

Miller, H. (1973). *The paintings of Henry Miller: paint as you like and die happy.* San Francisco: Chronicle Books.

Palmer, S. [Lovell], (1987). *"Creative art therapy and symbolic healing,"* in proceedings of the fourth international conference on the study of shamanism and alternate modes of healing. Ruth-Inge Heinze, (ed.). Madison, WI: A-R Editions.

———— (1988) *"When the bough breaks: cancer and the shamanic path as experienced by a creative art therapist,"* in Proceedings of the Fifth International Conference on the Study of Shamanism and Alternate Modes of Healing. R.-I. Heinze, (ed.) Berkeley: Independent Scholars of Asia.

Wadeson, H. (1987). *Dynamics of art psychotherapy.* NY: John Wiley.

Authentic Movement

Adler, J. *Who is the witness? A description of authentic movement.* Contact Quarterly, Winter 1987: 20-9.

———— (1991). *Body and soul.* Keynote address, American Dance Therapy Conference, San Francisco, Ca. Tape available through ADTA.

———— (1986). *Free movement and sexuality in the therapeutic experience..* Unpublished manuscript.

———— (1970), [Boettiger]. *Integrity of body and psyche: Some notes on work in progress.* American Dance Therapy Conference Proceedings.

Brooks, C. (1974). *The rediscovery of experiencing.* NY: Viking Press.

Chaiklin, H. (1975). *Marian Chace: her papers.* American Dance Therapy Association.

Chodorow, J. (1982). *Dance/movement and body experience in analysis.* Jungian Analysts, Murray Stein (ed). LaSalle, IL: Open Court.

———— (1991). *Dance therapy and depth psychology: The moving imagination.* NY: Routledge.

Frantz, G. (1972). *An approach to the center: interview with Mary Whitehouse.* Psychological Perspectives 3 (1). Los Angeles: C. G. Jung Institute.

Smallwood, J. [Chodorow] (date unknown). *Dance therapy and the transcendent function.* American Journal of Dance Therapy.

———— 1974). *Dance-movement therapy.* Current Psychiatric Therapies. 14. J. H. Masserman, ed. NY: Grune and Stratton.

Whitehouse, M. (1958). *The tao of the body.* Paper presented at the Analytic Psychology Club of Los Angeles.

————(1977) *Transference and dance therapy.* American Journal of Dance Therapy.

The Sand Tray and Art Therapy
by Betsy Caprio, M.A., M.Ed., A.T.R.

Betsy Caprio, M.A., M.Ed., is the director of the Center for Sacred Psychology in Los Angeles. She is the author of several books on psychology and spiritual development from the Jungian perspective, including Coming Home, At a Dream Workshop, *and* The Mystery of Nancy Drew: Girl Sleuth on the Couch. *Betsy holds masters degrees in transpersonal education and clinical art therapy, and is currently working on a doctorate in ministry with a focus on the creative arts. At present, she is a research fellow at Loyola Marymount University, where she is exploring the use of already created art in art therapy. She is a member of the Los Angeles Sandplay Association and the American Art Therapy Association.*

> *The sand tray…just a shallow wooden box half-filled with sand, standing amidst shelves of miniature people, buildings, animals, plants and other items—but what a powerful tool for self-discovery and healing!*

I came to the sand tray in the late 1970s, after hearing the late Dora Kalff of Switzerland lecture on it for the Los Angeles C. G. Jung Institute. Soon after, with my colleagues at the Center for Sacred Psychology in L. A., I set up a sand tray for use with our psychotherapy and spiritual direction clients. Later, during a year-long art therapy practicum, I conducted sand tray research with residential patients in a large psychiatric hospital.

By this time, our center had accumulated a wide range of miniatures, and arranged them on shelves by category, and set up the recommended two trays, one for wet and one for dry sand. We had also connected with sources of training and supervision both locally and in Europe.

The Sand Tray Process

The directions to a client for making a sand tray are simple: the person is shown the sand tray area—in our case, an alcove of a consulting room—the two trays are pointed out, and the person is invited to "make a picture in the sand." Most people use objects from the shelves to create a scene in one of the two trays; sometimes the sand alone is molded or swirled into a configuration which pleases the traymaker. Clients know when a tray is finished.

In the very nondirective Jungian style used at our center, the finished creation then is looked at carefully by the client and the therapist, who has been recording during the traymaking process. There may be questions and comments about the figures. For example, I might say to someone, "I wonder if that lion is tame or wild...," or "Is there anything in that treasure chest you put in the tray?" Sometimes the client will want to tell a story about the tray; the therapist may ask if the tray has a title, or which is the most important item in the tray. Other than comments of this sort, which stay within the visual metaphor, no interpretation is made of the finished sand tray.

A photograph is taken or a sketch made of the scene which has unfolded, and this is kept by the therapist. The tray is taken apart after its creator has left the room, at which time the therapist might hunt for any objects hidden in the sand. When a series of trays is finished—and this may be from a few to a great many, as dictated by the client's psyche—the trays are then reviewed by client and therapist from a more analytical and interpretive standpoint: "Let's see what the psyche had to say when given a space in which to say it." The traymaker almost always has comments to make about the process.[1]

My original intuitive hunches about the value of the sand tray as a therapeutic modality have been verified over and over. I am convinced that it is an exquisitely valuable tool with which the psyche can express itself, and I use it side-by-side with traditional art therapy techniques. Before considering the sand tray's use in therapy, let's take a very brief look at its background.

Sand Tray History

Margaret Lowenfeld, an English pediatrician (1890-1973), is recognized as the originator of the sand tray. Actually, she was quick to credit her young patients with its invention, as it was the children coming to her office at the Institute of Child Psychology in 1920's London who put together the miniature toys and sand and water there and developed what she named "The World Technique."[2]

In the 1950s, Dora Kalff (1904-1990), a Swiss Jungian analyst who was the first of that school to work with children, studied with Lowenfeld and adapted her World Technique to Jungian thought. Kalff termed her use of the sand tray "Sandplay," to distinguish it from Lowenfeld's style; she and her circle, now known as the International Society of Sandplay Therapists, have produced the bulk of the small amount of literature on the use of the sand tray in psychotherapy.[3]

Jungian theory is committed to the concept that the psyche, when given a safe place in which to speak, tends toward reparation or healing and health. The sand tray is seen in the Sandplay world as such a safe place: Kalff's "buzz words" have long been "a free and protected space."

Therapists of persuasions other than the depth psychologies have also, more recently, explored and written about the sand tray, so that today the two traditional styles of using it are being supplemented by a variety of other approaches. In addition, there are many articles in the literature on sand tray use by classroom teachers and other educators.

Is the Sand Tray Art Therapy?

The sand tray—clearly a visual modality—has grown up separately from the many techniques which come under the art therapy umbrella, and yet it is surely related to them: in a finished tray there is the picture which has been created, the use of an earth material which has much in common with clay, and the use of pre-formed images, as in collage.

However, there are differences between the sand tray and the art therapy modalities. Here are some of them:

• The sand tray is easier and more playful for the client than even the simplest of art therapy methods and, therefore, potentially more regressive. This can be a plus or a minus, depending upon the client and upon the treatment plan of the psychotherapist.

• Similarly, the sand tray doesn't carry the negative school-oriented attitudes clients so often bring to "making art," i.e., being graded, not being able to draw. It is such a benign means of expression that client resistance is often non-existent. Again, this may be a plus or a minus, for some clients very much need to maintain their defenses.

• The sand tray is a multi-media technique. Instead of just one medium, there is moldable material (the sand), there is the means of changing the material's consistency (through adding water), and there are the little miniature objects that create the scene. A rough comparison to art therapy might be that the sand tray has some of the qualities of clay, finger paints and collage/assemblage rolled into one. This is a big advantage—but can also be a disadvantage if it overwhelms the client; the structure provided by the box, the sand tray area of the office, and the relationship between therapist and client is what prevents the client from retreating very often.

• On the other hand, the traymaker is, ultimately, limited by the choices on the therapist's shelves. This can be a disadvantage, or not as clients learn to adapt themselves to and use the resources of this particular therapist, which happens in any therapeutic relationship.

• Because a sand tray is so simple to make, and because the images contained within it are mostly of professional quality, the traymaker usually has a very high level of satisfaction with the finished product. Of course, this may also be true with art therapy products, and when it is not true, the struggle with the media and a client's dissatisfaction can then be grist for the therapeutic mill. The bottom line with sand tray work, usually, is a great sense of achievement and aesthetic satisfaction with the finished visual product. I see this as a plus, and have been moved many times by clients' expressions such as "I just love my tray," or "I couldn't get my last sand tray out of my mind."

• Finally, the history of the sand tray marks it indelibly as a means of connection with the unconscious. Both Margaret Lowenfeld and Dora Kalff, who in many ways were not unlike the "founding mothers" of art therapy, were firmly rooted in the tradition of depth psychology. They both saw the tray of sand and the figures as a way to elicit visual images of unconscious psychodynamics (and, the Jungians would add, images of the archetypes of the collective unconscious).

The sand tray literature stresses the importance of the therapist's connectedness to his or her own unconscious, and an understanding of symbolism, much as in dream work. These, of course, are also the roots of art therapy, but since Margaret Naumburg and Edith Kramer first began teaching and writing, art therapy has found a home within many metapsychologies, some of them quite divorced from the unconscious and from symbolism.

And so, even though there is much the sand tray shares with art therapy, it has a history and a literature all its own. I look at them as first cousins, and encourage those who want to use the sand tray in their practices to have specific training and supervision in its use.[4]

Most-Asked Questions About the Sand Tray

Because the sand tray has been thought of for so long, in the United States at least, as a Jungian therapeutic tool, it's not very well known by the broader psychological community and is the source of many interesting queries. Here are some of the most-frequently-asked questions about its use (and my responses reflect the Jungian or Sandplay point of view):

• *Is there a standard size for the sand tray—and why this size?* Sand trays made to Kalff's specifications are 21" x 30" x 3". The idea is that the traymaker be able to take in the entire tray without moving his or her head.

• *Where do you find all the little things that go on the sand tray shelves? And, must I have a complete set of figures before I begin offering sand tray experiences to others?* As you might imagine, objects for the sand tray are everywhere—from our children's discarded toys, to the beach and woodlands, to toy stores and thrift shops and craft stores and cake decorating supply shops. Once one begins a sand tray collection, any tendency the collector may have toward obsessive-compulsive traits really becomes clear!

In the 1940s, Charlotte Buhler of Vienna, London and, later, southern California devised the "Toy World Test" which called for a standardized set of miniatures to be used with the sand tray for diagnostic purposes. Other than Buhler and her followers, however, sand tray practitioners have collected their own array of items for use in the tray—their "world"—and each collection is uniquely representative of the therapist who has put it together. When clients enter your sand tray space, in a way they're entering your psyche.

And, no, one doesn't have to get it all together before beginning. In fact, therapists who work at different sites or have no office space for a tray may develop portable arrangements of baskets or cardboard boxes of miniatures, which they carry about in a light-weight (usually plastic) tray.

• *Is the sand tray used just with children?* No. Shortly after its beginnings, those using it found the parents of their young clients wanting to make sand trays, and its use as a modality for all ages was established.

• *With which populations is the sand tray contraindicated?* The primary caution in using the sand tray, especially in an out-patient or private practice setting, is to be sensitive to the traymaker's reaction to it. If the person seems overwhelmed—as may happen with anyone but particularly with someone with weak ego structure, as in borderline personalities—the sand tray might best be used early in a session or foregone. Creation of a sand tray often provides very speedy access to the unconscious, and for the barely-coping client who has to leave our office and function in the world, our treatment plan will often call for sealing over and buoying up defenses, not eliciting a rush of material from the unconscious.

My experience with patients in a psychiatric hospital, however, where

311

their coping mechanisms had already given way and the hospital provided safety, was that—like art therapy—the sand tray provided a safe and healing means for the expression of the patients' deepest fears and longings. The structured, concrete nature of the sand tray, the ease of traymaking, the choices offered, and the soothing quality of the sand all make it a valuable adjunct to a hospital's therapeutic resources in the hands of trained practitioners.

• *Is the sand tray used for diagnosis—and if so, how?* Buhler's (1951) work focused on three types of trays which she interpreted diagnostically. These were aggressive sand worlds, empty worlds, and distorted worlds; the third category included closed worlds, disarranged worlds, and rigid worlds. When two or more such designations applied to any tray, Buhler (1951) postulated that emotional disturbance might be present.

Little formal sand tray research has been done, but the literature is full of anecdotal material about "red flags," warning signs to the therapist about possible psychopathology and even clues as to the etiology of the client's disturbance. A few of the more obvious indicators of problems are flooded wet trays, the inability of the traymaker to touch the sand, and double walls around all or any portion of the tray.

Kalff emphasized the importance not of diagnosis but of the process of making a series of trays. An important ingredient in both visual and non-visual Jungian work is the ability of the therapist or analyst to understand what the psyche is expressing; thus, the practitioner's own experience with his or her dreams, art work, the sand tray, and other ways in which the unconscious communicates is essential. Of course, since the use of any item in the tray may be overdetermined, one avoids reductionistic symbolic interpretations such as "that snake is a phallic symbol" (though it may well be).

• *Is the client given the picture taken of the finished tray?—and if not, why?* In the Sandplay style of using the sand tray, the client is not given the picture of his or her tray. The reasoning behind this is that the work is to be kept within, not without. The goal is for the client to leave "carrying" his or her finished picture internally so that the link to the unconscious may be maintained.

In addition, the pictures are needed for the therapist's ongoing consideration and the final review by client and therapist.

The same reasoning explains the lack of interpretation of trays along the way. Trays "too understood" cognitively may detach the client from the processes of the unconscious which, in Jungian thought, hold the keys to healing and development.

• *Do the findings of art therapy research translate to the sand tray?* This is an intriguing question, and one that has just begun to be addressed. My limited research showed that psychiatric patients' sand trays mirrored what we would think of as typical manic art and typical depressed art: i.e., overflowing and chaotic trays for the manic patients, and barren, lifeless, colorless trays for the severely depressed patients. However, the sand tray ideation in both cases was less florid than that of the same patients' artwork.

The artwork of schizophrenic patients is, as we know, often full of image salads and bizarre ideation. My expectation before seeing any sand trays made by schizophrenic patients was that their trays would be similar. This was not the case; the sand tray seemed to elicit a healthier side of these patients, and their trays were barely distinguishable from those seen in private practice. Patients diagnosed as paranoid schizophrenic, however, favored watchtowers or mountains made in the sand from which they could keep an eye on the goings-on in the tray (Caprio, 1989).

• *How about the use of the sand tray with groups, couples, or families?* The sand tray grew up as a modality for use with individuals. There is some literature describing experiments with its use in group process and in conjoint therapy (e.g., Spare, 1981). From the Sandplay point of view, this makes little sense, as a finished sand tray is viewed as a picture of the intrapsychic contents of the traymaker, not of interpersonal dynamics (although these too may show up in a tray). My own feeling is that the former use is so well served by the sand tray that its tradition and strengths should not be watered down by other uses...we shall see what lies ahead.

• *Are there other rules for the use of the sand tray?* Yes and no. There are many important guidelines which have been left to us by Lowenfeld and Kalff and their first generation followers. It is important to point these out to trainees, without decreeing a set of "rules" carved on stone. What seems most important to me is that each practitioner who decides to incorporate the sand tray into his or her work has a firm rootedness in some metapsychology (or combination of theories). In this way, questions about the use of the sand tray in practice—just like any other practical therapeutic questions—can be examined in the broader light of "what am I doing, and why—and how does my theoretical background help me answer this specific question about the use of the sand tray?"

Sand Tray Training

The traditional basic requirement for using the sand tray with others is to have had the experience of making one's own series of sand trays. This is particularly true in the Jungian or Sandplay world. When members of the helping professions come to our center seeking sand tray training, the first question we ask is, "Have you made your own series of trays?"

One of the interesting developments at our center has been the attraction to the sand tray of people in helping professions other than psychotherapy and education. We have now used it for more than ten years in spiritual direction, that religiously-oriented one-to-one work rooted in the guide-seeker relationships of old. And now, we also find among our basic and advanced trainees speech pathologists, physical therapists, pastoral counselors, physicians' assistants and rehab counselors, all trying to develop ways of translating this intriguing mode of expression to their disciplines.[5]

I have also discovered, both in my own supervision and with those who come to our center, that the sand tray seems either to appeal greatly to practitioners and clients—or not at all. This makes me wonder if there isn't a "typical" sand tray therapist. The common denominator among those I know who use this valuable tool seems to be some antecedent, often from childhood, which predisposes them for this work. With some, it's happy memories of beach days; with others, it's an early love of miniatures or doll houses or of stories of little people, like those in "The Borrowers" books and "Gulliver's Travels."

And, speaking of antecedents, in 1911 the novelist H. G. Wells wrote of the games he and his sons played with miniatures on the floor of their home in England. When Margaret Lowenfeld remembered his book she knew that, without calling it such, Wells had discovered a therapeutic tool; she found a historical precedent for her work, and might also have cited earlier ones such as the healing sandpaintings of the Navajos and the Tibetan Buddhists.

And so, we have the sand tray...a deceptively childlike, yet enormously powerful means of access into the depths of the psyche, a visual modality that makes a powerful first cousin to art therapy.

References

Ammann, R. (1991). *Healing and transformation in sandplay.* LaSalle, IL: Open Court.

Bowyer, L. R. (1970). *The Lowenfeld world technique.* Oxford: Pergamon.

Bradway, K. (1979). *Sandplay in psychotherapy.* Art Psychotherapy, 6(2), 85-93.

Buhler, C. (1951). *The World test: manual of directions.* Journal of Child Psychiatry, 2, 69-81.

Caprio, E. (1989). *The sand tray and its relationship to art therapy.* Unpublished master thesis. Loyola Marymount University, Los Angeles.

Currant, N. (1989). *Room to breathe.* American Journal of Art Therapy, 27 (3), 80ff.

Dundas, E. (1978). *Symbols come alive in the sand.* Aptos, CA: Aptos.

Friedman, H. (1986). S*andplay: an approach to the child's unconscious* (audio tape). Los Angeles: C. G. Jung Institute.

Kalff, D. M. (1980). *Sandplay: a psychotherapeutic approach to the psyche*; original German, 1966. Santa Monica: Sigo Press.

Lowenfeld, M. (1967). *Play in childhood*; first published 1935. NY: John Wiley.

Lowenfeld, M. (1979). *The world technique.* London: George Allen and Unwin.

Rhinehart, L. and Englehorn, P. (1987). *Sand tray dialogue.* Santa Rosa, CA: Rainbow Bridges.

Shaia, A.J. (Spring, 1992). *When men are missing.* Northern California Sandplay Society Newsletter, 1-4.

Spare, G. (1981). *Are there any rules? (musings of a peripatetic sandplayer).* In Sandplay Studies: Origins,Theory and Practice. San Francisco: C.G.Jung Institute.

Wallace, E. (1987). *Healing through the visual arts—a Jungian approach.* In Rubin, J.A. (ed.), Approaches to Art Therapy. NY: Brunner/Mazel.

Weinrib, E. L. (1938). *Images of the self: the sandplay therapy process.* Boston: Sigo.

Wells, H. G. (1911, 1975). *Floor games.* NY: Arno Press.

Notes

1. The basic text for use of the sand tray from the Jungian point of view is Kalff (1980). Guidelines for Sandplay are offered by Jungian analysts Weinrib (1983), Friedman (1986), and Ammann (1991), with additional information in Dundas (1978).

2. See Lowenfeld (1967 and 1979), and Bowyer (1970).

3. Jungian therapist Alexander Shaia (1992) of California's Bay Area reports that in a personal interview with Kalff, just before her death, she said she wished she had chosen the name "sand therapy" or "sandwork" to distinguish her approach from the play therapists.

4. Among the few who have considered the sand tray within the context of art therapy are Jungian analysts Kay Bradway (1979) and Edith Wallace (1987), as well as Currant (1989) and myself (Caprio, 1989). Art therapists Rhinehart and Englehorn (1987) have developed a sand tray dialogue technique rooted in Gestalt therapy principles.

5. The semi-annual *Journal of Sandplay Therapy* is available from Sandplay Therapists of America, 331 Thistle Circle, Martinez, CA 94553.

Images from the Past:
The Life Review Scrapbook Technique with the Elderly
by Celeste Schexnaydre, M.A.

Celeste Schexnaydre worked with geriatric patients at San Gabriel Valley Medical Center. A native of New Orleans, she received her Master's Degree in art therapy from California State University, Los Angeles and is currently working at a psychiatric hospital in Louisiana.

" . . What a weight has been lifted by telling you this!"
                                    65-year-old woman

" . . This scrapbook has helped me more than any other therapy
I've tried."   *88-year-old man.*

" . . I feel ready to go forward with my life."
                                    82-year-old woman.

Introduction

The subject of art therapy with the geriatric population is one which has not been explored a great deal. Although there has been recent interest in the treatment of the elder population, there are not many specialized techniques. Combining art therapy with the Life Review Scrapbook is one such technique which has proved useful.

My interest in the geriatric population began during fieldwork for my Master's Degree in art therapy. My initial feelings toward this population have changed dramatically. In the beginning I found myself fearful of approaching the many aged patients in wheelchairs. I realize now that I was faced by my own mortality and found myself thinking "I don't ever want to reach this point." I found myself changing my attitude and what I discovered was rewarding. Instead of looking at these people as faceless, enfeebled bodies, I began to see the true beauty in each individual. I realized that underneath the shrinking figures was a wealth of knowledge and stories they were aching to tell. For many of these people, the stories were all they had left.

I realized the need for a sound art therapy technique designed to help the elderly, and in the beginning of 1991 I began a study designed to test whether art therapy techniques, combined with the life review scrapbook (Butler, 1963) (Appendix A), could lift depression in the elderly. The results were significant. The study indicated an an average sixteen point improvement on the Beck Depression Inventory (Beck, 1961) within the experimental group (Schexnaydre, 1991).

Reminiscing Through Art

The life review scrapbook combines art therapy theory with the concepts of life review and reminiscence in relation to the elderly. This technique involves the purposeful seeking of memories and images from one's past and present in order to compile them into scrapbook form. The memories are transformed onto paper by writing, drawing and collaging. The life review scrapbook is a concrete form of memory for the past, present and future. It connects the older person to tomorrow and affirms their existence to future generations.

Uniqueness of Geriatric Population

"The aged," "senior citizens" and "the elderly" are all terms we use to refer to persons over 65 years of age. By the year 2030, it is estimated that approximately 20% of the population will be over the age of 65 in America (Conklin, 1985).

The elderly, in the course of a lifetime, experience an overwhelming amount of loss. They are subject to the loss of spouses, children, friends, and relatives. Many are also subject to the loss of their homes and must adapt to living in convalescent or retirement homes. The elderly encounter decreased income, loss of visual and auditory acuity, and loss of what our society terms as beauty and status. The geriatric patient suffers disproportionately from depression.

In the later years of life, it is important for people to remember times when they felt strong and capable, overcame problems, and made difficult choices on their own. The challenge in old age is to use the skills and resources that have been gathered throughout a lifetime to enhance one's present life. "It is possible that the past provides a reservoir of identity upon which to draw. Encouraging the elderly to maintain contact with the younger, functioning person they once were can be extremely beneficial and can not only boost self-esteem but can also help lift depression" (Dewdney, 1976).

Art Therapy Goals

Art therapy provides a place for the elder population to explore, express and reflect upon their lives. It enables them to reminisce about their past, understand who they are and how they have become their unique person.

Therapeutic goals for the geriatric client often differ from goals set for other client populations because of the tremendous losses usually experienced by the elderly. By providing a framework in which one can succeed, the art therapist helps the client deal with these losses and heighten self-esteem. Feeling successful about expressing oneself creatively helps the elder preserve a sense of dignity and pride.

Art therapy with the geriatric population is used to revive memories from the past, resolve past or present conflicts, boost self-esteem and confidence, increase attention span and communication skills and stimulate cognitive functioning. The creative process assists elders in gaining new perspectives through the sharing of their feelings, thoughts and memories. It enables them to create from their sense of being (Weiss, 1984). Other goals include promoting socialization and improving cognitive functioning, lifting depression, and helping the elderly person become more self aware and approach death and the final developmental stages with a feeling of integrity rather than despair (Erikson, 1963).

Resistance

The elderly are often resistant to art therapy. They shy away from art therapy because they are intimidated, feel they must be sufficient artists to participate and are suffering from low self-esteem. Many have not picked up art materials since they were children and need much encouragement to get started.

There is a definite reward in store for those who sample art therapy. Art therapy allows the elderly client to express himself in a new way, providing an outlet for feelings of confusion, helplessness, anger and depression. *The goal in providing art therapy to the elderly is improvement in the quality of life rather than emphasizing psychodynamic processes and is usually supportive in its nature.*

Life Review Theory

Life review with elderly people was first addressed by Robert Butler in 1963 when he described the life review process as a naturally occurring and universal mental process in which past experiences progressively return to consciousness. "Life review is not synonymous with, but includes, reminiscence..." The recurrence of memories from the past may be due to the purposeful seeking of them or to the unexpected return of them. An important aspect of the life review is the resurgence of unresolved conflicts and the opportunity to examine and reintegrate those experiences back into one's life (Butler, 1963).

Butler believed that the life review process usually occurred in early old age and was brought about by the realization of approaching dissolution and death. He described the life review as a normal process, spontaneous and unselective, and he felt that if unresolved conflicts and fears were successfully reintegrated, they could give new meaning to the elder's life (Butler, 1974).

Life review has a positive, therapeutic capacity, in that the individual reflects on his life in order to resolve, reorganize and reintegrate what is troubling or preoccupying him. The emotions which accompany the life review vary and many times an element of pain and discomfort arises as memories resurface. The resolution of past conflicts and the opportunity to reexamine one's life and to make sense of it is what is so rewarding about the process. Psychotherapy of all kinds is often painful with the realization and acceptance of one's faults, flaws and mistakes which have occurred over a lifetime. It is this type of cathartic experience which restores balance and harmony. Butler maintains that the life review is a natural healing process, which represents one of the underlying human capacities.

Impact of Art Therapy Combined with Life Review Theory

Both art therapy and life review therapy are valid, potent therapies with the ability to bring to mind images of the past, uncover hidden conflicts as well as aid in boosting self-esteem. They complement each other—life review therapy helps to bring the imagery out and through art therapy an image evokes a memory.

Unlike art therapy alone, life review therapy is usually a less difficult technique to introduce to the elderly client. One reason may be that the life review process has already begun naturally and all the therapist need do is step in, listen and encourage. If the client has not begun the process by himself, it is usually very easy to get him involved in it.

Life Review Scrapbook

The life review *scrapbook,* an art therapy technique aimed at achieving these goals through combining the use of art therapy and life review theory, allows the patient to experience the benefits from both these theories simultaneously. *The wide variety of sensory experiences offered by the media, such as the color, texture and smell of paints and glue, the sound of scissors cutting through paper and the visual imagery and organization of collage stimulate and evoke memory. Often images which cannot be recalled voluntarily can arise spontaneously through the contact of the senses with the media.*

The life review scrapbook is actuated by compiling images, drawn and found, with an autobiographical sketch of the client's life. The therapist assists the client in reminiscing by asking trigger questions and genuinely listening to the details of the important memories of the client's life. The therapist also helps the client find images in magazines or asks him to draw a memory from the past. The process of finding or making images in a creative environment often sparks old memories and allows for the resurfacing of feelings from long ago.

The art therapist must tread carefully, being aware of the power of memory and imagery. *Careful listening that supports and encourages without interpreting or judging the many images and memories evoked is essential.* The art therapist is primarily concerned with creating a safe, nurturing environment which allows for life review process and the resolution of the past, present and future. Each client finds his own meaning and identity and the art therapist follows, listens and assists.

Selecting Appropriate Candidates

While the success of the life review scrapbook depends on many factors, it is mainly determined by the emotional energy put into the process by the client. Naturally, the elderly client who already appears to be reminiscing a great deal on his own would be suitable and also any person who is ready and willing to resolve some problems from the past. Persons who might not benefit from the life review process are people who avoid the present and greatly emphasize the future, those who have consistently exercised the human capacity to injure others and those who may best be described as "characterologically arrogant and prideful" (Butler, 1963).

Other considerations for choosing candidates would be that they possess a moderate level of cognitive functioning and a fairly intact remote memory. Some elderly do suffer from poor short-term memory but not remote and long-term memory loss. If the client appears appropriate but is unable to do the artwork because of a physical disability, he may still be able to find images with assistance. Clients suffering from organic brain syndromes such as dementia or Alzheimer's may be appropriate depending on the stage of the disorder. The therapist must assess this and decide what the client is capable of achieving.

I have found that most elderly folks show their personality traits quite readily, and I am usually able to distinguish their appropriateness within a few quick meetings. Most older people have been the same throughout their lifetime; they just become more intense in their personality traits.

There are two ways to turn if you are faced with uncertainty about appropriateness. The first is bring the idea to the client and see how he reacts. If he feels there has been too much pain and he would rather keep the past in the past, then let it be. You may find once they have had time to consider, they decide they have led decent lives which deserve to be told. The second way to decide appropriateness is to ask a family member about using the life review scrapbook with their elderly relative. Usually the best source for the decision lies within the therapist's intuition.

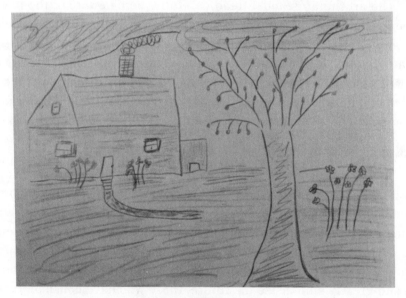

Fig. 1 Early Memories

Beginning the Scrapbook

Once the client has been interviewed and chosen, I introduce the idea of the scrapbook to them. I usually say "You really sound like you've had an interesting life. I wonder if you would like to make a scrapbook about it." The client is usually flattered at the interest in his life, and I go on to describe the process of the life review scrapbook. I tell him that I would like to help him make a scrapbook about his life and, while we cannot include every detail, we can try to highlight those important memories of his life-time. I explain that he would be expected to find and draw pictures to illustrate the pages of the book and of course that he could also include some real photographs if he likes. Sometimes the depressed client needs to be gently encouraged by hearing the genuine interest of the therapist in the details of his life. Simply asking a few prompting questions can help the client realize how significant a life he has lead. Gentle persuasion and genuine interest by the therapist generally encourages the client to participate in this unique opportunity.

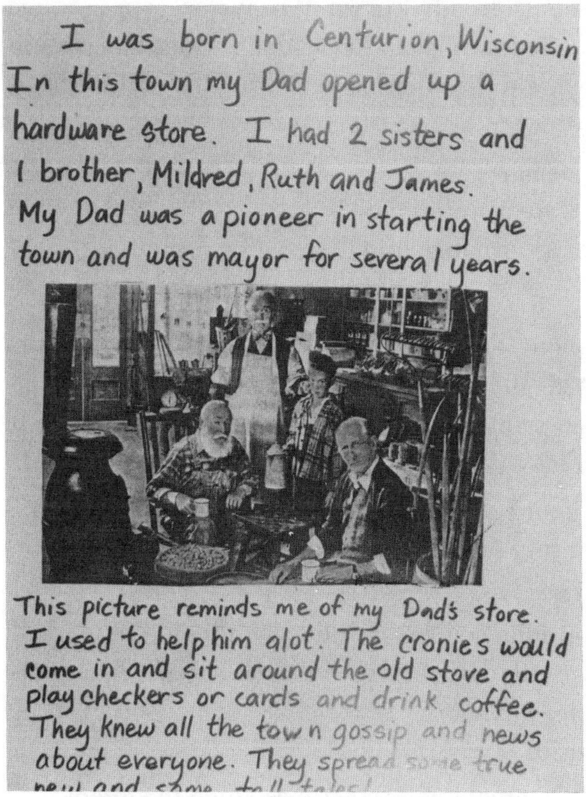

> I was born in Centurion, Wisconsin
> In this town my Dad opened up a
> hardware store. I had 2 sisters and
> 1 brother, Mildred, Ruth and James.
> My Dad was a pioneer in starting the
> town and was mayor for several years.

> This picture reminds me of my Dad's store.
> I used to help him alot. The cronies would
> come in and sit around the old stove and
> play checkers or cards and drink coffee.
> They knew all the town gossip and news
> about everyone. They spread some true
> news and some tall tales!

Fig. 2   Photos to stimulate recall of early memories

The life review scrapbook can usually be completed in about eight one hour sessions over a two- to three-week period, depending on the resolution process of the client. I have helped clients who only required five sessions and those who required twelve. The scrapbooks average about 14 pages in length. It is important to allow the client to reminisce freely, but also to provide a structure to follow.

I have found it easiest to start at the first memory moving up until the present. Often one memory will trigger another and although the memories may not seem related to the listener, it is important to remember that this is the time the patient has chosen to revive the memory. Throughout the scrapbook process, the art therapist must continually explore the feelings that specific memories bring up and explore why the memory has resurfaced. Omission of certain areas or people from a client's reminiscing can typically signal an area which needs to be looked into and resolved, as well.

Executing the Life Review Scrapbook Technique

Session One is verbal and exploratory. I try to collect as much general information as I can. Sometimes I already have a well-rounded idea about the client. For instance, finding out where the client grew up, if he ever married and if he had any children are important facts to inquire about in the beginning session if this is not already known. Always ask open-ended questions when possible and maintain good eye contact. Once some foundation has been built, you can aid the client in reviewing his childhood by asking questions like:

- "What is your first memory?"
- "How many people were in your family?"
- "Did you like school as a young child?"
- "What was it like?"

By writing down brief notes and key words, you can help the client in finding pictures to represent his life and also help yourself remember important details. The first session primarily gives the art therapist a chance to assess the client's life and areas in need of resolution.

Session Two. Collect more detailed information about the client's childhood and then move on into the later years of adolescence and adulthood.

I may begin looking through some magazines with the patient or ask the patient to draw about a particular memory. *A drawing of the first house* the client lived in or *the first schoolhouse he remembers* is a good exercise which brings up many memories (Fig. 1).

When helping to find pictures, I will sometimes guide the client if he cannot get started. For example, if the client remembers a train ride out west, we will look for a train, or if he remembers how tasty his mother's apple pie was, we will look for a picture of pie. Some clients do not need much direction and may simply let the pictures remind them of things. It is surprising how well the magazine pictures can describe and stimulate memories. Clients frequently find pictures of people that remind them of their family, especially their grandchildren.

It is important to stress early on that the pictures and drawings need not and probably will not be perfect replicas. The pictures are there for

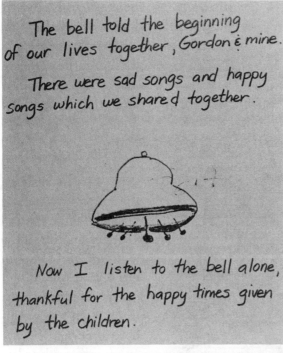

The bell told the beginning of our lives together, Gordon & mine.

There were sad songs and happy songs which we shared together.

Now I listen to the bell alone, thankful for the happy times given by the children.

Fig. 3   A poem for her deceased husband

illustration and mainly stimulation of old memories. After the second session I sometimes suggest the client look through some old magazines for pictures and I tell them I will do the same.

Session Three. I bring all my supplies in for session three. These include: magazines, scissors, glue, markers, 8 pieces of 12" by 18" drawing paper which is folded in half for now (I bind it when completed) and a file of folders containing cut-out magazine pictures (Fig. 2) grouped by subjects such as houses, people, children, animals, outdoor scenes, hobbies and miscellaneous. In this session, the making of the scrapbook proceeds beginning with the earliest memory of the client's life.

The front page of the scrapbook will be the title page. I suggest that we work on this last because I feel the client will have a better summation of his life after the scrapbook is completed. Therefore I turn to the next page and we begin with the introduction. Occasionally the client may be unable to write because of nervousness and shakiness due to medication, depression, stroke or a disease such as Parkinson's. If this is the case, I offer to act as the scribe and the client dictates in statement form what he wishes to be written down.

In the Beginning...

Normally the client will begin the scrapbook with a general opening statement, such as, "I was born in New Orleans, Louisiana and this is a drawing of the house where I spent my childhood." The next page might include some memories about family members and favorite things done in childhood with pictures representing the memories and so on. The first few pages often move slowly because of the client's unsureness of how the scrap-

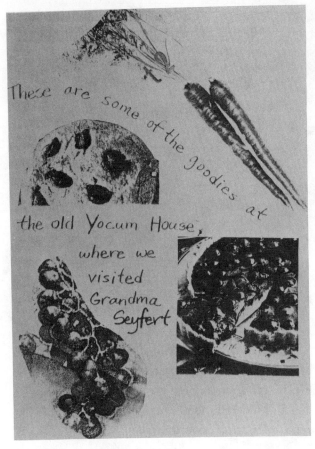

Fig. 4 A photo for each memory.

book should actually look. Once the first few pages are accomplished, the process moves more quickly and the client becomes increasingly more involved and dedicated.

By this session, the client is usually nearing the later adult years of his life in the storytelling. Keep in mind that the client continues to reminisce throughout the scrapbook process. However, hearing the life story once from start to finish in the beginning is important because the therapist needs to be able to determine in which areas to concentrate.

Long forgotten memories may not appear until the fifth or sixth session. As I go along, I am always looking for clues. However, usually the client will just come out with it. One of my first clients revealed during the fifth session that she had endured forty years of beatings by her husband and had never told another human being. She told me afterward that she had never felt as relieved as when she finally told me about this abuse.

The Client Leads

Sessions Four-Eight. The number of sessions needed to complete the scrapbook vary from client to client. While some require more time for simply getting everything down on paper, others need extra time to work through issues and resolve them. By the fourth session, the client is leading the way and I assist him.

Normally I allow the client to include or exclude anything they wish, but if something is excluded or merely touched upon which seems important, I will inquire about it, saying "I notice you have not mentioned your father. What was he like?" or "Why do you think this is?" While the client may still not want to share any more information, I am almost certain that he will in the future when he is ready.

Omissions

Many times a client will unconsciously leave events out. When this is brought to their attention, they are given the opportunity to explore the reasons why and begin the resolution of the life review process.

On the other hand, there are also clients who consciously recognize what parts of their lives have caused them pain. Therefore they know what areas do or do not need to be resolved. One of my clients had chosen to leave out some rather difficult memories about her relationship with her daughter. A few sessions later, she decided she would include these memories because she felt she needed to accept their occurrence.

I always encourage clients to cut and paste all their pictures even if they are unable to write. If they are unable to draw, I might encourage them to write poetry. One of my clients wrote a poem as a tribute to her deceased husband and concluded her scrapbook with the poem (Fig. 3). I normally like the client to try to find a picture for every page and memory. Sometimes they are able to find many pictures to represent a memory (Fig. 4). I have also had clients who have included pictures of themselves from childhood which gave the scrapbook an added dimension (Fig. 5).

Significance of Symbols

As the client chooses pictures to represent his life I will ask him why he chose the picture, and we can further explore the possible symbolism behind them. The images chosen generally are quite revealing and open up the possibility for a wide range of heretofore unconscious feelings to emerge. One of my clients chose a picture of a clown to adorn the title page of her scrapbook. After much resolution, she admitted that the clown was a self-portrait and it represented the mask of happiness she had always felt she had to hide behind (Fig. 6).

Session Nine. During this session the final touches are added to the scrapbook and the nearing termination of the art therapy sessions is discussed. The final pages of the scrapbook should bring the client's life up to the present. Usually there are a few pages left blank in the scrapbook and I encourage the client to fill these in at home with pictures of his family and

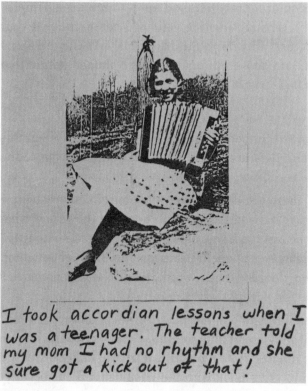

I took accordian lessons when I was a teenager. The teacher told my mom I had no rhythm and she sure got a kick out of that!

Fig. 5 Photos from childhood

future events to come. It is important to stress that their lives hold quality and significance. The only task left is for the client to find a picture to adorn the cover and title the scrapbook. The picture chosen can be anything the client wishes, but the title should be one which is meaningful. This is sometimes a cause of distress for the client because of the difficulty of titling one's life. Simple titles are best, but before I suggest anything, I let the client think about it a while.

At the end of the session, the scrapbook is completed. The client and I discuss his feelings about the process and its termination. We recap the events and the resolutions which have taken place. The client is usually excited about seeing the final product. I tell him I will bring it in to our last session together, bound and completed. Then I cover the scrapbook with construction paper, punch a few holes down the side and tie it together with some pretty, cloth ribbon. The client may wish to help with the binding, in which case I will punch the holes and allow him to tie it off in session ten.

Session Ten. The finished life review scrapbook is given to the client. The client and I are able to discuss the overall process at length and tie up any loose ends. We often talk about the benefits and effects of making the book. Resolutions of issues which occurred or are possibly still occurring should be touched upon.

At this point the client generally expresses gratitude and compliments me. I usually commend the client as well, telling him how rewarding it is for me to have shared in the experience of his life and the success of

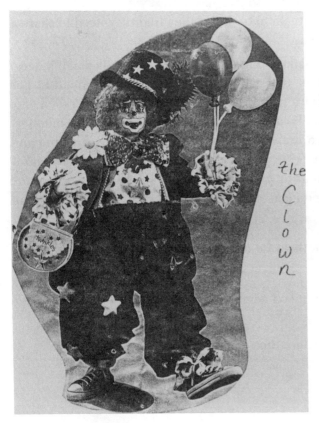

the *C l o w n*

Fig. 6 Mask of happiness

the scrapbook. Often he will ask me to sign the scrapbook. This has proven to be a nice way to end the session and finalize the process.

Making "Now" Significant

Making the present better for the elderly client is a significant accomplishment. Skillful use of the strategies that facilitate reminiscence and enhance life review can contribute to life satisfaction in the elderly population. The life review scrapbook helps the elderly client evaluate the meaning of his life and live for a better today. He has a renewed interest in life and creativity as he undergoes the process of the life review scrapbook. He is given the chance to examine and make sense of his life; he comes to understand his flaws and strengths and is better able to tolerate conflict and confront death. The quality of the present and the time remaining is emphasized rather than the quantity of time or the future.

The life review scrapbook is a tangible record of the elder's life; it serves to maintain self-identity and provides memory retraining. It also helps the elder to deal with issues of change, adaptation and death. As the elder works on his scrapbook, he creatively puts his life back into order.

Different Populations and the Life Review Scrapbbook

Art therapy combined with life review therapy also works well with other age groups alone or in groups. Following are topics which stimulate reminiscing.

First, I start my groups by stating that this is a group where everybody is to reminisce and share old memories with each other. I also say that it is often difficult to remember good memories, especially when a person is feel-

329

ing depressed. I encourage them to try but if they find they need to share a bad memory, that is also okay.

I bring in plenty of markers and drawing paper (usually small pieces) ,and I give the group a topic and ask them to draw a picture about it. For example, I ask them to draw a picture of one of their favorite toys when they were children. This is usually an easy task which takes about five minutes. After everyone is finished drawing, each person shares his drawing and memory. Generally someone else will have something to comment on regarding each reminiscence creating great group cohesion. The meaning of the art can also be explored and I can often learn a great deal about each patient for future exploration.

Topics and Questions for reminiscing with the elderly

First house

Map of childhood neighborhood

Favorite toys

Favorite leisure time activities

Vacations

Favorite foods and recipes

Holidays

What is your very first memory?

What was your life like when you were a child?

What were your parents like?

Did you have any siblings?

What was school like and did you like it?

Did you ever receive any honors, medals or special gifts?

What was dating like?

What was the first job you ever had?

How did you meet your spouse?

What was your wedding like?

How many children do you have?

What did you enjoy most about raising your children?

What did you enjoy least?

What are your favorite hobbies?

What might you change about your life

Summary

My study included seven experimental participants and seven control participants, all over 65 years of age and diagnosed with major depression at the facility where I am employed. The experimental participants completed the Beck Depression Inventory before and after the life review scrapbook (Beck, Ward, Mendelson, Mock & Erbaugh, 1961). The control participants simply completed the Beck Depression Inventory upon admission and discharge. All participants also received treatment team therapies.

The hypothesis posed was that the experimental group would show a significantly higher improvement in the Beck Depression Inventory than the control group through the use of the life review scrapbook. This hypothesis was confirmed with significant findings attesting to the magnitude of improvement in the experimental group. The experimental group improved an average of over 16 points on the Beck Depression Inventory, whereas the control group improved an average of only 4 points. Critical levels for an f-test were established and were significant. The life review scrapbook was found to be a sound and valid art therapy technique.

References

Beck, A., Ward, C., Mendelson, M., Mock J., & Erbaugh, J. (1961). *An inventory for measuring depression.* Archives of General Psychiatry, 4, 53-63.

Butler, R. N. (1963). *The life review: An interpretation of the aged.* Psychiatry, 26 (1), 65-76.

Butler, R. N. & Lewis, M. I. (1973). *Aging and mental health.* St Louis: Mosby.

Butler, R. N. (1974). *Successful aging and the role of life review.* Journal of the American Geriatric Society, 22 (1), 529-535.

Conklin, C. (1985). *Why a psychogeriatric unit?* Journal of Psychosocial Nursing, 23 (5), 23-27.

Dewdney, I. (1976). *An art therapy program for geriatric patients.* American Journal of Art Therapy, 15 (2), 249-254.

Erikson, E. (1963). *Childhood and society.* NY: W. W. Norton.

Schexnaydre, M. C. (1991). *An experimental study designed to lift depression in a psychogeriatric population through the use of the life review scrapbook and art therapy.* Unpublished master's thesis, California State University, Los Angeles.

Weiss, J. C. (1984). *Expressive therapy with elders and the disabled: touching the heart of life.* NY: The Hayworth Press.

The Art of the Sun Wheel
by Lillian M. Rhinehart, M.A., A.T.R, M.F.C.C.
and Paula Engelhorn, M.A., A.T.R.

Lillian M. Rhinehart and Paula Engelhorn combine over 40 year' experience in the fields of teaching, counseling and the arts. They have published articles in the American Art Therapy Association's Art Therapy Journal, Arts in Psychotherapy, and the Proceedings of the International Conference on Shamanism and Alternative Modes of Healing. They have given workshops extensively in the United States and Canada, and are co-founders of Rainbow Vision Circle, a non-profit corporation dedicated to growth and healing through the arts.

The Sun Wheel is an ancient rainbow wheel of color. It is a circle containing individuation concepts helpful to the therapist. Three archetypes form the basis of the Sun Wheel: 1) the circle or mandala as a representation of wholeness, 2) the rainbow color spectrum and 3) a numerical system of one, four, twelve. In combination these archetypes form a powerful base. The Sun Wheel offers a way to growth and healing through *ceremony and the art process.* Art therapy experiences are an integral component in working with the Sun Wheel.

Introduction

Jungian psychology, gestalt therapy concepts, color and ancient American wisdom are integrated in our work. We find these concepts best illustrated through the Sun Wheel, an ancient medicine wheel, a rainbow wheel of color. The Sun Wheel introduces the therapist to an individuation process and a way to apply this process within a therapeutic framework. Ancient wheels of the past provided ways for people to seek balance (Storm, 1972), and the return of the Sun Wheel in a time when the Earth and its people are in need of balance is providing a way for individuals and therapists to explore the quest for wholeness.

The concepts of the Sun Wheel encompass the following elements: 1) the circle or mandala as the greatest representation of wholeness; 2) the rainbow color spectrum; and 3) a number system of one, four, twelve. The circle, the rainbow and the numerical formation of the Sun Wheel are all ancient archetypes. Archetypes are synonymous with the word prototype and mean original model. Jung said, "Archetypes were and still are, living psychic forces that demand to be taken seriously"(Jung,1950). The archetypes of the Sun Wheel are a powerful foundation for individual and collective growth.

The Sun Wheel Archetypes
1. Circle
There are many legends in our Native American heritage of the circle as a path to wholeness. Perhaps the greatest of these is Black Elk's account. The holy man of the Sioux spoke eloquently of the circle: "You have noticed that everything an Indian does is in a circle, and that is because the Power of the World always works in circles, and everything tries to be round . . . even the seasons form a great circle in their changing, and always come back again to where they were. The life of a man is in a circle and so it is in everything where power moves" (Niehardt, 1960).

In *Memories, Dreams, and Reflections*, Jung spoke of mandala drawings and the goal of the development of the psyche in the following way, "I know that in finding the Mandala as an expression of the Self, I have attained for me the ultimate" (Jung, 1961). The Sun Wheel is also a circle or a mandala, and, like a mandala drawing, it is a statement of wholeness and represents a path to individuation.

2. Color
The Sun Wheel is a rainbow wheel of color represented by six hues. It is based on refracted light theory, where all the colors together form white light (Birren,1961). In the Sun Wheel, psychological and physical life begins on the circumference of the wheel. There are twelve major places around the perimeter, each represented by one of the six rainbow colors. The Sun Wheel functions similarly to an astrological wheel. Just as people enter the astro-

logical wheel at a particular sign, every person enters the Sun Wheel at a particular color. From their beginning color place at birth, each person starts the process of growth.

The twelve major places in the circumference of the Sun Wheel represent twelve Tribes or twelve different stages of growth. These stages each are a rainbow color. We come into the world as a member of a particular Color Tribe. The Color Tribe or home place on the Sun Wheel is easily identified by the individual. Because color is a known conscious or unconscious factor in everyone's life, home color places can readily be identified by walking around the Sun Wheel. Once individuals learn as much as they can in this beginning color place, they can travel around the wheel learning from all the other color positions.

The ability of individuals to choose personal color was clearly evident at a presentation we gave at an American Art Therapy Conference. During the presentation we correlated the four colors related to Jung's Four Psychological Functions with the Myers-Briggs in the following way:

Red was related to the function type, *feeling*
Blue to *thinking*
Yellow to *intuition*
Green to *sensation* (Jacobi, 1943).

We asked participants to choose their primary color from the four colors presented. Then we asked each participant to take the Myers-Briggs Type Indicator (Myers-Briggs, 1962). Though the numbers were small (30), the percentage of those identifying primary or auxiliary Functions through the four color choices was 70%. Our continuing work with the Sun Wheel and color identification is based on this strong implication that people can choose their color of origin.

Color surrounds us. It is a natural source of healing, it emanates from our bodies, and is above our heads and under our feet. The Sun Wheel unites the colors above our heads with the colors under our feet into a full circular rainbow. The Sun Wheel is a continuing circle of six distinct hues. All of the colors constitute a multiplicity of gradations from the deepest to the palest of shades. When meanings of colors and each of their shades can be explored in the art process, the personal work of growth and healing has begun and individuals are ready to move within the greater circle of color, the greater circle of consciousness.

3. Numerical Formation

The Sun Wheel structure is based on a number system of One, Four, and Twelve.

335

One represents Light, consciousness, the *Self* archetype.
Four represents the *Cardinal Directions*.
Twelve forms the circumference of the wheel representing the color
    places, or *Color Tribes*.

Nature and history give us many examples of these numerical patterns.
In one year, there are four seasons and twelve months. There is one God,
four archangels, and twelve signs of the zodiac. This particular numerical
order is no mere coincidence, but rather an archetype of consciousness.

The center of the Sun Wheel represents the Light of Consciousness or
the Self archetype. The Self (Jung, 1950) is the central archetype in the collective unconscious, just as the sun is the center of the solar system. It is the
archetype of order and unification, harmonizing all the archetypes. It unites
the personality, giving it a sense of "oneness." The major objective of the Sun
Wheel is to provide a way of working toward "oneness" or individuation.

The four places surrounding the central point on the Sun Wheel represent the Four Cardinal Directions. Native Americans have recognized and
named the powers of the Four Directions, and have assigned them four colors,
usually *yellow, white, red,* and *black*. One of the reasons the Four Directions
are powerful is because they have been identified over centuries as holding
great properties and are important resources for archetypal information.

The Four Cardinal Directions provide a source of psychological development. In the Sun Wheel, growth through the Cardinal Directions parallels
the idea of growth around the medicine wheel; one grows by exploring and
learning about the personal meanings associated with the four Cardinal
Directions (Storm, 1972). Another parallel to growth through the Cardinal
Directions is the Jungian typology system (Jacobi, 1943). In typology, *one way
of perceiving reality is given at birth and the remaining three ways are to be
developed as a way toward personal wholeness.* The Sun Wheel works in much
the same way. *We are born in one place on the wheel and in the growing
process, we move around the wheel and learn through the meanings of the
four Cardinal Directions.*

The twelve places marking the circumference of the Sun Wheel are
divided into two distinct groups, six Earth Tribes and six Sky Tribes. The
six colors of Earth and Sky are the same. The Red Earth place on the wheel
is exactly opposite the Red Sky place. Next is the Orange Earth Tribe opposite the Orange Sky Tribe, and so on until the six major colors of the Rainbow are completed and magnified by one.

These two distinct halves represent *psychological polarities*. The polarities are united in the center of the wheel, repeating the psychological truth

336

that *opposites must be reconciled for integration or individuation to occur.* The Gestaltist speaks of polarities and uniting the opposites through awareness or integration (Perls, 1969). Jungians also speak of uniting opposites. Many of these opposites can be integrated within the circle of the Sun Wheel. The Color Tribes in each of the two separate halves of the Wheel can represent any polarity: masculine and feminine principles, light and dark, spirit and matter.

Each of the twelve Color Tribes have four distinct smaller circles connecting them with the Center of the wheel, the place of consciousness. These distinct color places are lighter shades of each of the major Colors Tribes. The grouping of four smaller circles represent guides to the Center. In sequence, from the circumference to the Center, they depict the four kingdoms: *mineral, vegetable, animal, and human.*

The Sun Wheel and Art Therapy

The creation of art is essential to the healing process and to the understanding of symbols that arise out of any Sun Wheel activity. In the quiet contemplative process of creating the symbol, the personal meaning and message begin to be understood. Jung was an early advocate of creating symbols in art form, knowing the art helped unlock the mystery of symbolic meanings. Throughout his lifetime he constantly produced drawings, paintings and stone carvings of symbols which came out of his art process (Jung, 1960).

When we work with groups we place a representation of the Sun Wheel on the floor in the middle of the room, made of round circles of colored paper (Fig. 1). This simple depiction of the wheel becomes the focal point for the group experience. We ask people to bring their art expressions to the wheel. We sit in a circle around the wheel and process the work. Energy is high and awareness is facilitated. Suggestions are made for progressive steps that might be taken with another art activity to further develop additional insights.

The workshops we give are designed for a healthy population, such as graduate students, creative arts therapist, or individuals seeking growth and healing. They are designed to last an afternoon, a day, a weekend or as long as a semester. The longer the time, the deeper and richer the art experiences become for the participants. The Sun Wheel Individuation possibilities can be modified for use with many different populations in a variety of settings.

Other Audiences

The examples of adaptations have confirmed our sense of expansion for this way of working. In Quebec, a group of creativity instructors took the concepts of the Sun Wheel into a summer cancer camp for young patients and their families. The children responded and found new avenues for self expression through their work around the wheel.

We took the Sun Wheel to a residential treatment center for teenage boys. They reacted to the art activities in a very positive way. The creativity of the individual art therapist will add to further exploration and expansion of the wheel as a factor for growth and healing in many settings and with many different populations. We know whenever any of the major archetypes of the Sun Wheel are activated, the art therapy process is enhanced. Even the simple act of placing groups of people in a circle to talk about their art experiences activates the archetype of the circle and all the circle holds for growth.

A Wide Range of Art Materials

We find it important to offer groups a large assortment of art materials, everything from paints, clay, and pastels, to leather scraps, feathers, beads, art tissue and found objects. A large variety of all sorts of media helps the creative process. We display the art materials to stimulate the participants, increasing their potential for creativity and growth.

We begin Sun Wheel workshops by asking people to walk around the paper color representation of the wheel, or by asking them to walk around an Earth stone wheel. When we have led groups of over a hundred people around a Sun Wheel, the individuals in these groups always find their home or Tribe Color.

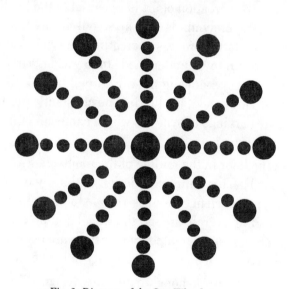

Fig. 1: Diagram of the Sun Wheel

Imagine a large wheel with six rainbow colors represented on each side of the wheel and then imagine people walking around that wheel until they find their color place. The archetype of circle and color immediately begin to interest groups of people.

We ask each person to find a color they sense is their home color, or a color they feel is needed in the now for growth and healing. Often participants find one color quite acceptable and the identical color on the opposite side of the wheel unacceptable. This acceptance or non-acceptance relates to the

Earth or Sky position of the color. Sometimes individuals feel strongly that the two identical shades of each color are different. For instance they might be absolutely sure one red place on the wheel is different than the other red place. The color positions echo where each person is in their individual growth process.

Art Therapy Exercises and the Sun Wheel

Once individuals in a group have found their home color, we ask participants to take an hour and, using any of the materials provided, explore the personal meaning of the color. We deliberately keep the directions as open-ended as possible to allow individual expression of each participant. At the end of the exploration, we always ask people to bring their work back to the wheel, and we process each experience. By focusing the work around the wheel we connect the person and their art expression to the circle. Our questions center on individual experiences of color, what the color means and what insights, gifts or surprises are revealed through the color exploration.

Another art activity we have done with large groups is to form family or Tribe units based on the same color each participant has selected. Through the art process, these groups then explore what that color means, or what they have in common as a color family. We sometimes have groups come back together after working all afternoon and present a group art activity to represent the color. These presentations often incorporate song, dance, movement and art work. The variety for personal and group exploration through the Sun Wheel is inexhaustible.

After participants have discovered a deeper relationship with their personal color, we teach about the qualities held within the Cardinal Directions. These Directions hold a vast amount of information. Directional knowledge is related to the path of the sun.

East, the place of the rising sun, holds the *quality of illumination.*
South, place of the noon day sun, is filled with *innocence and childlike wonder.*
West, where the sun sets, is the place of *maturity.*
North, place of the night sky, is the home of *wisdom and transitions.*

When participants have a basic sense of some of the qualities held within each direction, we ask them to relate the personal color choice to the Direction their color is near. Almost always the color chosen and the Direction the color is near has a deep significance for each participant. For instance, if someone finds their color is in or near the East they often have a sense of new beginnings.

We can see people nodding their heads in agreement as the qualities of each Direction are explained and they connect their color choice with those qualities. We see people get tears in their eyes as they respond to the Direction of their life in the moment. There is an acknowledgment given when individuals begin to feel connected to a far greater circle than themselves. This is the nature and the strength of archetypes. Circles function in us, Directions function in us, color functions in us, whether we know it or not.

The art activities suggested to explore the personal meaning of a Cardinal Direction center around the qualities of these Directions. Participants are asked to explore the Direction, and to integrate those qualities with their color choice. As with most of the art exercises we suggest, any and all media are available to help express the individual's ideas. Before the work is brought back to the circle for processing, we sometimes ask people to write a poem or a statement about their art product. We explore through media and metaphor the beauty of these strong archetypes influencing our psyches on a daily basis.

Exploring Opposites

As we explore the four Cardinal Directions in the art process, we can also investigate the relationship of the Earth or Sky position each participant selected in the original walk around the Sun Wheel. What does a drawing or art production look like coming from the Red Earth position; does it look different from Red Sky art work? We have asked participants to explore the

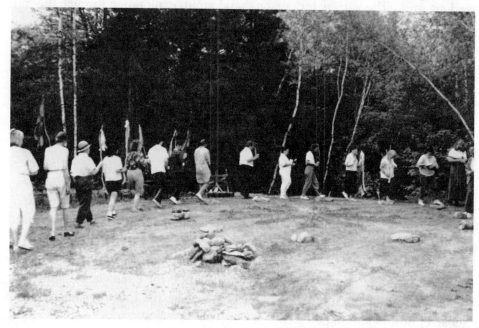

Fig. 2: Ceremony at the beginning of a Sun Wheel

340

opposite side of the wheel. If they chose Earth, what does it feel like and look like to be in the Sky? We can also ask people to explore their home position, and to add the opposite of Earth or Sky. These art activities help the *opposite feelings*, represented by Earth or Sky positions, to be integrated into the individual psyche.

Once we have done art processes to teach about color, Directions and Earth and Sky positioning, people are excited. The wheel is no longer an abstract idea; it has become a living reality. The inner circle of each participant is responding to the Sun Wheel in the room, and the participants are feeling the connection between all the circles: the sun, the moon, the Earth. We, as leaders, simply facilitate the *natural cyclical nature* of each of our beings. We are born, we mature, we die. On a psychological level, we repeat this cycle over and over again throughout our lives.

The Four Kingdoms

When the wheel becomes alive for participants, there is no end to growth through art that can arise out of its deep archetypal depths. For instance, the Four Kingdoms (*mineral, plant, animal, and human*) represented by the four stepping stones of the Sun Wheel, offer an endless source of personal information for growth and healing. Each time guided imagery is done around the Sun Wheel, the individual can choose a different color place from which to experience the meditation. Twelve different color places, each with four different possible guides offer an immense amount of potential information. Even if an individual completed all twelve positions in order, the next round of information would offer another set of guides for further explorations. The personal growth potential through this process is tremendous and never ending.

In the following art exercise, the Four Kingdom guides can be explored for growth. We ask participants to find a comfortable place around the wheel. One of us drums while the other leads guided imagery. In the guided imagery, we ask the participants to enter the wheel on their ray of color and seek a guide from one of the Four Kingdoms. Because we find animal guides to be wonderful teachers, we suggest in the beginning exercise to seek an animal guide. When the guided imagery is over, the group is instructed to create their guide in clay. If people are not visual and do not see a guide during the meditation, we say "*trust your hands*," so that they allow their hands to create the animal. We have not found anyone who cannot create an animal guide, either through the imagery experience or the direction to "*trust your hands*." Once the animal guide has been created, we deepen the experience through a written dialogue process and ceremony.

341

The guides most often represent personal psychological stages of development. Following the guided imagery, the art process amplifies the symbols and guides coming out of the Four Kingdoms. *Manifesting the symbols and continuing a dialogue with the guide is a key component to the powerful information which flows out of the Sun Wheel.*

The Beginning and The End

We explore the center of the wheel as a beginning focus for a long workshop, or to end a workshop. The center represents consciousness, mystery and the Self archetype. It is the balancing point for all polarities. When we begin with the center, we ask participants to create a three dimensional art form to represent their personal commitment to growth, or what they hope to achieve through the time of the workshop. It is a thought-provoking exercise allowing individuals an opportunity to look within. In the ceremony, we place the finished art products in the center of the wheel, asking each person to make a concise declaration about what they hope to activate through this art expression. It is a moving and effective way to begin a long term workshop.

Another art activity to close a workshop is to bring participants back to the center of the wheel, back to the center of themselves. We ask participants to relate parts of themselves to the center: the color they chose, the position of Earth or Sky, the Direction, all are woven into one statement. At the close of this exercise, we ask such questions as, "How

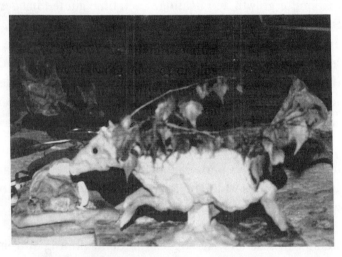

Fig. 3. Horse guide placed near the sun wheel

did the work come together," "How do you relate to the center" or "What was the inner dialogue that went on while you did the work?"

The process of the Sun Wheel offers many art explorations. It is an endless source for information, readily accessible to any who seek growth and healing. A one day workshop will allow the opportunity to explore one or two of the myriad facets of the Wheel. In a day, usually the personal color choice and the Direction can be explored. Week-long workshops are better. A semester to teach the art of the Sun Wheel is ideal.

Conclusion

The Sun Wheel Individuation process presents a way to work toward consciousness and healing. Through the activation of three archetypes *circle, Rainbow and numerical formation*, it offers an opportunity for groups to discover and claim individual unconscious parts of themselves and to integrate opposites within. The process depends on the art experience to help people find their own wisdom and inner balance. The Sun Wheel process offers art therapists a focal point for the growth inherent in the art experience.

The principles of the Sun Wheel are based on the belief that the Self archetype must be activated in each individual if growth is to occur. The Sun Wheel's foundation is the knowledge that once the Self archetype has been activated, co-creativity between man/woman and Spirit is achieved and the individuation process moves forward.

Our conviction is that only clients, patients or groups who touch and experience the central archetype can begin to find healing. Reflecting upon a dream about the center of a mandala, Jung said, "Through this dream I understood that the Self is the principle archetype of orientation and meaning" (Jung, 1961).

Working with the Sun Wheel has given us a deep appreciation of the three archetypes personified in its structure. Circle, color, and numerical formation are a rich base for continued growth producing exploration through the art process. Many art therapists have commented on the alive, creative energy emerging from the art of the Sun Wheel. We, too, have made the same observation and have experienced the creative flow and level of energy present in the work. The creative forces released through working with the Sun Wheel are representations of the Self Archetype.

We begin each workshop around the Sun Wheel and end each workshop with the wheel of rainbow color. Ritual and ceremony become a natural next step to the art of the Sun Wheel. We close a workshop with ceremony and invite all participants to honor each individual and the living symbol represented in the art work, acknowledging the presence of the Self archetype of healing. At the close of a Sun Wheel workshop the art productions are all held within the wheel. Each participant sees his or her work in its uniqueness, and also as a part of the whole, a part of the great collective circle.

References

Birren, F. (1961). *Color psychology and color theory*. NY: University Press.

Jacobi, J. (1973). *The Psychology of C. G. Jung*. New Haven: Yale University Press.

Jung, C.G. (1950). *Collected works*. N. J.: Princeton: Princeton University Press.
—— (1960). *The structure and dynamics of the psyche*, vol. 8 of the Collected Works. Princeton: Princeton University Press.
—— (1961) *Memories, dreams and reflections*. NY: Pantheon Books.

Myers-Briggs, I. (1962) *The Myers-Briggs type indicator*. NJ: Educational Testing Services.

Niehardt, J. G. (1961). *Black Elk speaks*. Nebraska: University of Nebraska Press.

Perls, F. (1969). *Gestalt therapy verbatim*. UT: Real People's Press.

Storm, H. (1972). *Seven arrows*. NY: Ballantine Books.

Women and Art Therapy
by Ellen Speert, M.Ed., A.T.R.

Ellen Speert is a registered art therapist in private practice in San Diego and past president of the San Diego Art Therapy Association. She teaches art therapy at the University of California in San Diego and in Switzerland, at Institut de Perfectionnement.

> *Psychological theory, like any other cultural institution, reflects the larger Western patriarchal culture in the unexamined assumption that the white, middle class, heterosexual "paradigm man" defines not just his own reality but human reality. Thus, without a critique of patriarchal bias in existing approaches to "human development," the experience of the "paradigm man" will be reified as "truth" while that of others will be distorted for not conforming to patriarchal dictates.*
>
> *from* Women's Growth in Connection

In exploring the topic of women and art therapy, my goal is to provide an expanded context for the theoretical as well as for the practical work we do as therapists. I am not suggesting that the traditional constructs of human development upon which most psychological training is based are wrong, but merely limited. They need expansion in order to embrace the emerging research on female growth and development. I will be speaking in generalized terms about "women" and "men," but please keep in mind that this refers to the "feminine" and "masculine" in each of us. This paper is intended to widen our perspective, not substitute one sexist view for another.

I will first present a brief overview of some of the new theoretical work on women's psychological growth and development. This research is being conducted by women whose purpose is to break out of the psychological constructs of the "paradigm man" referred to in the opening quote. In the second part, I will discuss the use of this feminist perspective in art therapy and show how other art therapists (both male and female) work from this paradigm. The third section presents the voice and images of a client who, over the course of two years of group art therapy, exemplified this female model of growth. I choose to present her own words rather than describe her process. This illustrates the principle of shared power and knowledge in place of the traditional, hierarchical model of therapist/client knowing in which the therapist presents her/his "more objective" perspective of the client. The last section provides some guidelines and directives.

1. Women's Psychology

The art therapy profession is practiced predominantly by women and the majority of our adult clients are women. In fact, to a great extent, we are the founders, clinicians, researchers, writers, and leaders as well as the consumers in this field. Despite this, our training programs and the structure of our research continue to reflect a framework based on psychological theories constructed by men, utilizing studies of male subjects (Wadeson, 1989, Talbott-Green, 1989). It is my feeling that trying to evaluate and treat women within these male constructs is no more appropriate than trying to sculpt a woman's body from a male model. There is more to it than adding breasts and deleting the penis...there is needed, in fact, a different basic structure upon which to build.

Similarly, we must base our therapeutic approaches on studies and theoretical constructs based on female development, sensitizing ourselves to the unique (although often pathologized) attributes inherent to women. Thanks to the recent writings emerging from the Stone Center colloquia, as well as the work of Jean Baker Miller (1976), Carol Gilligan (1982), Emily Hancock (1989) and others, we are able to broaden our perspective to include women-based models and thus more appropriately shape the therapy we practice as women, with women.

A. Development: A Look at Differences

The value our Western culture places on individual accomplishments and the emphasis we put on development of the self is reflected in and reinforced by our psychological theories. The developmental stages outlined by Freud, Erikson and many other male researchers are structured by the concept of increasing levels of separation from others. Erikson (1950) saw human development begin with the establishment of basic trust in infancy and then move through the progressive stages of autonomy, initiative, and industry (all solo tasks) before the issue of relationship (intimacy) reemerges in the young adult years. Freud (1905) also saw our development as a struggle for basic self mastery (over impulses), with relationship viewed in terms of drive gratification. Jean Baker Miller (1981), on the other hand, found that from infancy there is an emerging sense of self as "being in relationship," a dynamic interplay between caretaker and infant. She posits that corresponding to Erikson's stages of autonomy and initiative in boys, girls are developing "new configurations" and new understandings within relationships, based on greater levels of relationship complexity. From the quality of her emotional connections, a young girl's sense of self esteem, competence and effectiveness develops.

Adolescence, a time when boys are expanding into the world, tends to be a period of contraction and conformity for girls (Hancock, 1989). Despite an earlier sense of self confidence, creativity and vitality, the early adolescent girl finds herself trying desperately to conform, hiding her individuality and subverting her self confidence. Yet during this time, her sense of competence and self worth come from her ability to take care of relationships even at the expense of developing more individualistic skills (Kaplan, Klein & Gleason, 1985). Late adolescence is an important time of relational growth. During this period, greater flexibility, sensitivity, adaptability and tolerance for relational conflict is achieved in normal female development.

This new construct confronts the assumptions of female deficiencies as measured by the previously held standards of separation, individuation and autonomy. It is interesting to note that while certain qualities are societally encouraged in the adult female (care-taking, putting the needs of others above one's own and having weak boundaries), these are the same features we label "co-dependent" since they deviate from the male norm. This illustrates the need for the construction of new models of healthy female development which will differ dramatically from the ones presently held.

B. A New Developmental Paradigm

In defining female identity, Miller (1976) identified the ability to form and maintain relationships as the organizing principle. Out of this paradigm, a body of theoretical work has emerged from the Stone Center colloquia and is collected in their book, *Women's Growth in Connection*. In this book Janet Surrey states that a female-centered theory would "...trace the development of identity through specific relationships and relational networks...to examine the nature of cognitive and emotional internal capacities." She goes on to specify that this theory would not be based upon "developmental crises or fixed states" as in the male-based theories of Freud and Erikson (p. 38-39). She thus moves the model from "object-relations," based on human separateness, to "subject-relations" or a "self-in-relation" model.

This new paradigm, with its emphasis on interpersonal connection, leads us to explore more deeply the quality of empathy, both as a measure of maturation and as a significant factor in treatment.

C. Empathy

Most clinical theories are based on the concept of ego strength which emphasizes the development of firm ego boundaries. Though seldom discussed as a criterion in the measurement of psychological maturity, empathy is also dependent upon a high degree of ego strength. Judith Jordan writes, "in order to empathize, one must have a well differentiated sense of self in addition to an appreciation of and sensitivity to the differences as well as the sameness of another person," (p. 89). She also describes the sequence of steps necessary for an empathic relationship. These are:

- cueing in to verbal and non-verbal affective states of others
- surrendering to this affective arousal and identifying with this affective state as if it is one's own and
- resolution—regaining a sense of separation and understanding

Therefore one must have ego flexibility to be able to relax and then restructure the boundaries to accommodate an empathic response. Adolescent girls tend to involve themselves in the development of these skills, while their male peers are working on more externally focused tasks.

A second dynamic which tends to manifest itself differently in males than in females is one's relationship to power.

D. Power >> Empowerment

The perspective of power as reflected in the traditional male paradigm is that of power over something or someone in the quest for self actualization. The female perspective of power has more often been lived out through the nurturance and empowerment of others. This has been seen most clearly in the traditional care-taking role of the home-maker.

Another relationship to power, and the basis on which I structure my therapeutic approach, is that of mutual empowerment. Through this, each person feels more real, more energized, more able to respond and act. Mutual empowerment allows both people to feel greater personal clarity and affirmation. Janet Surrey (1986) writes of the creativity and energy aroused by mutual affective connection which leads to increased knowledge and awareness of both self and other. This concept of mutual empowerment is central to my focus on a group therapy format in working with women. I will say more about this in section two. I will now present the concepts of empathy and empowerment as they are reflected in the therapist-client relationship.

E. Therapeutic Distance

The traditional stance, which has determined our view of the appropriate amount of distance between client and therapist, has been based upon two assumptions. The first is that we must remain objective, unemotional, relatively impersonal and not too involved. The second is to avoid gratifying the patient, in that frustration and deprivation lead to growth. This stance is based on a patriarchal perspective which places the therapist in the parental and, therefore, inherently superior role (Stiver, 1985).

The feminist model of treatment challenges these two assumptions, creating instead a relational matrix. It allows us to open ourselves to the client's experience, responding more authentically to their relational needs, reducing the neutral, objective position while expanding the frame of reference. One must, of course, continue to place the needs of the client as the focus of treatment. I believe that sharing ourselves to create a relational context often does just that. It has been my observation that empathy and connection meet a greater need than adherence to traditional roles, and add richness and depth to the experience for both client and therapist.

2. Art Therapy from a Feminist Perspective

In this section I will discuss specific applications of women's psychology within the practice of art therapy. We will look at:
a) perspectives on symbol interpretation
b) therapeutic distance and use of self in treatment and
c) the group therapy format

A. Symbol Interpretation

In striving to be viewed as valid within the greater psychological community, many art therapists have, consciously or unconsciously, internalized the belief that validity of assessment, intervention and research must be based upon standardized, measurable graphic productions. A depersonalized approach to symbolic interpretation has logically ensued. In some cases, this even includes the analysis of images in isolation from the artist and the artistic act. How can this serve the need for connection, empathy and empowerment which we have seen is integral to women's psychological development? A non-patriarchal perspective in the practice of art therapy has been

349

reflected in the writings of male as well as female art therapists. Shaun McNiff (1989) and Bruce Moon (1991), for example, both refuse to label pathology or base their treatment on the dissection of imagery. As Moon (1991) writes, "Those who force visual symbols into verbal constructs may be guilty of 'imagicide', i.e., the murderous destruction of an image" (p. 28).

Indeed, our profession has long struggled over the accuracy with which we can assess an image separate from its creator, and yet we continue to conduct our research following traditional parameters in our quest for objectivity. Harriet Wadeson (1989) points out the irony that in our female-dominated field, we strive to emulate the male models of research and therapy(separating, cataloguing and quantifying), despite the inappropriateness of this approach. Marlene Talbott-Green (1989) enumerates the reasons for the exclusion of feminist psychological research in our journals (which in turn keeps it out of our practices).

My position, as an art therapist as well as an art therapy educator, is to de-emphasize the interpretation of symbols for and with clients. Instead, as a group, we connect with these symbolic expressions, breathing them into ourselves, rather than taking them apart. This joining is an empathic response to the art as well as to the artist. It also reduces the tendency to create "flat-feeling," easy-to-label, clichéd representations of feelings, since emphasis is not placed on the verbal explanation of the art's meaning. I do value the story each woman tells as it emerges from her art creation, but words never seem to fully honor or convey the depth of the actual art-making. I see the creative act carrying the healing, often telling the story without words, and truly connecting us. As Moon says, "Meaning is located in the context of relationship to others" (p.31).

B. Therapeutic Distance

The second point of departure from the traditional therapeutic model is reflected in my perspective on therapeutic distance. In the art therapy groups I lead I am a full participant. I work on my own pieces and discuss them to the depth of my own understanding. My guidelines for this are:

- to use the group's needs to shape the themes within myself which I choose to explore
- to stay conscious of how my creations interact with theirs and
- when my issues are incompatible with those of the group, I save them for my own time outside the group

By participating on this level I attempt to "stay honest" with the process, modeling as well as giving permission to truly enter the art. I am not asking others to explore themselves in a way I, myself, would not. And, as Bruce Moon (1990) writes, "I believe that the most validating experience I can offer my patients is to respond to their (art)work with works of my own that resonate with and illuminate their struggle" (p. 62). This reduces the patriarchal structure, that of a therapist who is above or removed from the group. It also diminishes the sense that I am spying on the participants, although I do observe both the individual art-making and group process closely.

Pat Allen (1988) writes of a third significant factor, the issue of transference. She states, "In art therapy, remaining true to the art process can offer an alternative to transference as the operative principle" (p. 118). The art pieces, rather than exclusively the therapist, contain the transference, and thus the therapist is free to join the group in a more authentic way than the traditional transferential relationship would dictate.

Martha Haeseler (1989) examines the appropriateness of therapists creating artwork alongside their clients. Although she sees many advantages (increased client participation, enhanced therapeutic alliance and mirroring), she also notes the countertransference problem. I find that this last factor further fuels authenticity and deep connection but requires experience and skill (and is greatly aided by supervision) in order to be utilized effectively.

C. Group Work

Although in my practice I do see individuals and couples, I strongly believe in working with my female clients in groups whenever possible. Yalom (1975) has written at length of the advantages of group treatment. For women, this model becomes even more useful, based on the issues discussed in part one. I feel that the structure of our therapy should parallel the context of our lives as women. New self images emerge based on relational learning, which in turn throws light on previous relationships, enhancing further relational growth. "The more frequent mirroring, mutual identification and more accurate empathy may all strengthen the girl's sense of relatedness, connection, and a feeling of being directly, emotionally understood," says Jordan (p. 34).

The group naturally structures itself in a circle, within which each woman travels, starting with a sense of isolation, gradually growing into connection with others, but then moving into a deeper appreciation of her own individuality. We have labored under the misconception that creativity is a solo act, yet the response of one image to another within the group, and the rituals that emerge from our group process, are more creative than the sum of our individual expressions.

Now I would like you to hear C's story and see some of her images as she describes her experience over a two-year period in a women's art therapy group.

3. C's Story

"When I began art therapy, the core difficulty that I faced was my unwillingness to participate in life. "Destroyer/Creator" (Fig. 1) expresses some of that struggle. This two-canvas image is a portrait of myself—both nurturing and devouring, in pain and in strength—and of my view of the universe—giving life and taking it away.

"Not wanting to be responsible for the consequences of my existence, I imagined other people and outside circumstances to be responsible. This posture gave me a strange form of negative power, but at the expense of my sense of self definition and, ultimately, of my self worth. "Nature Abhors a Vacuum" (Fig. 2) is the image that unveiled my awareness of the destructive 'power' I had generated by my posture of escape and resignation.

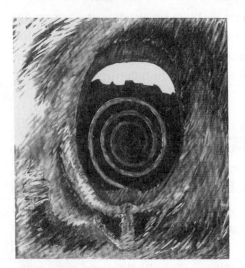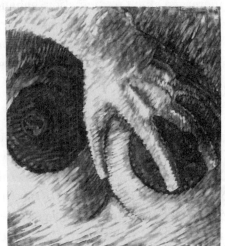

Fig. 1 Destroyer/Creator

"My abdication also resulted in not wanting to be responsible for, or even connected to, my body. A finger-painting (Fig. 3) revealed this dislocation to me. The central figure (in red) is surrounded by flames (also red), except for her head, which is protected by a green 'helmet'—the ultimate mind/body split. In the upper right-hand corner I created a 'dream' image of what I was seeking/hoping for. It is all green—an integrated body, its posture transformed from 'hands thrown up in despair' to 'hands extended in strength,' within a ring of green flame.

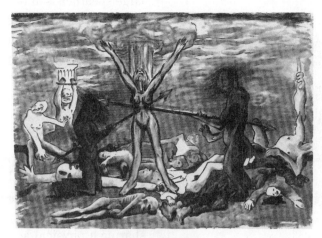
Fig. 2 "Nature Abhors a Vacuum"

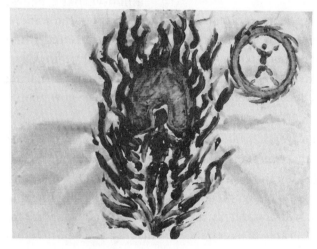
Fig. 3 Fingerpainting of my abdication from my body

'I also held myself away from genuine relationship by withdrawing from other people. The image (Fig. 4) of a woman with her back to a telephone illustrated this for me. I had turned away from human interaction (symbolized by the telephone) in fear, depression (the 'helmet' in this picture is black, not green), and also in anger.

"My posture of self-abandonment also obscured any sense, for me, of personally chosing a direction in life. The painting (Fig. 5) of a partly 'invisible' and unconscious woman reclining on a couch showed this lack. My anger/power is evident in the threatening figure hovering in the background and in the 'invisible' attacking dog next to the unconcerned dog.

"As I was able to internalize and transform the information in these (and other) images, I created a picture (Fig. 6) where the woman is able to materialize, awaken, and take some control (saying 'STOP' and collaring the dog).

"From that image I was able to readdress the issues in "Nature Abhors a Vacuum" (Fig. 1). In this new drawing, 'Yes' (Fig. 7), the central figure, is now embracing life in all its horror (not giving up in the face of it), she is owning her own anger/power (the nuclear explosion), and recognizing her connection to everything (the umbilical cords). A subsequent image (not shown) of a woman with

353

large spearheads at her waist, but not piercing her, and with a stream of water flowing through her from the starry sky onto the earth below, was ultimately cleansing and empowering.

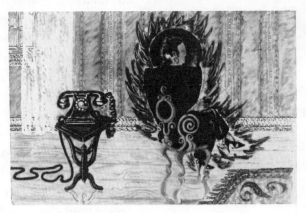

Fig. 4 A woman with her back to the telephone

"In the group art-making sessions I was able to form a bond with others by sharing a physical act, a non-verbal process, with them. Then I was drawn more and more into speaking about the work—no longer out of obligation—but giving myself permission. I found I had something to say. This transformation came about because of many things, but two of the more important were, first, from experiencing regular group sharing of personal concerns and, second, from a growing awareness of how people express themselves through art.

"Meeting weekly in a small circle, telling one another about our lives through our art was a powerful experience, and I realized that I was not so isolated. I began to see patterns in our 'stories,' not just random events, and this new vision imparted a kind of significance to life. Watching other people make objects and then discover how deeply meaningful those objects were for them was also powerful. I was able to experience art-making as a self-defining process—not just making a beautiful object.

"Finally, I want to stress the importance of the group context. Within a respectful, supportive non-invasive group environment, created by a sensitive therapist, I was able to define my own art and, consequently, myself. It allowed me to

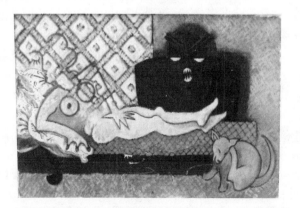

Fig. 5 Abandonment of a personally chosen direction in life

reconnect with my childhood feelings of well-being, to go on to establish better relationships with the people in my life and to establish and accomplish my personal goals of full-time art-making and a mutually supportive marriage."

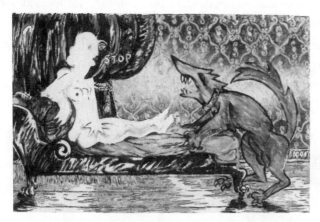

Fig. 6   Woman materializes and starts taking control

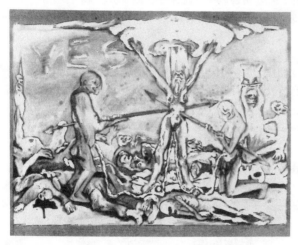

Fig. 7   'Yes' is now embracing life in all its horror

After writing her own 'story,' C. and I reviewed the great volume of artwork she had created and chose some to illustrate her journey. We thus become even more connected as we reflected upon the distance we had come together. Therefore our process in creating this chapter paralleled that of group art therapy. We began with a shared purpose, then created alone, but finally came back together to share what we had made, both being enriched by the experience

4. Directives and Guidelines

Following are a few guidelines to help you on your way to creating a feminist art therapy environment.

- Pursue your own personal therapy and art so that you can safely join in the process with your clients and not get lost or overwhelmed.
- Design the physical therapeutic environment to accommodate comfortable interaction, reducing a sense of separateness. I choose to

355

work on the floor, which is covered with industrial carpet and pillows. This affords a sense of shared open space and comfort. Tables seem to set boundaries between us.

• Provide materials which access the creativity, strength and playfulness of the young girl within. These include, but are not limited to, feathers, glitter, nature objects, colored tissue, pipe cleaners, finger paint and jewelry bits, as well as the standard clay, paint and drawing materials.

• Be sensitive to and encourage the emergence of group themes, stories and projects, as well as respect the uniqueness of each woman. Realize this may take a non-verbal form.

• Encourage the creation of group ritual. These rituals may be different for each group of clients and carry rich significance.

"In imagery, women's world may be viewed as a web of connectedness in which a woman would attempt to mend tears."   Wadeson

Conclusion

Intuitively, many male as well as female art therapists have been working with and responding to their clients within the feminist paradigm of connection, empathy and mutual empowerment. Yet we as a field continue to formulate our research and treatment models on the traditional patriarchal psychotherapeutic designs. This chapter has outlined some of the elements inherent in women's growth and development and has illustrated how art therapy can reflect this model. Many thanks go to C. for adding her voice and images, deepening my experience as we worked together.

References

Allen, P. B. (1988). *A consideration of transference in art therapy.* The American Journal of Art Therapy. 26 (4), 113-118.

Ellis, M. L. (1989). *Women: the mirage of the perfect image.* The Arts in Psychotherapy. 16 (4), 263-276.

Erikson, E. (1950). *Childhood and society.* NY: W. W. Norton.

Gilligan, C. (1982). *In a different voice.* Cambridge: Harvard Press.

Hancock, E. (1989). *The girl within.* NY: Fawcett Columbine.

Haeseler, M. P. (1989). *Should art therapists create artwork alongside their clients?* The American Journal of Art Therapy 27 (3), 70-79.

Jordan, J. (1984). *Empathy and self boundaries.* Stone Center colloquium paper, Wellesley, MA.

Jordan, J., Surrey, J. L. et al. (1981). *Women and empathy: implications for psychological development and psychotherapy.* Stone Center colloquium paper, Wellesley, MA.

Kaplan, A., Klein, R., and Gleason, N. (1985). *Women's self development in late adolescence.* Stone Center colloquium paper, Wellesley, MA.

Miller, J. B. (1981). *The development of women's sense of self.* Stone Center colloquium paper, Wellesley, MA.

Miller, J. B. (1976). *Toward a new psychology of women.* Boston: Beacon Press.

Moon, B. (1990). *Existential art therapy: the canvas mirror.* Springfield, Illinois: C. C. Thomas McNiff, S. (1989). *Depth psychology of art.* Springfield, Illinois: C. C. Thomas.

Stiver, I. (1985). *The meaning of care: reframing treatment models.* Stone Center colloquium paper, Wellesley, MA.

Talbott-Green, M. (1989). *Feminist scholarship: spitting into the mouths of the gods.* The Arts in Psychotherapy, 16 (4). 253-262.

Wadeson, H. (1989). *Reflections: in a different image: are "male" pressures shaping the "female" art therapy professions?* The Arts in Psychotherapy. 16 (4). 327-330.

Yalom, I. (1975). *The theory and practice of group psychotherapy.* NY: Basic Books

Clinical Art Therapy In-Service Education
Janet K. Long, M.A. MFCC, A.T.R.
and Linda Chapman, M.A., A.T.R.

Janet K. Long and Linda Chapman, leaders in the field of art therapy in the San Francisco Bay area, have given many art therapy in-service presentations to other mental health professionals. In the following article they summarize their thoughts for art therapists, who may be called on for presentations to non-art therapists, suggesting ways to make the experience productive and satisfying.

Part I
Tailoring Your In-Service Presentation to the Needs of the Facility
by Janet Long

Janet K. Long is adjunct professor, California College of Arts and Crafts, Oakland and in private psychotherapy and art psychotherapy practice. She is co-designer of and instructor in the post-masters Certificate Program in Clinical Art Therapy, University of California, Berkeley-Extension, co-author of The Windo Manual, *a therapeutic/educational resource tool, a consultant to agencies seeking art therapy staff training to meet their special needs since 1975, and a founding member of the Northern California Art Therapy Association (1973), receiving this organization's Distinguished Person Award in Education, 1990, and the Affiliate Chapter Member Award, AATA.*

After teaching art therapy at the college and university level for over twelve years, I have been sought out by social work agencies and hospital clinics to bring practical art therapy training to their trainee and permanent staff members. These clinics generally treat troubled children and their families, severely emotionally disturbed/abused or abandoned children, learning disabled/emotionally disturbed children and adolescents, and individuals and families with chronic illnesses/chronic pain and other trauma syndromes. The common cry from these clinics is, "Give us practical art therapy methods for assessment and treatment with our special population of clients/patients that we can learn and use now!!" They want easily accessible methods to help them assess and treat clients who do not respond well to other therapy methods.

What kind of training is appropriate? What can or should be taught in a limited amount of time to other professionals who usually have a great deal of general therapeutic knowledge, but very little about art therapy?

The following is a general outline of the type of presentation I make. It varies a great deal, of course, depending on the specific needs of the audience, and the amount of time available.

General principles

Art therapists offering their expertise as in-service training to other professionals need to clearly distinguish the practice of art therapy from these other professions. The clinical uses of art as an imaginative healing process encompasses unique attitudes, knowledge, procedures, and training—distinct from psychology, social work, marriage and family counseling, special education, or nursing.

I have learned to tailor the in-service presentation to the specific needs of each facility requesting the training. For example, one family service agency called me and requested that I provide a 9-hour training in child art therapy. They had no expertise in this area and could only afford 9-hours of training for their staff and interns. They wanted me to give a general presentation on the appropriate developmental uses of art media and processes used with different aged children and adolescents; then to present specific cases illustrating art therapy with depressed and anxious children, abused and traumatized children, pre-psychotic and psychotic children, and troubled teenagers; after this, to consult with the staff on their problem cases. A tall order in 9 hours!

I listened carefully to the director's description of what this agency wanted from this in-service education. I asked her about the kinds of cases her agency was struggling with. I also asked about the backgrounds of her staff members and about the type of on-site room space in which this training could take place. Fees were agreed upon both for my time and the art supplies needed to give such an in-service. With this information I could then design an outline of the theory, techniques and cases most relevant to this institution's needs. I could also then assemble the art supplies, handouts, and slides I needed to teach this group.

Each art therapist needs to define her/his area of expertise within the field of art therapy, e.g., child art therapy (sub-specialty: learning disabled, severely emotionally disturbed, trauma victims, foster children, hospitalized psychiatric populations, etc.) Once you have clearly defined your own areas of interest, point-of-view, and special skills and knowledge, then you are ready to prepare the materials from your professional work that fit this focused subject. It is important to be organized in your thinking and presentation style, in your knowledge of materials and their uses, in your references and high-quality visuals used to teach (charts, slides, videos, etc.)

Begin by giving in-service trainings in the institution in which you are employed. Building confidence and skill in teaching the ideas and methods of clinical art therapy comes with much practice over time. You might start by explaining what you are doing with your clients/patients/students at your worksite, perhaps to communicate to team meetings or to enlist support and interest from enabling staff. Most fellow staff members become fascinated with how the art itself speaks to the issues of a particular client. Showing a series of several clients' artwork and explaining the interactive/imaginative process between the client and his/her art and between the client and therapist is the most basic way to talk about the therapeutic benefits of art therapy in relation to given goals for treatment. Your enthusiasm and thoughtful preparation will carry your audience to a new understanding of your professional role, your dedication to your clients, and your unique contribution to the treatment of clients in that facility.

The style of presentation that serves me best after I have listened carefully to the needs of the host institution includes:

1. Introducing myself—my background and interest in this facility's needs; followed by staff members telling me what they would like from this in-service experience.

2. Giving general information about major theoretical ideas in the form of simple explanations and prepared charts hung on the wall (using a blackboard if needed to diagram or list various information).

3. Giving handouts to reinforce information given and reprints of articles that give depth to this particular topic in art therapy.

4. Demonstrating the essential art media and ways of presenting these art media to clients. Giving participants specific well-known methods and for-

mats that have proven effective within the field of art therapy for the population under consideration. Giving ways of presenting and using special art processes that I have developed in my own practice. Presenting these students with easy-to-control, low-frustration materials and methods will ensure their enjoyment of the process; these professionals are hungry to explore their own creative process while experiencing the art tasks you give them. The hands-on part of the in-service vitalizes the concepts presented.

5. Showing high-quality slides illustrating case histories that are relevant for this in-service; being sure to discuss the structured or unstructured process involved, presentation of media, outcomes as they relate to treatment goals and through which the client reveals issues that give the therapist cues for future sessions. I also show slides that illustrate theoretical/research ideas in my presentation (e.g., examples of art by abused children that correlate with research by other art therapists).

6. Taking questions from my audience; answering these with examples from my own experience and references to the art therapy literature.

7. Asking for feedback from my audience: Did my presentation meet their needs? Do they want more training? If so, discussing local courses being given and further readings. Asking if they want another in-service to further develop the topics under consideration, or if they would like on-going case consultation? (Eventually, if an institution finds the need for art therapy services, they think about hiring an art therapist for a staff or consulting position.)

8. The therapists involved generally have and express feelings of frustration and burn-out with individuals and families with such long-term problems. The art therapy in-service training that I design for each clinic has each therapist actually engaging in the creative process. They brainstorm about what they want from the training, discuss specific cases, (I visually diagram what they are saying on a chalkboard), but even more they learn about clinical art therapy paradigms and methods through hands-on art activities. This active participation in creative learning by "doing art" seems to restore these therapists' interest in their cases and helps revitalize their own energies. Some of the therapists find themselves so interested in art and art therapy after these trainings, that they enroll in further classes and certificate programs to continue the learning process.

Now some specifics.

Beginning Art Therapy Paradigms

After the therapists in each setting describe what they want from the art therapy training, I introduce basic art therapy paradigms that usually fit most groups' educational needs. Very few of these therapists have formal art training, and most have had no art experience since elementary school. Thus, my approach is to acquaint these beginners with art media and art therapy methods in the least intimidating way.

I begin by talking about art therapy principles, art media, and methods that will be presented in the training, using slides from my files of clients' artwork to illustrate the talk.

Slides are also shown of normal art development in children and adolescents (Kellogg, 1967; Kramer, 1972; Lowenfeld, 1939, 1975; Naumberg, 1973; Rubin, 1978; Uhlin, 1979), so that these therapists have a developmental frame of reference when looking at artwork (i.e., how most people develop the forms of people, trees, houses, cars, boats, and other objects and scenes from basic scribble and placement patterns). The language of looking at artwork (Furth, 1988) is also discussed, e.g., feelings evoked at first glance, what is central in the placement of the lines and shapes on the page, obvious additions or omissions to the figures drawn, transparencies, perspective, movement, color, context and content of the subject, and representational and abstract styles of conceptualization.

From this opening slide show and explanation of form in artworks, the creative process from a process and media perspective is discussed. The most complete system available, The Expressive Therapies Continuum (ETC), (Kagin and Lusebrink, 1978), is given to students in an outline form. This outline emphasizes that all creative activity starts with the kinesthetic and sensory ("K—S") experiences of the artist/client, then progresses to the perceptual and affective ("P—A") levels of experience, and then continues to develop at the cognitive and symbolic ("C—Sy") levels—all integrated progressively and culminating at the creative ("Cr") level. The development of this creative process theoretically comes from how our brains are vertically and laterally organized, and parallels theories of Piagetian cognitive development already familiar to most of the therapists attending these in-service trainings.

Each level on the Continuum is explained in developmental terms:

• How each person experiments with art materials at the "K—S" level (kinesthetic and sensory), using basic movement and sensation, experiencing little "reflective distance" in relation to the media itself (i.e., the artist is temporarily merged with the art materials).

• This basic experience moves the artist to perceive the structural properties/boundaries in forms and feel feelings that modify this inner organization at the "P—A" level (perceptual and affective), thereby experiencing more "reflective distance" in the creative process, a dialogue between the person and the art media.

• At the "C—Sy" level (cognitive and symbolic), the artist is able to cognitively describe and attribute intuitive-symbolic meaning to the lines and shapes of his/her artwork, performing complex interactions with the media.

• At the "Cr" level (creative), the art process comes to closure, where inner and outer reality become bridged in a synthesis, a whole expression of the artist.

The discussion of the structural nature of art materials comes from this review of the "ETC." Depending on the art media used, the artist/client can experience varying levels of freedom of expression, varying levels of emotional arousal, and varying needs for uses of ego defenses. Landgarten (1981, 1987) rates art materials on a 10-point continuum from the least to the most controlled:

Least controlled

1: Wet clay

2: Watercolor paints

3: Soft plasticene (colored modeling clay)

4: Oil pastels

5: Felt markers (thick tip)

6: Collage

7: Hard plasticene (colored modeling clay)

8: Felt markers (thin tip)

9: Colored pencils

10: Lead pencils

Most controlled

For purposes of training and developmental considerations, I present the *most controlled media first* to other therapists and then progress through the media list toward the least controlled media. I also present what I call "transitional media," those media embodying the range of resistive (most controlled) to fluid (least controlled), such as water-based aquarelles, (crayons that can transform into watercolors with the addition of a wet brush to the drawn surface).

The last major paradigms I present in these in-service trainings involve the theoretical orientation of art therapy methods presented. Art therapy has its roots in art, art education, psychoanalytic and analytic psychology, and has developed methods involving Gestalt, humanistic, phenom-enological, medical, visual thinking and imagery ideas.

My aim is to present a wide range of methods based on these theories, making the goal of the assessment and the aim of the treatment a priority. Different circumstances and goals require the use of more or less structured and directive methods. Each training group chooses whether the training will emphasize more pragmatic or interpretive approaches. This eclectic approach will be illuminated in the next section.

Actively Learning about Art Materials and Art Therapy Methods

First, I demonstrate a simple technique with the easiest to control media, e.g., crayons, markers, oil pastels and chalks. I usually introduce the *projective scribble technique* (Betensky, 1973), where each participant is asked to choose one color from the assorted media on the table, then to place this crayon or marker in the center of an 18" x 24" piece of white drawing paper, and, with eyes closed, to scribble freely on the page.

Next, each is asked to look at their scribble, turning the paper four ways to see their marks from four different perspectives. To get distance I suggest that they stand up at the table or put the paper on the floor as they move it to help them find a suggestion of "something," in what they have drawn.

As soon as they see something interesting in their scribbles, each is asked to take other colors and complete the drawing of "what they see." Projecting onto the scribbles uses basic principles of visual thinking (Arnheim, 1974), and allows for freedom to use imagination to form imagery within the lines of the simply-structured scribble. The group members show and discuss their drawings; emphasis is made of how each actually "looks" at his/her drawing—at the unique process of seeing into the scribble to distinguish a design, a pattern, a person, an animal, a whole scene, etc., and perhaps at the personal meaning this image has to its maker. At this juncture, I usually discuss how simple structure can help facilitate the production of imagery for those not comfortable with "making art."

This phenomenological method provides trainees with an example of the Expressive Therapies Continuum in action: from choosing and placing the crayon or marker on the page and making the kinesthetic scribble with eyes closed, to opening eyes and perceiving a form or forms and adding color/feeling to this form, developing the whole or part of the scribble into a conceptualized "picture." If the artist chooses to make a title for his/her drawing, these words then link the world of the image with the world of words. Theory is woven into the discussion of all art experiences, and brainstorming the potential use of each method with therapists' clients adds to the reality of this union of theory and hands-on art experience.

Adding Color to the Kinetic Family Drawing

Most of the psychologists, social workers, and family and child therapists attending these trainings are familiar with projective assessment techniques that use drawing activity, such as draw-a-person, house tree-person, Kinetic Family Drawing, draw-yourself-in-a-boat and draw-a-story. The nurses, doctors, and occupational and physical therapists present in some hospital and clinic settings are not very familiar with these methods and seem to benefit from seeing and discussing actual examples of such client drawings. I usually have each member of the training group make a Kinetic Family Drawing, but using the added dimension of color with markers and crayons. Burns and Kaufman's texts are used to illustrate the "reading" of such drawings to glean something about family dynamics (1970, 1972). Why art therapists prefer to use color in this exercise is discussed; color as representation as well as color as clues about feeling/affect are explained. Depending on the trainee group, I give training in the various theories of symbol formation at the end of each method's presentation.

Family Art Evaluation

Kwiatkowska's (1978) and Landgarten's (1987) "family art evaluation" drawing series are presented to the group by showing case examples; the importance of seeing family members engaging in an activity within the therapy room is emphasized. Seeing how members of a family actually reveal roles and attitudes via these processes encourages trainees to participate in this drawing exercise: Participants form dyads; then each partner chooses a different color marker and keeps this color throughout the exercise; one person is chosen to begin by drawing a simple line or shape; the other is then told to add to this beginning drawing any sort of line or shape with his/her own color; turns are taken in this way, back and forth, in silence, until each person feels finished with this interactive drawing; he/she then signs his/her first name to the drawing as a way of saying, "I am finished." This interactive drawing is then discussed, with each member of the dyad disclosing any personal thoughts about how the drawing unfolded, such as who took the dominant role in visually deciding the subject of the drawing, how he/she felt about the other person's interactive style, etc. A title is then created by each pair for their joint drawing.

Gestalt Family Collage

After the discussion regarding using drawing media to portray the family, I present another method, the Gestalt Family Collage (Rhyne, 1962). Here we use cut or torn shapes made of colored construction papers on a black construction paper background to represent self and family members. The colored shapes are easily seen against the black background. Each shape is cut or torn spontaneously, no pre-drawing encouraged or allowed; the shape represents the particular characteristics ("rounded," "soft," "jagged," "pointed," etc.) of the person being represented. Shapes are arranged to show the relationship of each to the other; thus, family members who are seen/felt as close to the client are literally close or overlapping, and family members who are seen/felt as more distant to the client are placed on the page to reflect this distance.

The Gestalt method employs visual thinking to intuitively problem-solve; in this method the dynamics of family relationships are shown via juxtaposed colored shapes. Since no drawing ability is required for successfully completing this task, most professionals find the process of collage, tearing, cutting and pasting, less anxiety-producing. Thus they find it easier to integrate this activity to what they already know about family therapy or other forms of therapy. See Figs. 1 and 2.

Gestalt World

Another Gestalt method shown in the slide presentation is the "Gestalt world," where members of the group/family create a world together on a common ground (round or rectangular) out of assorted construction papers and other collage/building materials. Fig. 3 is an example of a "world" made jointly by social workers and foster children under their supervision. The goal of the social workers was to actively assess the social skills of these children being considered for new home placements. This form of "group" assessment was common with this team at that agency; but they wanted training in more non-verbal, interactive methods that would allow the children some space to reveal less defended behaviors than was the case in primarily "verbal" assessment situations.

This group decided to use "a Neighborhood" as their theme. Younger children in this group (ages 4 to 10) preferred the colored modeling clay media over the construction paper, so most of this world was drawn and built with these younger children directing the action. The social workers took the children's lead, helping them cooperate and combine ideas so that this neighborhood would meet each person's needs. The result is a neighborhood of

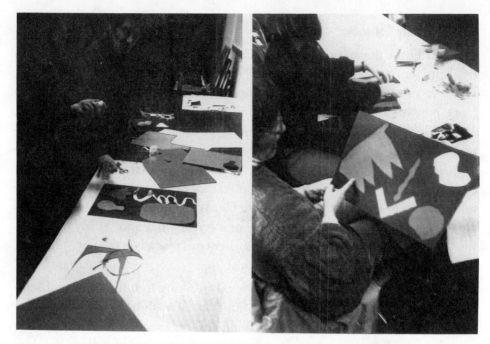

Figs. 1 and 2   Collage, cutting and pasting, is less anxiety-producing.

houses, roads and freeways and bridges, and several parks—nature retreats, an amusement park with rides and slides, and a lake park for ducks and children only! As the art therapist giving an in-service training with a mixed therapist/client group, I intervened to help with communication and art-media problems between groups of children and between the social workers and the children.

In Fig. 3 you will notice the concentration of clay in the upper left-hand corner; this was the starting point with all the children working together to build a nature retreat. It has trees, benches, a stream, and "hiding places" for children to play in. The theme of "hiding" seems common with this population of abused/neglected/abandoned children. There are only two houses and a tent structure that were built by three boys. None of the children made human figures; only ducks were drawn onto the ground paper. A bridge, in the lower right-hand corner, connects a road with an open field across the freeway. The roadways were organized by the social workers and the children as the process evolved.

In the closure discussion with the social workers, they commented on how much parental-type support was needed from them with these children, yet how absent any parental figures were in the landscape. When one therapist made a child figure out of clay and gave it to a 7-year-old boy to place in the "neighborhood," he blended this piece of clay into his house structure! This child could not accept the sculpted child figure as a positive gift from the therapist, a common theme with children displaced from their family of origin because of abuse issues. At the same time, this child's transformation of the clay into the house he was building was very animated, making the merging of the two figures a symbolic statement. Based on knowledge of the child's history, the therapist interpreted this as the child symbolically saying, "I am merged with family space—filled with painful past experience, but wanting a family for the future."

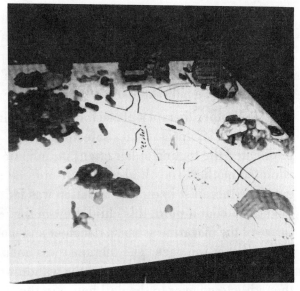

Fig. 3 A "Gestalt World."

Assessing each child's ability to bond is the task of these therapists. This process of seeing in action the psychological dynamics and interaction skills of the children using the art process provided each therapist with insights beyond the usual verbal interview.

Completion Collage

To develop further the individual themes developed by this child and other children during this "world" art experience, I suggested that the therapists use the completion collage method during their next individual sessions with these children. Choosing magazine pictures that might represent conflictual, ambivalent situations or emotional states that each child has experienced, the therapist then takes these intentionally "loaded" images and glues each down to a white, usually 12" x 18", piece of drawing paper. After choosing several of these pictures for each child, the therapist then presents these to his/her client saying, "Look over these pictures and then choose one that you would like to complete. You can use either drawing or collage materials to complete the picture."

The therapist who made the clay child figure mentioned above chose several images from *Parent's Magazine*; the image the child chose to develop was that of a father and son standing together, looking happy.

This child completed this picture with crayons, drawing a rainbow

369

over the heads of both father and son, then writing "I wish" on the left side of the page. The therapist asked if the boy could tell the story of his collage; the child responded by asking the therapist, "Do you think this boy can be happy?" The therapist answered with a "yes," which brought about squirming and a half-smile from this child.

Another therapist chose for her child client a magazine picture with the image of an upset mother screaming at her young daughter. This theme duplicated the feeling of her client's traumatic experiences with her drug-addicted mother. The child was court-ordered not to return to her mother's care; the therapist knew this situation was laden with ambivalence for her client. Without a word, this child drew in the rest of the page with a mirror image of the magazine scene, a daughter and mother arguing and then added tears all over the page. The therapist was amazed at the feeling and undefended level of disclosure this usually withdrawn child portrayed. They were then able to go over to the doll house in the therapy room and make some (child-directed) order to the inside of the house. The art therapy activity opened the door to this child's locked-in trauma.

Clay Family Sculpture

A method used to explore family dynamics, also well-received by non-artist therapists, is the wet clay or colored modeling clay family sculpture (Keyes, 1983). In this three-dimensional exercise, the client is asked to sculpt a figure to represent him/herself and each other member in the family. "Family" here can mean family of origin, current family, or any group that functions like a family in the client's life. Social workers enjoy learning this method by sculpting their own families, then sharing with their in-service peers anything they wish about their sculptures. Many different expressive styles are possible and totally acceptable in this exercise, among them both representational human figures or abstract-expressionistic figures that are arranged to replicate the feeling between members of the family.

Dialogue with the Figures

The in-service participants learn to dialogue with the figures, create transactional dialogue between figures (e.g., "The message you gave me as a child, Mother, was____, and I learned____ about myself from this message"), and to narrate the process of how they formed the figures and the meaning of the shapes and colors they used. For clients who are kinesthetic-visual thinkers, this use of clay might be a better choice of media than two-dimensional drawing or collage methods.

Finding Your Way with Clay

Some in-service staffs enjoy this clay exercise so much, and find it to be so successful for their clients, that they want more clay training and more ideas for using clay with clients. An exercise I give to these willing participants is called "finding your way with clay" (Berensohn, 1972). First, I have each person take a hand-sized lump of wet clay (red, yellow, and gray low-fire clays are available) and *roll it into a ball* using both hands; after each has a smooth ball, I have them put their thumb into the center of the ball and *pinch out an evenly-turned pinch-pot*; next, each *flattens out the pot* using whole-hands and sides-of-hands; after the clay is flat, each *rolls it up into a tight 'tortilla' shape*; each *rolls the clay roll into a coil*, getting it to be a *long 'snake-like' shape*; this coil is then rolled up and the *lines created by coiling the clay are smoothed*; then each flips the round, clay shape over and smooths the lines on the other side; and the last step before rolling the clay back into a smooth ball is to *roll up the sides of the clay into a bowl shape*. This exercise with the possibilities of molding clay challenges the novice to explore the fluid properties of wet clay and gives each participant a vocabulary for forming the clay.

One learns not to get too attached to any of the forms made during the process, but rather to experiment with the inherent nature of the molding clay. When the participants have again their round ball shape at the end of this journey with clay, I show them how to *pull out a five-part figure*: a head, two arms, and two legs. They then have the opportunity to form any "creature" they like, now having a new sensory repertoire of how to use clay. I encourage each to blend the colors of clays available on the table, mixing the red with yellow or gray, or adding red and/or yellow to the gray clay.

Participants find this journey with the clay liberating; the transformational nature of the art media speaks to the process of using art activity as the actual manifestation of the symbolic internal transformation. All art materials give to the "maker" a sense of mastery if the spontaneous experience is properly orchestrated. In-service groups learn through their own art experiences the advantages of starting with easy-to-control art media with simple, guided instructions, and then progressing to more fluid, not-so-easy-to-control art media, or multi-media with looser or no instructions. Inherent internal structure within a media (e.g., markers or modeling clay) gives the beginner the feeling that he/she is in control. With more fluid media such as paints or wet clays, the structure needs to come more from the artist-maker. Learning to gauge frustration tolerance within ourselves and our clients for various art media becomes part of the learning process in the in-service sessions.

371

The Theme of Mastery

The theme of mastery is not new to the staff members in attendance. Mastery as a psychosocial, developmental challenge and as a recurring challenge when we are traumatized by life cycle or unusual events, is well understood by social work and hospital professionals. Transferring this concept to the uses of art media seems a natural transition for most participants in the art therapy trainings.

Masks "Before" and "After" the Trauma

Occupational therapists in one training group devised a mastery art activity for their trauma victim clients. They helped their clients make rectangular and round clay slabs from which they formed masks representing life "before" and "after" the trauma. This mask making activity proved a very powerful intervention; the mastery over the clay paralleled the mastery needed to cope with the trauma experience.

Medical Art Therapy

A pediatric childlife specialist in a hospital training group designed and built a model MRI (Magnetic-Resonance-Imaging) machine and then used this model in play therapy with children preparing to encounter this machine as part of their treatment. This type of play is meant to provide mastery experiences for hospitalized children. After playing with the doll in the model MRI machine, a child would then be encouraged to make a drawing of any remaining fear about anticipating this test or a drawing of having mastered the experience in the play.

In other hospital training groups, in-services illustrating the use of medical art therapy with patients have been well received. The staff is given the assignment of drawing, painting, collaging and/or sculpting their "pain" or "illness" to learn this method. The metaphoric representation of the internal experience of the pain or disease process using art media is in itself transformational. By expressing this subjective experience, putting it outside the self and looking at it from this distance, each person can then begin the process of changing the experience by revisualizing it. This process evolves with each piece of artwork added to the "pain" series.

Hospital professionals are amazed at how personally involved they get with their own images! They see others dialogue with their drawn or painted or sculpted images, and they learn how different subjective experience is from standard medical definitions and procedures. Allowing the time for this expression becomes a priority; they experience the relief this sort of art therapy gives. Slides are shown of artworks by cancer, arthritis, headache and back pain, asthmatic and cardiac patients to illustrate the medical art therapy process (Long, Chapman, & Appleton, 1989, 1992). Basic theories of imagery in healing (e.g., Achterberg, 1980) are given to provide a framework for understanding the connections of our nervous and immune systems with the visualization-imagery experience.

Goals and Outcomes of these Specialized Trainings

The goal of these in-service trainings is to acquaint these clinical professional staff members with practical art therapy methods that can be utilized within the context of each specialized institution. An introduction of basic theoretical paradigms within the field of art therapy is followed by slides of methods and cases, then hands-on experiences of methods suited to the needs of each clinic. Cases are presented by the participants, who then brainstorm which methods would be best suited to these particular cases. The instructor interjects additional methods which complement the needs of each actual case.

The goal of these trainings is not to train allied professionals to be credentialed professional art therapists, although some of those in attendance pursue more art therapy training as a result of the in-service. It is emphasized that the art therapy methods involve art materials that have structures and properties best understood through much experimentation and practice.

Professionals in these trainings seem to benefit personally from the art expression; they become more interested in their work with clients/patients, feel less frustrated and burned-out, and experience stress reduction as they play with the art materials offered. As they gain skill with the art media and methods, their confidence and creativity grows. The cohesion within some groups of trainees also increases as members share their experimental art and concerns about their cases.

Follow-up sessions with trainees serve as forums for the discussion of the art therapy methods tried with clients/patients. The instructor continues to brainstorm art therapy treatment plans with the trainees. Questions are answered about procedures in handling art materials with clients, about the specific steps in some art therapy methods, and about the suitability of certain techniques with specific clients. Meanings of symbols, of specific forms of imagery, and of color are discussed from psychoanalytic, analytic, Gestalt and other frameworks. Administrators in attendance at these discussion groups are continually impressed with the depth of understanding and sensitivity the therapists use in discussing the art of clients.

373

Sometimes presentation of very specialized art therapy diagnostic tools is requested by social work agencies that see abused, emotionally troubled children and adolescents in follow-up sessions. These therapists are now ready to concentrate on comparing the cognitive and emotional styles of these children, mainly to assess ego strength and coping abilities. The Levick Emotional and Cognitive Art Therapy Assessment (LECATA) is often formally presented at this time. Several follow-up sessions are needed to master this assessment tool (Levick, 1983).

Consulting in this way sometimes results in on-going part-time work for the instructor. I have written grants that fund my work in hospitals after these institutions have decided that there is additional need for art therapy expertise on staff. Presenting these in-service trainings thus creates the need for professional art therapy services within these institutions.

References

Achterberg, J. (1980). *Bridges of the bodymind.* Champaign, Illinois: Institute for Personality and Ability Testing.

Arnheim, R. (1974). *Art and visual perception.* (rev. ed.). Berkeley, California: U. of Cal. Press.

Berensohn, P. (1972). *Finding one's way with clay.* NY: Simon & Schuster

Betensky, M. (1973). *Self Discovery through self expression.* Springfield, Illinois: C. C. Thomas.

Burns, R. C. and Kaufman, S. H. (1970). *Kinetic family drawings.* NY: Brunner/Mazel.
———(1972). *Actions, styles and symbols in kinetic family drawings.* NY: Brunner/Mazel.

Furth, G. (1988). *The secret world of drawings: healing through art.* Boston: Sigo Press.

Goldberg, F. A., Coto-McKenna, S. and Cohn, L. (1992). *Creative arts group process evaluation tool: implications for clinical practice and training.* The Arts in Psychotherapy, 18, 411-417.

Kagin, S. L. and Lusebrink, V. B. (1978). *The expressive therapies continuum.* Art Psychotherapy, 5(4), 171-179.

Kellogg, R. (1967). *The psychology of children's art.* NY: Random House.

Keyes, M. F. (1983). *Inward journey: art as therapy.* San Mateo, CA: Open Court Press.

Kramer, E. (1972). *Art as therapy with children.* NY: Schocken.

Kwiatkowska, H. Y. (1978). *Family therapy and evaluation through art.* Springfield, IL: C. C. Thomas.

Landgarten, H. B. (1981). *Clinical art therapy, a comprehensive guide.* NY: Brunner/Mazel.

Landgarten, H. B. (1987). *Family art therapy, a clinical guide and casebook.* NY: Brunner/Mazel.

Levick, M. (1983). *They could not talk and so they drew: children's styles of coping and thinking.* Springfield, IL: C. C. Thomas.

Long, J. K., Chapman, L. and Appleton, V. (1989, 1992) *Medical art therapy, a comprehensive text for defining the field.* Unpublished text.

Lowenfeld, V. (1939). *The nature of creative activity.* London: Routledge and Kegan Paul, Ltd.. (1975). Creative and Mental Growth. NY: Macmillan.

Lusebrink, V. B. (1990). *Imagery and visual expression in therapy.* NY: Plenum Press.

Naumberg, M. (1973). *An introduction to art therapy: studies of the "free" art expression of behavior problem children and adolescents as a means of diagnosis and therapy.* NY: Teacher's College Press.

Rhyne, J. (1962). *The gestalt art experience.* Palo Alto: Science and Behavior

Rubin, J. A. (1978). *Child art therapy.* NY: Van Nostrand Reinhold.

Uhlin, D. (1979). *Art for exceptional children.* Dubuque, Iowa: Wm. C. Brown.

Part II.

An Outline for Presenting an Effective Art Therapy In-Service
by Linda Chapman

Linda Chapman, M.A., A.T.R., is Director of the Art and Play Therapy Program on the Pediatric Unit at San Francisco General Hospital. A past president of the Northern California Art Therapy Association and board member for twelve years, Ms. Chapman was a 1990 recipient of a NCATA Distinguished Person Award for leadership in the organization and a second award for innovative work in the field of medical art therapy. Currently co-authoring a medical art therapy book, Ms. Chapman lectures and teaches in the area of child art therapy and physical and psychological trauma.

The following is a concise guideline for giving an art therapy in-service presentation. It can be limited or expanded in any area to accommodate the needs of the facility and the goals of the presenter.

I. Questions of Facility

    A. Time available

    B. Number of participants

    C. Education and experience of participants

    D. Philosophy of facility

    E. Population served

    F. Space available

        1. Tables

        2. Floor, carpet

        3. Light

        4. Shades for windows

    G. Equipment available

        1. Projector, screen

        2. Art materials if applicable

H. Needs of facility, what do they want to learn

I. Financial arrangements, contract.

II. Questions for Self

A. What are goals for in-service

B. Own strengths and weaknesses

III. Things to Remember

A. Written presentation

B. Slides

C. Business cards or information for future contact

D. AATA info

E. Local Art Therapy Association information

F. Handouts

G. Bibliography

IV. Introduction

A. Education and training

B. How you came to field of art therapy

V. History of Field

A. 30's Margaret Naumberg

B. 50's Edith Kramer

C. 40's-50's Hannah Kwiatkowski

D. 60's Janie Rhyne

E. 60's first graduate art therapy program, Hahneman Medical School

F. 70's first meeting of AATA, national organization monitoring education and training of art therapists

G. 80's art therapy widely accepted for assessment and treatment

H. 90's certification

VI. Personal Definition of Art Therapy (to be personalized to fit you)

A. Using skills as artist with training in psychology and psychotherapy as art psychotherapist

B. Therapeutic goal to encourage, clarify and extend associations and ideas without imposing own projections, participating in the process

C. Works with unconscious content to facilitate expression via metaphor

D. Uses images and imagery as healing process

E. Uses verbal associations in conjunction with non-verbal

F. Concrete projections can be referred to without misinterpretation

G. Process fosters independence, autonomy in client's ability to interpret own work

H. Supports ego, contributes to psychic organization

I. Portrays many things at once

J. Shows progression and regression

K. Enlivening and fun

VII. What Art Therapy is Not

A. Art skills not necessary

B. Not a conscious process (art, drama, dance, and music therapies), conscious processes are therapeutic, but different (OT, RecTx, Activity Tx)

C. Although many clinicians use art in therapy, this is not art therapy

VIII. Materials

A. Not randomly selected

B. Structured/unstructured

C. Aggressive

D. Expressive

E. Materials elicit different responses

IX. Assessment

A. Must understand development

B. Must understand normal graphic development

C. How art therapy used in assessment

D. Slide examples

X. Treatment

A. How art therapy is used in treatment

B. Slide examples

XI. Techniques

A. Specifically designed, directive, goal oriented

B. Non-directive

XII. Art Experiences as Part of In-Service

A. Time must be realistic

    1. Explain technique

    2. Discuss self-disclosure issue for the setting

    3. Art making

4. Process time

5. Questions

B. Should not be designed to elicit deeper material but to give participants a positive, non threatening experience with art making

C. Don't encourage people to "act roles," work with what emerges and is appropriate for setting

D. Do not leave, be mindful of what is going on in room, listen carefully and be aware of what is coming up for participants

XIII. Slides

A. Slides must be good quality

B. Art therapy release required for all slides

C. Stress confidentiality

D. Participants may be profoundly affected by some images, be sensitive to viewers, allow for debriefing time

E. Examples, not entire slide collection

1. Assessment

2. Treatment

a. Short treatment

b. Longer treatment

c. Normal graphic development

3. People typically ask many questions about slides, so monitor time

XIV. Questions

A. Be sure to allow time for questions and watch time.

B. Note questions for information to add to your presentation

C. Keep answers brief to allow for more questions

XV. Ends

A. Get feedback from facility/participants to assist in improving in-service

B. Ask for letter if applicable

C. Send thank you note for invitation to present in-service

Grant Writing Skills Create Jobs
For Art Therapists
by Doris Arrington, Ed.D., A.T.R.

Dr. Arrington is professor and director of the art therapy program at the College of Notre Dame, Belmont, California.

Since 1980, graduate students at the College of Notre Dame in Belmont, California, have had the option of writing a grant in lieu of a thesis. This chapter discusses some thoughts behind the establishment of this unprecedented option, some of the successful projects, as well as guidelines for novice grant writers. The discussion illustrates how viable an activity grant writing can be for *clarifying the role of an art therapist* and for the creation of *art therapy jobs*.

Introduction

Ten years ago, most Americans had no idea what a pita fajita was. But with a bombardment of advertising it has become an understandable phrase to anyone who watches TV or eats at Jack In the Box. Metaphorically, grant writing can be viewed as a pita fajita.

It sounds different, could be interesting, maybe fun to say, has a foreign connotation and is definitely unknown. So, how do you get the public to try something "unknown"? You say it and describe it over and over and over.

History (or getting the public to taste the pita fajita)

In 1979, when the art therapy program at the College of Notre Dame was established, the purposeful use of art to meet psychological needs (Ulman, Kramer, Kwiatkowska, 1977) was over forty years old, the

American Art Therapy Association (AATA) was ten years old and the Northern California Art Therapy Association, (NCATA), a young nine year old, was a diverse group of approximately 75 creative and skillful people located from Sacramento to Santa Cruz. The knowledge of who art therapists were and what they did was, however, still unknown in the San Francisco Bay area. We were unknown to the extent that when art therapy was discussed, even educated individuals asked if art therapists repaired paintings.

Demographics in 1979 indicated that there were three registered art therapists south of San Francisco, all trained out of the area. The good news was that the field was wide open. The bad news was that it appeared that too few knew what professionals in the field actually did. Selling the profession was the number one priority for anyone in the field.

As president of the Northern California Art Therapy Association and the director of the newly established art therapy program, I was not alone in my belief in the power of art therapy and in the potential of the art therapist. I may have been unique, however, in my belief that art therapists could get paid as well as other mental health professionals.

Administrators at the College of Notre Dame had become interested in art therapy as a program offering first in 1976 when I taught an elective class, "Art as an Inner Experience", to undergraduates in the Behavioral Science Department. Art therapy had more positive exposure when "In Touch Through Art," the first art therapy art show, was presented at the local Belmont art center (1976, Eslinger, Virshup and Arrington). But, even with the support of the College and interested students, no art therapy program will survive unless the graduates get jobs.

Art therapists know that an on-site art therapist supplements assessment, communication and treatment options for a school, an agency, or a hospital. But the challenge in 1979 was how to find jobs for art therapists, without job descriptions. The task was more difficult because shrinking public funds and social service cutbacks precluded hiring anyone. My goals for the program included curriculum development, well-supervised practicum experience and art therapy exposure. Our program would be only as good as our employed graduates. The program objective had to include graduate employment. If the program was to become viable, its mission had to include not only educating art therapists but also educating the mental health community and the public about art therapy.

As a younger professional, I had been an educational curator for a contemporary arts museum. Knowing that museums are built on patrons and grants, I learned that a good project needed good people supporting it. Therefore, if the right patron knew about the right project at the right time, the project had a good chance of being funded. Or, if I could write a grant to interest a foundation in a project, then I could get grant funding. Because art, used as and in therapy, is a visual expression of "internal images, feelings, thoughts, and sensations" (Lusebrink, 1990) and can be used as a second language, I reasoned that once the staff in an agency had experienced a creative and skilled art therapist trainee, that agency would want to keep the person on the job. Furthermore, if art therapists could receive funding for their jobs through grants, they would be even more valuable to agencies because they could write grants.

From its inception in 1979, the art therapy program offered students the *option of writing a grant that furthered art therapy in lieu of a thesis.* History has proven this to be a successful paradigm for the art therapy program. It has also been successful for the many art therapy graduate students who have written grants, and for the larger community that continues to benefit from art therapy services funded through grants first written as graduate research projects.

With the press of practicum training and course work, the first graduates from the program found the grant option more palatable than writing a research paper. Five of the first eight graduates wrote grants. All were application grants and one included a research component.

The art therapy application grants included two grants to school districts where the art therapist trainees worked as teachers. David Anderson was funded to provide after-school art therapy groups in San Francisco. Although Gordy Loughlin's grant to establish art therapy support in a classroom for seriously emotionally disturbed adolescents was not funded, the school district, once apprised of the advantages of art therapy with this population, used their own supplementary funds to establish such a program (Anderson & Arrington, 1986a).

Jennifer Fields (ahead of her time) wrote a grant to use art therapy to reduce stress. Her grant was not funded. Cathy Malchiodi moved out of the area and wrote a grant to introduce herself to her new location. She wrote a proposal for using art therapy with battered children to increase self-esteem. This was the first of several grants funded by the YWCA for Malchiodi. As a result of her work with battered children, she wrote *Breaking the Silence: Art Therapy With Children of Violent Homes*, published in 1990 by Brunner/Mazel.

Valerie Appleton wrote an application and a research grant to continue her practicum experience with burn patients in a San Francisco hospital. This grant was funded and refunded for many years and became the focus for her professional development. In 1985, Appleton became the first graduate student in her doctoral program to receive a prestigious scholarship from the University of San Francisco for continuous service and dedication to research for her work using art therapy with burn patients. In 1989, Appleton's doctoral dissertation, *Transition from trauma: Art therapy with adolescent and young adult burn patients,* was published. In 1990, Appleton received the Distinguished Person Award from NCATA for her research and clinical work with burn patients. Today, eleven years after writing her first grant to work with burn patients, Appleton is considered an expert in the field of PTSD. She presents at conferences and teaches at colleges and universities in both the United States and Canada.

From this robust beginning, writing a grant in lieu of a thesis was established as a viable option for College of Notre Dame graduates. Over the past twelve years, one fourth of the graduates have written grants. Although only a little over half of those have been funded, more often than not, "when people go through the rigors of preparing and submitting a grant, jobs have often resulted, even when the particular grant proposal was not successful" (Anderson & Arrington, 1986a, p. 36).

Demystifying the process

Students view grant writing as either a creative challenge or a mystical and threatening bafflement. Often grant writing gets lost in the masses of information that must be included within the art therapy and marital and family therapy programs in California. The program attempts to link each experience to the next in the chain of College of Notre Dame graduate education. Ideally, every class, assignment, project and discussion assists graduate students in their professional journey. The faculty tries to make each hoop students are expected to jump through meaningful. In order to demystify the process, introduction to the advantage of grants begins the first time the applicant is on campus whether it is for the "Evening of Information" or the first interview. From the beginning, students know that the option is theirs and the possibilities are unlimited.

It cannot be emphasized too strongly that all grants, even those that have not been funded, can supply information for future study. Theses and grants, funded and not funded, often contain the most current information on a particular topic and therefore may include a base of information on art therapy. Sometimes the grant topic is just ahead of its time or may need just a different slant. All metropolitan areas have large community foundations that provide comprehensive libraries and grant writing classes. Anyone thinking of writing a grant should visit one of these foundations to review a the vast amount of information available, usually free, to anyone.

Identifying Areas of Interest

The first thing that potential grant writers must do, even before visiting a community foundation, is to *identify an area of interest* they would like to pursue. This is where creativity begins. Funding agencies want to fund innovative ideas and they are interested in positive exposure. Often the ideas funded are those that meet a need of the agency or show the agency in the most positive way. *Because of its visual nature, art therapy or the process of art therapy is a natural for communicating a point.* For example:

Maggie Conroy, an artist and art therapist, believed that the process of artistic creation comes naturally to children and non-controlled expression was important in a child's emotional growth. Conroy proposed to the *Apple Computer Child Center* that art could be therapeutic in calming an active child, in releasing energy and in giving children an added ability to communicate. She further proposed that the children in the center be given the experience of producing artwork with quality materials and their art works be displayed in a special way in their center. Apple funded the proposal which resulted in:

- Six different showings in other Apple divisions and buildings within the company prior to returning the show to its home in the Apple Child Care Center.
- A request from a parent advisory group for a second show involving the work of older children of Apple employees.
- An original art piece by a 4-year-old hangs in the office of a senior vice president.
- An exchange of children's art with representatives of other countries.
- Interest in applying the "process over product" principle by other preschools in the area.
- Exposure for the children and (slight) fortune for the grant writer who presented many workshops and traveling lectures about the art, the artists and the show (Arrington, 1990, p. 126).

Anne Reidy works at the Veterans Administration Hospital with

383

Vietnam Veterans with Post Traumatic Stress Disorder (PTSD). Art therapy has been an integral part of this unit since 1981. During that time, over 1500 drawings and paintings done by veteran patients have accumulated. Reidy proposed that she be given release time to systematically organize the art and develop a computer data base for storing and retrieving information as it relates to imagery and stress disorders. The VA approved the proposal which could be the basis for future art therapy research in areas of PTSD (Arrington, 1990, p 126).

Connie Holmlund interned at the state hospital with children and experienced the emotional trauma communicated by the children in their artistic expressions. She believed that publication of the children's art work would be a concrete validation of the children and their artistic efforts. In addition, she believed that the publication would serve to educate others about art therapy and give credence to the power of art as means of expression for children with psychiatric problems (Arrington, 1990, p 126). Holmlund proposed publishing an appointment calendar featuring color photographs of art work created by children who are patients at the state hospital. Fully funded, this calendar was sold throughout California and at the AATA conference in Washington. In its second edition, the calendar is self supporting and provides funds for Holmlund to work part-time with the children at the state hospital.

Roberta McGovern worked as an art therapist in a convalescent home where Alzheimer patients suffered in their loss of meaningful relationships. McGovern wrote a grant for funds to purchase materials so that the patients could work with their families to create a book of memories. This foundation-approved grant has been a success for the convalescent home, the patients and their families.

Sponsor

The second thing that the person writing a grant must consider is what agency might sponsor his or her project.

Hospitals. Hospitals often have in-house funding. Valerie Appleton's grants were funded within the hospital. Another art therapy student, Nadine Blaschak, interning at the hospital with Appleton, wrote a grant to include art therapy in an area of the hospital not currently served by art therapy. After Blaschak completed a pilot study in this new area, the hospital funded her proposal. Her funding has been renewed yearly.

Corporate Funding. Conroy went to her husband's employer for funding. Beverly Stone paid for her education by working as office manager

384

for an energy corporation. Like most corporations, they fund local charitable projects yearly. The firm, in support of Stone and her career goals, funded her proposal to run an art therapy group for sexually abused females at a psychiatric center for children.

Community organizations. The local arts council funded half of the expenses for Holmlund's proposed Children's Calendar while requiring the other half to be matched. The Hospital Volunteer Service Group matched the funds within a week.

Diane Young and Amy Horn went to a community foundation in the Bay area with their proposals for using art therapy as treatment with children of battered women and children of alcoholics. Separately, they were both investigating funding sources. The agency, after reading their proposals, funded both projects.

National interest groups. Jennifer Woods worked with an AIDS patient in a hospice setting. When he died, she and his sister organized his art and photography into an art exhibition titled *"An Inside Look: Living & Dying with AIDS."* She received funding to display the work both locally and in Washington, D.C., concurrent with the display of the Names Project Memorial Quilt.

Nuts and bolts about putting a pita fajita together.

When writing a grant you want to address something that can be accomplished within a reasonable amount of time for a reasonable amount of money. This process usually begins with the following ingredients:

Summary

The summary should be clear, concise and specific. It should include some information about who you are in relationship to the grant and why you should be given the money. It should also include the scope of your project and its projected costs. When you go to an agency for the first time, the summary "is probably all you should give out (but have the rest in your pocket, just in case the agency or corporation wants to see it)." (Anderson & Arrington, 1986a)

Introduction

The actual proposal should always begin with an introduction. This introduction builds your credibility. It should address you, your organization or art therapy and include your beginnings, your uniqueness, your accomplishments and your other supporters. Kiritz (1988) suggests that you start a "credibility file" which you can use in this section. It should include newspaper clippings, articles from magazines and literature references. Often potential funding sources select your grant because of you. This was the case in Stone's grant. They may also select it because of your topic and population. This was the case of Horn, Holmlund, McGovern, and Young. Some may select it because it enhances their setting. This was the case of Appleton and Conroy.

Limit the introduction to one page and use large type. It will be helpful to begin with the following statement. (You fill it in!)

You.. (your hospital or institution)

seek $.. from Corporation

for .... (Specify what: a program, an

evaluation, an arts festival, etc): for the time period......to......

Matching funds will come from...

(Examples: Board contributions, NCATA, California Arts Council) "This project follows.....number of years of successful............" experience. (Anderson & Arrington, 1986.)

Problem

The problem statement or needs assessment comes next, and addresses the specific problem you want to solve through the program you are proposing. First document that a problem exists and then discuss how your proposal can solve it. Here you want to be specific to your program. For example, if you were selling pita fajita, you would talk about the pita fajita, not other foods that are also for sale.

Objectives

Next your grant will include program objectives which are the expected results. "If you have defined a problem, then your objectives should offer some relief of the problem" (Kiritz, 1988).

Methods

Now you are ready to address the methods of how you intend to accomplish the objective you mentioned above. This includes a specific "plan of action, treatment plans, and timeline for accomplishing the project" (Anderson & Arrington 1986a). Be sure that you have done your homework and know what other models are out there. You may want to identify why you are using your specific model (White, 1975).

Evaluation

Your evaluation process can be either *formative* or *summative*. A *formative evaluation* is used to make changes and adjustments in your program as it proceeds. As an art therapist, you may do this by using an on-going art-based assessment process (Arrington, 1992), serial drawings, observational checklists of clients' skills, or behaviors, staff and/or parent observations, etc.

A *summative evaluation* determines how effective you were at reaching the objectives that you established. A summative evaluation may include the results of pre- and post-tests, art-based assessments alone or in combination with paper and pencil assessments, serial drawings, observational checklists of clients' skills or behaviors, staff and/or parent observations, etc.

> "...remember that a funding agency wants to see some tangible results of its funding of your program. You want to provide good public relations for art therapy, your specific program and the funding agency. Therefore, you should also include how you will disseminate information about the program. This can be done by including some outcome such as: an art exhibit, a videotape, a national presentation or a published article (Anderson & Arrington, 1986a p. 37).

Sometimes it helps to start writing your grant by using a chart like the one below (Kiritz, 1988). Start with your objectives, make them clear, specific, measurable and obtainable. Next, define the problems that you are trying to solve and the methods of how you will solve them. Finally, include how you will evaluate how well you have met your objectives. Complete one idea under all four headings. Then complete a second idea under all four headings and then a third, etc.

Objective	Problem	Methods	Evaluation
1.			
2.			
3.			

Budget

Remember! Programs are funded, not jobs. So sell your program and your job will be included. The first budgetary item should be personnel, if your budget includes payment for someone's time. You may be the personnel. If personnel is part of the budget, you should include both wages and fringe benefits. Fringe benefits must include FICA (Social Security) and Workman's Compensation. They may include health insurance and/or retirement. Our students often include personal liability insurance. Personnel may also include consultants. Our student often include their supervision by state licensed or registered art therapy personnel.

Non-personnel budgetary items include: indirect costs, space cost, equipment costs, consumable supplies, any travel, telephone, postage, and tangible outcome costs, such as film, or monograph publication.

> "Give a detailed accounting of all items. Be sure that you check on actual costs of items and briefly explain why you have included items in your budget. It will also be important to list the value of *'in kind'* contributions (any support other than actual dollars such as space, use of office equipment, secretarial help) after the rest of the budget. Do not hesitate to include ALL possible *in kind* contributions. This accounting makes your project look better— that is, the agency knows what you are really giving them" (Anderson & Arrington, 1986a p. 37).

Indirect costs are paid to a host institution in return for their assuming responsibility for overseeing the project. These indirect costs include bookkeeping, payroll, etc. (Kiritz, 1988). Indirect cost may range from 1% to 15%. In days of tight money, host institutions may waive the cost rather than not get the grant.

Future Funding.

This is an area that needs to be thoroughly thought out so that you include realistic plans. If your proposal is successful, client fees may be available for future services. Other funding agencies may also be interested in your project. If possible, you want to include support letters and/or even written commitments.

Conclusion

In the last three years, over one half of the grants written by College of Notre Dame students have been funded. But more important than the money received are the lives that have been significantly changed because of the grants written. There is no way to describe the rise in self-esteem or the change in view of the graduate student who interns one year and, because of grant funding, directs a program the next. There is no way to estimate how many clients have benefited and how much clients have gained from art therapists being able to work with them because of grant monies. And, there is no way that any of this would happen if people were not interested and willing to go through the process of writing grants.

Grants written about art therapy not only provide jobs for art therapists but they promote the field of art therapy. They also establish personal feelings of success and competence as they allow art therapists to take charge of their professional direction and to actively involve themselves in personal issues of concern.

You know that grant writing has lost its mystery when, like the pita fajita, the grant writing sounds good enough to try, you try it and then you try it again and again. My hope is that after reading this chapter you will still find the idea of grant writing interesting and fun to think about doing and maybe even different from what you are used to doing. I would also hope that it no longer sounds so foreign or unknown and definitely is no longer a mystical and threatening bafflement. Perhaps it is something you've thought about for a long time and now will put on your *"To Do"* list.

I hope that you are sold and will join in the process.

The author would like to thank Frances Anderson, Ed.D., A.T.M., H.L.M., who, in 1985, encouraged her to publish information on the unique graduate research option of grant writing available at the College of Notre Dame.

References

Anderson, F. and Arrington, D. (1986a). *Grants: Demystifying the mystique and creating job connections.* Art Therapy 3 (1), 34-38.

———(1986b). *The Grants Manual.* Normal Ill., and Belmont, Ca.: Available from either author.

Arrington, D. (1990). *Grants: demystifying the mystique and creating job connections—Part II.* Art Therapy.7(3), 126-127.

——— (1992). *Art-based assessments.* The Research Manual. IL: American Art Therapy Association.

Arrington, D. and Anderson, F. (1992). *Grants: a structure for research.* The Research Manual. IL: American Art Therapy Association.

Eslinger, S., Virshup, E. and Arrington, D. (1976). *In Touch Through Art.* Los Angeles.

Kiritz, N. (1988). *Program planning & proposal writing.* L. A.: Grantsmanship Center.

Lusebrink, L. (1990). *Imagery and visual expression in therapy.* NY: Plenum Press.

Ulman, E., Kramer, E., and Kwiatkowska, H. (1977). *Art therapy in the United States.* Craftsbury Common, VT: Art Therapy Publications.

White, V.P. (1975). *Grants, how to find out about them and what to do next.* NY: Plenum Press.

The Creative Process:
A Heuristic Blueprint for
Training, Research, and Practice
by Leslie Howard, M.S., A.T.R.

Ms. Howard received her art therapy education at the College of Notre Dame, followed by a teaching assistantship at California State University, Northridge. Currently she is doing art therapy with terminally ill AIDs and cancer patients at St. Vincent's Hospital, and group art therapy for elderly deaf adults in an independent living center. She is in private practice in Westwood.

> *For it was not so much by the knowledge of words that I came to the understanding of things, as by my experience of things I was enabled to follow the meaning of words.* Plutarch

Becoming a psychotherapist demands more than simply acquiring the theory and technique necessary for competent clinical work. It calls for socialization into a field and a way of life for which mastery is an ever—evolving process. The core issue is described by Bugental (1987) as "accepting—even welcoming—the constant challenge to move past where one is and explore where one is becoming." *Heuristics* is defined as learning, discovering, or solving problems on one's own—by experimenting, evaluating possible or solutions, or by trial and error.

The primary resource that psychotherapists bring to the treatment session is themselves, the people they are, and not simply the skills they possess. Who one is as a person is a central variable in clinical practice. No therapist can truly delve into experiences that he or she is unwilling to address or explore personally.

Psychotherapy research indicates that effectiveness among therapeutic modalities is basically equal. No one therapy approach has been found to be superior. The research does indicate that therapy is more effective than no therapy, suggesting the presence of an eminent quality in the therapy, namely the personhood of the therapist (Luborsky et al., 1975, Sloane et al., 1975). This implies that the person of the therapist has a more significant impact than the specific theoretical orientation or technique of the therapist.

The use of self is recognized as the primary element of influence in the therapeutic enterprise. "Understanding other human beings," writes Storr (1979), "therefore, requires that the observer does not simply note their behavior as if they were machines or totally different from himself, but demands that he make use of his own understanding of himself, his own feelings, thoughts, intentions, and motives in order to understand others" (p. 168).

Experimental findings led Strupp (1958, 1959) to assert that although the therapist's contribution is both personal and technical, no amount of expert technique would favorably tip the scales toward psychodynamic growth without the emotional matrix. It follows that adequate functioning as a therapist demands a deep commitment to the development of the self.

Commitment to personal development is transmitted to others by a central grounding in the self. Trungpa (1983) believes that the essential work of psychotherapists, "...is to become full human beings and to inspire full human—beingness in other people who feel starved about their lives" (p. 126). Full human—beingness is defined by him as wakefulness. To be awake is to be stirred by one's senses. The question then is how to wake up. What activities bring the senses alive?

An answer may be found by observing young children as they openly explore the world. Vivid sensory and emotional interest is at an unmatched peak during the period from infancy to early childhood. No other period can compare with the curiosity and zest with which we engage the world. Here, we begin acquiring knowledge by a gradual accumulation of sensory data.

This free play of sense perception, thought, feeling, and action characterizes creative experience. The creative experience transports one to these early childhood roots where direct subjective experience dominates.

"...The creative experience," notes Erikson (1988), "demands of us only that which is genuinely our own, and all that we do have that is genuinely our own is our personal, accrued store of sense data. That is what we really know. The rest is all secondhand and debatable" (p. 26).

It is evident that the core of the creative process, the activity of shaping and externalizing experience, is imbued with healing properties. An understanding of the essential qualities and tasks of the psychotherapist may be developed by addressing the nature of the creative process. The essence of creativity is change and transformation. This connects psychotherapy and creativity at a fundamental level. To be creative is to be involved in acts for which consequences are unknown. The therapist, like the artist, may be seen as an explorer, stepping into uncharted territory, willing to risk losing the way and becoming lost for the sake of finding meaning.

What better method to actualize the transcendent quality of the healing process than to immerse myself in a creative exploration and see what is revealed? I looked to my passage into the profession as an opportunity to initiate a method of inquiry which would honor and support my personal evolution. This investigation is about discovering and finding my own questions and answers by being involved in my own experience. My aim was to create a forum within the ordinary circumstances of my life for the subtleties and complexities of my psyche to emerge.

The project may be seen as an initiation or rite of passage into the psychological life. Like a vow, it is a committed symbolic action, revealing a personal investment in experiential learning. The inquiry became an integral aspect to my first year of clinical practice as an art therapist.

Essential Therapeutic Qualities

Use what language you will, you can never say anything but what you are.   Ralph Waldo Emerson

Empathy is considered a focal quality in the person of the psychotherapist. Experiencing and understanding the feelings and thoughts of another person without explicitly having them is the action of empathy. The empathic process is accomplished by the projection of one's own person into the person of another. The literature contains many references to the nature of the empathic process, an experience Kohut (1959) terms "vicarious introspection." As a vital therapeutic disposition, empathy may be seen as a condition to be nourished.

Several authors have emphasized the essential role of congruence. This is the condition of being without facade, openly attuned and true to one's continual flow of inner experience (Rogers, 1962). Congruency implies transparency or the willingness to be a real person devoid of a professional screen (Truax and Carkhuff, 1965). This assumes that a degree of self exploration has taken place in the therapist. The capacity to be fully present is the cornerstone to therapeutic creativity. Continued commitment in the face of failure invites innovation and improvisation (Jourard, 1967).

Wholeness of presence and willingness to risk oneself are considered by Bugental (1967) to be the central attributes of authentic commitment and therapeutic effectiveness. Primary attention to the subjective realm of the client via the therapist's own subjective experience characterizes the experience of authenticity and sets the stage for the empathic process.

Subjectivity is defined by Bugental as "...that inner, separate, and private realm in which we live most genuinely. The furnishings or structures of this realm are our perceptions, thoughts, feelings and emotions, values and preferences, anticipations, and apprehensions, fantasies and dreams, and all else that goes on endlessly night and day, waking and sleeping, and so determines what we do in the external world and what we make of what happens to us there" (Bugental, 1987, p. 7).

Much of the theoretical literature emphasizes the need for the therapist to be *self-aware*. It is not suggested that the therapist be "perfectly analyzed" (Silverman, 1985, p. 175), but rather that he or she be deeply committed to the development of the self and the process of becoming. Corey (1977) highlights the value of the therapist's willingness not to become a "finished product" (p. 234).

This is not to imply that there is no place for theory and technique in the practice of therapy. Jourard (1967) sees the commitment to study theory and technique as proof of the seriousness of one's purpose. However, the person of the therapist is the determining element in the nature and quality of the therapy offered. Rogers (1962) points out that no amount of theoretical and diagnostic knowledge will make the trainee more effective in relating with others.

Specific qualities in the therapist have been underscored as a primary element in the therapeutic process. This suggests that experiences which foster *self-development and creativity* ought to be given a place of prominence in psychotherapy training and on-going practice.

Art and the Art Therapist

By descending far down into the depths of the soul...the artist attains the power of awakening other souls.   Ralph Waldo Emerson

Dissanayake describes art as a behavior which is as distinguishing and universal in humans as speech and the manufacture and use of tools. She calls this proclivity *making special* because the act of expression or response to an artifact is achieved as one creates or acknowledges a special-

393

ness that without one's activity would not exist. The activity or object is thus placed in an out of the ordinary realm. *Making special* acknowledges and embodies the alternative reality, creating "an intimate connection with a world that is different from if not superior to ordinary experience, whether they choose to call it imagination, intuition, fantasy, irrationality, illusion, make-believe, the ideal, dream, a sacred realm, the supernatural, the unconscious, or some other name" (Dissanayake, 1988, p. 94-95).

Making special is what makes art therapy special. One of the primary therapeutic strengths of art—making is its unique potential to contain polarities and ambiguities. It does this by providing a format for the organization of inner and outer experience into a coherent form. Engagement with art materials becomes a way to dwell within emotional realms that might otherwise be overwhelming.

The activity of giving shape was not, early in its evolution, a leisure activity, but a way of comprehending the world. Dissanayake sees this as a demonstration of the human propensity for finding and making meaning, and a testament to the fact that humankind cannot bear senselessness. Art offers an avenue for the exploration and expression of otherwise incommunicable aspects of ourselves. "If all meanings could be adequately expressed by words," wrote Dewey (1934), "the arts of painting and music would not exist. There are values and meanings that can be expressed only by immediately visible and audible qualities, and to ask what they mean in the sense of something that can be put into words is to deny their distinctive existence" (p. 74).

Art therapy training programs which do not address the kind of knowledge developed by a first-hand experience with art materials encourage what Allen (1992) identifies as a "Clinification Syndrome." This is a process whereby the art therapist comes to hold the skills of other clinicians while simultaneously withdrawing investment from the practice of art. Allen makes an impassioned plea for a sustained involvement in art making by practitioners of the field. She contends that an immersed interest in the phenomena of art-making and its effects on human behavior is necessary to develop theoretical depth and halt the stunted development of the field of art therapy as a discipline in its own right.

Characteristics of the Creative Process

Education for creativity is nothing short of education for living.
Erich Fromm

The creative act calls for one to move into close rapport with oneself. Receptivity and appreciation for the inherent limitations of one's medium pro-

394

vide clues to the art of living life. The creative cycle has been conceptualized as consisting of four phases, generally known as preparation, incubation,
illumination, and verification (Patrick, 1955). They will be presented here
as distinct entities, although in practice they are rarely so distinct, but are
more likely fluidly traversed during the process.

Preparation begins as the seed of creation brings a notion of something to be done. An investigation of possibilities is begun as the creator questions, collects and explores. In this way the initial idea may be transformed.
Fromm (1959) regards this as *a capacity to be puzzled.*

Incubation describes the period when the unconscious takes precedence as the ideas *"go underground"* (Kneller, 1965, p. 51). Here, unexpected connections are made. This phase is often experienced as chaotic,
causing one to lose sight of the original goal. Ehrenzweig (1967) calls this
the "schizoid" stage, where fragmented parts of the self are projected into
the work. These aspects of the self are seen as alien.

The third phase elucidates the moment of *illumination* when a solution to the problem is grasped. *A solution is found amidst a sense of joyful exul-
tation, bringing some integration to the chaos.* This "manic" phase initiates
unconscious activity toward integration (Ehrenzweig, 1967). He likens the
work at this stage to a receiving "womb" which contains and integrates the
fragments into a whole.

Finally, *verification* occurs when cognition and judgment bring the raw
material into finished form. A sustained analysis of the elements help the creator distinguish between what is valid in the material and what is not (Kneller,
1965). This is Ehrenzweig's (1967) stage of *re-introjection*, where part of the
work is taken back into the ego.

Fromm (1959) puts forth several conditions which he sees as central
to the creative process. Initial puzzlement evolves into an ability to concentrate and focus on one's task as the most important thing in life at that
moment. Here, the self is experienced as the central core to one's world. And
finally, being that conflict is deeply rooted in the human condition, the ability to accept the conflict and tension which result from polarities can become
a source of wonderment from which strength is developed. He refers to the
condition of creativity as

*"...the willingness to be born everyday. Indeed, birth is not a single
process taking place when the child leaves its fetal existence and starts to
breathe by itself... Every act of birth requires the courage to let go of something;
to let go of the womb, to let go of the breast, to let go of the lap, to let go of the*

hand, to let go eventually of all certainties, and to rely only upon one thing: one's own powers to be aware and respond; that is one's own creativity" (p. 53).

Conditions for Creativity

> *On leaving your home, do you not often change your route without thinking about it? Do you cease to be yourself on that account? And do you not get there anyhow? And even if you don't, does it matter?*
>
> Pablo Picasso

The creative process requires an interaction between conscious thought processes and unconscious emotional processes. The elements that nurture the birth and growth of the creative impulse have particular relevance for mental health practitioners who are engaged in a creative process aimed at nurturing the creative process in others.

The need to be receptive to oneself is fundamental, writes Kneller (1965). Ideas must be attended to and given significance, or they will be lost. May (1975) writes, "We cannot will to have insights. We cannot will creativity, but we can will to give ourselves to the encounter with intensity of dedication and commitment. The deeper aspects of awareness are activated to the extent that the person is committed to the 'encounter' " (p. 46).

Arieti (1980) talks of *aloneness, inactivity,* and *daydreaming* as attitudes fostering creativity. Listening to the inner self, making contact with oneself, and opening up to unusual paths in one's dreams, provides relief from social convention, while expanding one's inner realms.

Vaughan (1987) identifies the importance of accepting the indeterminate. Some surrender of control is necessary if a creative process is to develop. Rogers (1976) touches upon this with his concept of extensionality, in which *openness to experience, tolerance for ambiguity, and permeability of boundaries* invite what Ghiselin (1952) calls a *"commerce with disorder"* (p. 14).

The Cultivation of Creativity

What nurtures the birth and growth of the creative impulse?

The lives of inventive people share a number of similar characteristics. These are not inborn virtues, but rather hard-earned habits which can be acquired through practice.

Writers on creativity often refer to the fact that inspired individuals are always primed for the experience. "If inspiration is indeed an abandonment and a transcendence, it is nonetheless impossible without groaning effort, without the painful winning of skill" (Grudin, 1990, p. 11).

Grudin (1990) suggests that personal habits and patterns of thought may cultivate the creative impulse, and articulates a collective code to the creative life. He describes the following practices to nurture:

The Passion for Work—Passion for and identification with one's work allows one to view the work as an expression of one's own character. Whereas social convention relegates leisure in opposition to work, the creative life transcends this distinction, and leisure and work come to complement each other.

Love of the Problematic—Our educational system stresses linear solutions to problems. The open-ended glory of the process is given little emphasis as compared to the end "find." To behold problems or things that don't fit is to celebrate the mystery of the unknown.

Boldness—"To think creatively," he writes, "is to walk on the edge of chaos" (p. 15). Following an idea in spite of its unfamiliarity and strangeness takes bold, inner courage. Being open to original ideas means that poor ones may emerge as well.

Consequence—Reverence for the process of one's project is defined by Grudin (1990) as consequence. This means that the interludes are seen as a part of the process, rather than as isolated periods where nothing is happening. Consequence provides the longevity and fuel necessary to persistently pursue the thread of a project into the weave of the future.

Innocence and Playfulness—The innocent consideration of a new project takes place when preconceptions are set aside, resulting in direct interaction with one's emerging insight. The ghosts of tradition can otherwise stand in the way of real contact. He terms this innocence because it reminds him of babies who experience new objects in their world. The objects are tasted, felt, and seen, without a known purpose or mental image of rightness. It is as if the object is being actively redefined from minute to minute. To set aside one's preconceived notions is to invite a redefinition of oneself with relation to the data.

Suffering—There is inherent pain in creative work, which is a symptom of the process itself. There are such things as failure, criticisms, enduring contradictions, reorganization of material occur—often requiring discarding material, and the awareness at the beginning of any creative venture that these experiences may be expected. Facing these experiences sensitizes one to life.

Openness—Each school of thought has had its innovators and heroes, causing the world of inquiry often to be perceived as a closed, heavily popu-

397

lated place. A room which is filled to capacity doesn't leave room for new possibilities. Inventiveness blossoms in an open environment. The sparsely furnished room of inquiry calls one to play with the possibilities—ideas have room in which to move.

Liberty—Popular assumptions about the world must be overturned and investigated. Rather than accepting the status quo, inventive people see the world as limitless, and capable of innumerable configurations.

Vaughan (1987) proposes four conditions for the creation of a fertile working environment.

Avoid Drifting with Circumstance—This is achieved by concentrating one's personal energy. Examples include: practicing meditation, learning a new skill, or working on a project of one's own choice.

Read—Reading sparks new ideas, and re-associations may be made with previously established ideas. Unexpected knowledge about oneself may be released.

Association with Colleagues—Continual association with others who are equally interested in personal searches provides reinforcement, encouragement, and inspiration. Vaughan (1987) writes, "New ideas are like newborn babies, weak and in need of support" (p. 307).

Live Symbolically—Keep a record of ideas, thoughts and feelings to be searched regularly. Finding what accords best with one is tantamount to finding the art of life. This involves personal experimentation and searching.

When concentration is used to still the mind, according to Vaughn (1987), it may have the effect of lowering the activity of the left hemisphere, thereby allowing the right hemisphere to dominate, releasing creative seeds which may have been incubating. Kneller (1965) calls for immersion in one's subject. This implies *commitment*, which is a necessary condition for prolonged concentration of energy. He pairs commitment with *detachment*, because too close a focus may narrow one's range of vision, stifling creativity. Detachment provides the necessary distance, allowing the work to be seen whole, so that it may respond back to the creator.

Active imagination means that one is personally involved (Vaughan, 1987), suggesting a passion for the work at hand. This condition must be balanced by the rigors of judgment and discipline (Arieti, 1980). Creativity, writes Kneller (1965), "...consists largely of rearranging what we know in order to find what we do not know" (p. 59).

The ability to surrender opens one to the involvement of the personality at different levels. This allows one "...to learn how not to push, to let things grow, to be able to know when to walk away, to be able—once you have the inspiration—to build rather than jump from one thing to another..." (Robbins, 1973, p. 10).

Finally, *learning to treat one's errors with respect* may suggest surprising new paths. There is often an intuitive truth to one's errors because they are the voice of the unconscious. This paves the way for the creator to submit to the work, allowing it to express itself (Kneller, 1965)

Creativity cannot be trained, but conditions may be cultivated to spark its emergence. The definition of psychotherapy as a creative enterprise asks us to draw on our ingenuity and intuition in our struggle to assist our clients.

The Inquiry

When we express what occurs to us, we do not always know what we are saying. Theodore Reik

For this study I initiated a fifty-two week visual dialogue with my art.

I wished to deliberately discard my conditioning to know, for the experience of delving into and living with my own mysteries. I wanted to embrace a course of action without knowing where I would go, reflecting the essence of being alive. Most importantly, I hoped that the establishment of a consistent and rigorous framework would offer the terrain in which I could cultivate the qualities and conditions essential to the practice of art psychotherapy.

My investigation may best be described as *heuristic*, a way of learning through one's own exploration, or in this case, an exploration of my art and myself. This form of inquiry has been hailed by Douglas and Moustakas (1985) as a way for researchers to develop their own questions by using a process that affirms intuition, imagination, and self-reflection in the quest for knowledge. Heuristics is an effort to know an aspect of life through a personal and passionate involvement in the study problem. One may address the richness of human experience by allowing the subjective realm to inform the research. Unlike traditional research models which seek to prove or disprove variables, the object of this approach is to uncover and articulate the nature of variables as they are.

Scientific inquiry is generally founded on a dichotomy between reason and emotion. This approach operates on an assumption that observation is most accurate when emotions are not involved. However, May (1975) notes that data from Rorschach responses indicate that people who are more emotionally involved can more accurately observe. When the emotions are engaged, things are seen more sharply (p. 49). Thus, reasoning ability may actually be more finely tuned when emotions are present.

Quality of experience is honored by heuristic research, which as a conceptual framework offers an attitude but does not impart a methodology. Instead, each heuristic study may be seen as a unique creative challenge aimed at revealing some essence of reality by using methods most fitting to the particular investigation. "Learning that proceeds heuristically has a path of its own. It is self-directed, self-motivated, and open to spontaneous shift. It defies the shackles of convention and tradition. With distinctive energy and rhythm, it pushes beyond the known, the expected, or the merely possible (Douglas and Moustakas, 1985, p. 44).

This touches the very roots of psychology. The Greek origins of psyche are related to breath, life and soul. Psychology is typically perceived as the scientific study of mind and behavior, but its classical roots suggest a poetic concept which is deep, mutable, and mysteriously elusive. Field (1934) wrote:

"When I considered anything that happened to me in terms of science, I had to split it up into parts and think only of those qualities which it had in common with others so it lost that unique quality which it had as a whole, the "thing-in-itselfness" which had so delighted me in wide perceiving. I wondered whether this was why sometimes, when I came out from reading in a scientific library, the first whiff of hot pavement, the glimpse of a mangy terrier grimed with soot, would make me feel as though I had risen from the dead. For this "dogness" of the dog and "stoneness" of the pavement which I loved so, were simply non-existent in abstract "dog" and abstract "pavement." It seemed to me then that science could only talk about things and that discussion broke up and killed some essential quality of experience" (p. 201).

The project acquired a shape of its own, distinguished by three phases: A fifty-two week visual dialogue, an exhibition, and a written phenomenological exploration of the resulting art objects.

The Visual Dialogue with Art

The idea for the visual dialogue developed as I sat under a tree drinking from a cup. The cup spoke to me as a symbol for the therapeutic holding environment, for the exchange within the therapeutic relationship, and as a metaphor for myself. I looked up into the tree and saw other aspects of myself. Later, I sculpted a paper mache form using a cup as a base and an aspect of the tree as a metaphor for myself.

It struck me then that this kind of visual dialogue continued on a weekly basis for one year, would create a setting in which I could experience and externalize the rhythm of my life. As I make day to day choices (What will I

400

make today? How will I make it? What materials will I use? What colors will I mix? How will I juxtapose the elements?) I project my point of view and am brought into direct contact with the responsibility for my life condition. The things I experience and reveal in the process of creation are inevitably some dimension of my life. London writes, (1989) "What we are is what we do. How we put our life together is how we put our paints together" (p. 25). This is the site for the dialogue—the place where I meet the materials with my senses (cup, modeling compound, paper pulp, organic debris, acrylic paint). I see what evolves. I do it once a week for a year.

The Exhibition

To view the art products—remnants of my year long investigation—is to see something of the character of my unfolding. The objects now stand as a portrait, reflecting the nature of lived experience. "Think of what it is like to dwell before a painted portrait," writes Nozick (1989) "and to let it then dwell within you. Think also of the ways this differs from reading a clinical description of a particular person, or a general psychological theory" (p. 12).

The Dialogue/Methodology

It is evident that the core of the creative process—the activity of shaping and externalizing experience—is imbued with healing properties. Potent meaning is found or further enhanced when images are re-experienced using another language system, thus utilizing both cerebral hemispheres. For this reason, I established a framework to enter into active participation with each art object. Rather than read extraneous meanings into the imagery through the interpretation of symbols contained within the work, my goal was to experience the work by seeing the phenomenon anew.

The framework that I established incorporates ideas from Betensky's (1987) phenomenological approach, Nucho's (1987) Psychocybernetic model, Gestalt Therapy (Perls, Hefferline & Goodman, 1951), and the wisdom of child's play. Schachtel (1971) notes the main functions of exploratory play. First, an acquaintance is made with the object by directly relating with it. A discovery of connections to oneself is then made by finding out what can be done with it, and how it might fit into one's world.

The dialogue framework is a process of inquiry which becomes progressively more concentrated. As I look at what has been produced, I note the Objective Qualities by naming what I see, and observing what stands out, or what is central. I answer the underlying question "what do you see?" (Nucho, 1987).

This question holds two fundamental principles of the phenomenological approach (Betensky, 1987). The phenomenological emphasis on individual perception and meaning is underscored in the question itself. It asks for my perception, which does not need to match the way others perceive. Thus, the subjective value of reality is emphasized. The other concept revealed in the question, "What do you see?" concerns phenomenological evidence. Rather than making interpretations culled from pre-established theory, my focal point is on that which is seen in the art expression itself (p. 159).

2. *Experiencing the affective qualities* is the next stage of the inquiry (Nucho, 1987). Here, I express the feelings I experience now as I look at the product. This may be different from the feeling I was experiencing when I initially made the object, or even from the feeling I had intended to convey. Thus, surprises may be noted here.

3. Then a dialogic exchange, which is based on gestalt theory, solicits what Nucho (1987) calls a *distillation of meaning* (p. 163). This is a technique to expand awareness, and experience a dynamic interchange between polarities (Zinker, 1977). The gestalt approach is concerned with the active exploration of the self. Hazy reminiscing gives way to the "here and now" where everything comes to life (Perls, Hefferline & Goodman 1951). Meaning is distilled by allowing it to coalesce through a direct experience with the object itself. Thus, I ask myself what the object would say if it could talk, or what I would like to say to my art object.

4. Finally the dialogue concludes with a response to the preceding answer.

Results

> *To produce is to draw forth, to invent is to find, to shape is to discover. In bodying forth I disclose...The work produced is a thing among things, able to be experienced and described as a sum of qualities.*
>
> Martin Buber

"Reality is not something inflexible and unchanging, but is ready to be re-made..." (Perls, Hefferline & Goodman, 1951, p. 246). By moving into active participation with the art products, I could essentially recreate the work, thereby re—absorbing it. Ehrenzweig (1967) notes that the establishment of a relationship with one's own work teaches one to communicate with submerged aspects of one's personality. Thus, I am less interested in what was occurring during my life, one year ago when I created the art products, then I am about what can arise now as I engage and recreate each piece.

Art objects are seen by McNiff (1989) as "companions, helpers, and records of involvement" (p. 105). The data now stands as a description of the texture and shape of my lived experience. More than a method to illuminate my underlying psychological and spiritual conditions, it became an opportunity to engage deep dimensions of my inner being. Patterns of meaning suggest themselves and reveal complex aspects about what I am, what I have been, and what I might become. The following seven examples are taken from the beginning, middle, and end of the project, to reveal how the experience may be engaged on many levels.

Week Two

Objective qualities: The spiny root system catches my eye. It is visually enticing, yet tactually forbidding. I wonder if it is as jagged as it looks—will it hurt me to touch it? Although it looks jagged, the color says something feminine. The color goes from light pink at the top to dark pink at the bottom— beckoning to the color inside. I remember how hard it was for me to get the roots to attach.

Affective Qualities: I feel fragile as I look at it now. It looks delicate and undernourished. It brings up a desire in me to protect it from harm—to shield it. I didn't plan it to be so delicate and jagged.

Distillation of Meaning: The cup speaks: You work so hard to make me appear interesting. I guess you don't believe I'm worthwhile without your additions. Yet in the end you make me appear untouchable. We both know that my roots aren't sharp— that they're actually soft and pliable—but I appear sharp. I'm sad that you do this because if keeps people from me.

Response: Without me, you wouldn't be compelling or inviting. Don't you see that without me your inner vitality wouldn't be seen. I think you need my addi-

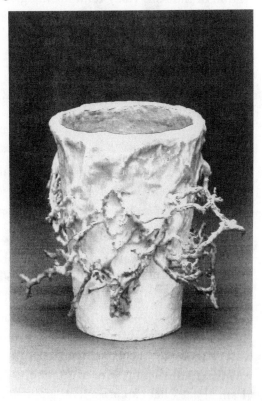

Week Two

tions to avoid being lost in the crowd. I help draw people to you.

Week Four

Objective Qualities: The wiry-looking branches which reach above the form and hover over the cup opening capture my attention. They extend every which way. There is a jagged and fragile quality to them. The form is divided evenly with two bands of color which are blended in the middle. The lower half is lighter.

Affective Qualities: The feeling I get now as I look at it is a cautious, uneasy feeling. It looks undernourished and shaky. Even the inside gives off a dried blood melancholia. My sensations about the branches are complex—on the one hand, they are humiliating

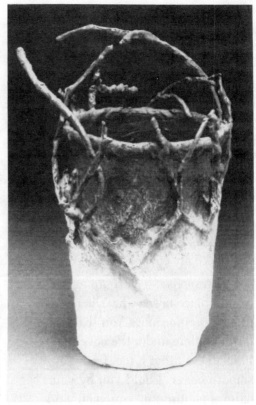

Week Four

because they are so fragile they look like they will break off. Yet this is right where my eye goes. It creates a lively play with the space above the cup—there is a visual irony: the darkness of the upper part brings my eye down, but the liveliness of the extended branches brings my eye up.

Distillation of Meaning: Speak to the cup: I have an urge to break off your branches because they are so fragile looking. I just know they are going to break, so I want to do it. I even feel lik e destroying you. Although you extend out and up, you hover protectively. You are somehow menacing.

Response: I can't count on you to hold my fragility. Why not think of ways to strengthen me. I feel threatened by you. I'm not yet able to extend with the solid grace of my trunk. Look how much energy I'm using to convince you not to break me.

Week Nineteen

Objective Qualities: The contrast between the smooth green outer surface and the black and pink undersurface is striking. The roots are under cover. My eye is most drawn to the texture and color of the lower half. It beckons.

Affective Qualities: Oceanic calm warms the upper two-thirds of the form. The dark and tangled lower portion rattles in all directions. Tranquil and smooth above, bewildered and brittle below.

Distillation of Meaning: The cup speaks: My smooth cover isn't long enough to cover me. My bottom section is without cover. I don't like hanging out like this. I'm brittle, I might break. Why did you make my cover so short?

Response: I left an opening—a place to see what's here—a place to come out. You'll never develop there under the cover. But I must admit that I, too, favor your smooth cover. I hold you by your calm smoothness, your soft and soothing blue-greenness, and I withdraw my touch from your dark

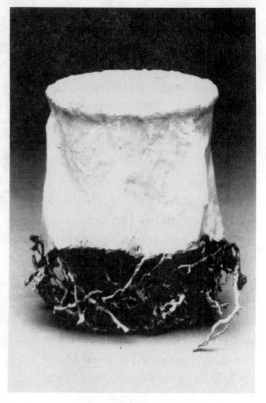

Week Nineteen

and brittle ways. I don't hold your bewilderment.

Week Twenty-One

Objective Qualities: Pink glows brightly from the surrounding darkness. Three textural slabs cling to the inner form. The perspective drastically changes as the form is turned from side to side.

Affective Qualities: Eagerness jolts from the muddled dark exterior—as if it were tickled out. The uneasy exterior goes around an affectionate opening. It speaks of desire.

Distillation of Meaning: Speak to the cup: You have different sides. Your rough thickness surrounds your thin darkness. Your thin darkness surrounds your bright hollowness. Nothing you do distracts me from your inside. In fact, your outside looks like a distraction which no longer fits—it hangs on you. You hang onto your own dark exterior. What does this feel like to you?

Response: Uneasy. I am stifled and weighted down, yet bewilderingly exposed. I am in-between. I am wedged. I am attached to my dark exterior.

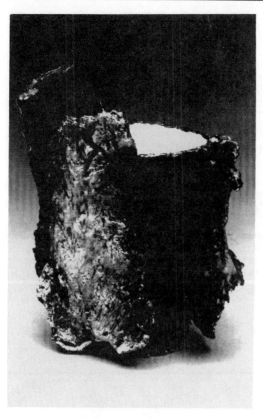

Week Twenty One

Week Twenty-Three

Objective Qualities: Two central breaks or tears in the outer covering immediately catch my eye. A series of fractured and sharp fragments are pushing for visibility—they jut out of the torn outer surface. The outer cover bulges with the form of something underneath. The outer layer is cool in color tone, whereas the inner layer is hot and dark.

Affective Qualities: I experience an active sensation now as I look—a rumbling movement. There is no stopping this. Although it looks like it could be unruly, it captivates me.

Distillation of Meaning: The cup speaks: Why are you always so compelled to lay these covers on top of me? My sharpness is not smoothed by your cover. That's not what I need. I need to be jagged and sharp and see what happens from that. I want to continue rumbling in my jaggedness even though I can't promise you that anything will come of it.

Response: When I go to touch you I am aware of my difficulty in accepting you, because I see you as untouchable. I cover you to make you feel more appealing.

Response: No, the cover makes you feel better. I am working against its weight. Besides, it's obvious by my sharp protrusions that my smoothness is just a cover.

Week Thirty-Seven

Objective Qualities: The form looks like it has exploded open. The mid-section exposes a different layer than the top and bottom sections. The outer surface looks weathered, like it has been exposed to the sunshine. The inside is dark, pink, and pithy.

Affective Qualities: I see a burnt, spent quality. The surfaces look

405

charred...like they've been in the center of a hot fire, but they're not burned up. I see potential here in the darkness.

Distillation of Meaning: The cup speaks: Wipe off that black darkness, I have pink emotion underneath. When you added the black on top, you obscured my pink. I am completely exposed to a new place around my entire mid-section, and you go and cover me. What's your problem?

Response: You looked too bright. I remember how compelled I was to darken your brightness. And I was equally compelled to lighten your colorful outside. I darken my vitality, and I lighten my impact.

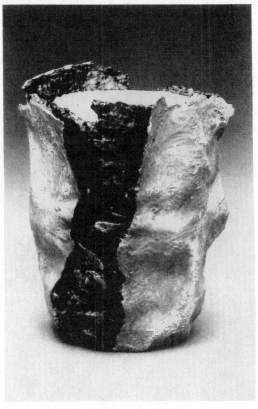

Week Twenty Three

Week Fifty

Objective Qualities: The trunk rises to a wide and fanciful leafy network reaching into the surrounding space. One part bends and branches back into the center of the cup. The fleshy trunk emerges solidly from a dark ground.

Affective Qualities: With triumph and exuberance, the form arches up and extends out. It moves buoyantly and confidently.

Distillation of Meaning: The cup speaks: When you shaped me, you attended to all of me. There is not a part of me that is left deprived, nor is there a special part. I am nourished from head to toe.

Response: Maybe that's why I'm having trouble engaging you like I did with number thirty—nine. Am I just tired now, or is it me and you, and the way you are so cordial and evenly dispersed. You don't seem like you need me. This is new territory. Our relationship is not based on need. You are nourished. How can I be with you in your satiated state? It's like learning a new dance.

406

Discussion

About the experience of life—most people are under the illusion that they can be happy only if something especially good happens. Oddly enough, there is only one phrase I know to express that life is good per se, that just being alive is good—the French expression, joie de vivre. *Joie de vivre simply means that just being alive is an extraordinary experience—It is immaterial what goes on, except for the fact that you are alive. It does not mean that you are very happy with the way you live. You can even be suffering; but just being alive is a quality per se.*   Rene Dubos

Learning to suspend judgment to allow for a natural unfolding is part of the ongoing work of the therapist. Shainberg (1983) writes, "…it is in the mutual participation of discovering the essential quality of the patient that the healing takes place" (p. 164). This has to do with learning how to become aware of one's own awareness.

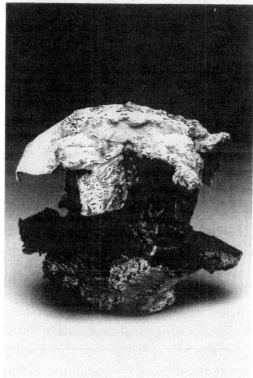

Week Thirty Seven

The open-ended nature of the fifty-two week dialogue demanded an open and searching attitude from me. Creativity is most likely to occur within this kind of adventurous mental set. The framework was a frontier in which I could exercise my emotional experiences, encounter existential strivings, and by following the work wherever it led me, cultivate the conditions and habits most pertinent to creative work.

The rigors of the exploration have furnished me with a concrete operational method for the development of qualities deemed most essential to therapeutic practice. My investigation became a portrait of my existence, showing me that being authentic depends on how I am with myself and with what is, rather than with what I do to improve myself. Authentic well-being means being fully awake.

Periods of change are characterized by higher levels of anxiety. As new meanings emerge, they must be integrated into the personality. The acquisition of skills and knowledge in graduate training must be integrated into a new personal and professional identity—a complex process which may be buttressed by a transitional relationship. If through the process of creation I was expressing some of the challenges and conflicts in adjusting to the vicissitudes of the profession, the creation may then come to be used for purposes of maturation and self-soothing, as a "transitional object" (Winnicott, 1971).

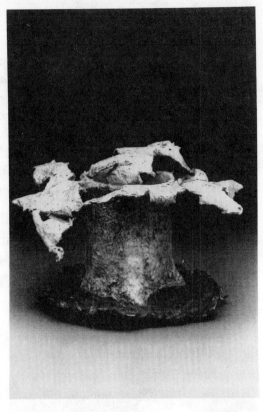

Week Fifty

The expression of my experience became a sort of reconstruction of my evolving personal and professional identity. By staying within the bounds of my own observation, assuming nothing that did not stem from my own experience, I sharpened my focus, becoming more openly attuned to my awareness. A key transformation occurred in my clinical practice when I became more open to observing the client as he is, releasing static notions about how the therapy exchange is supposed to occur. When I allow this to happen, I experience my presence as the medium in which, Shainberg (1985) writes, "the being is the doing" (p. 175).

As I viewed the work in its entirety, the transformation was reflected in the art forms themselves. Object relations which had been externalized were mirrored back to me, allowing them to be experienced and gradually re-assimilated—a process which continues to evolve. The forms progress from an applied-looking and decorated condition to appearing as if the form and color emerge from the forms themselves. Simultaneously, my relationship with the art forms evolved. My initial experience of them as "other" grew to an experience of them as being a part of me, to being something in themselves that I can see as "other" but carry with me.

The experience became a bridge for the development of two significant mentor relationships. A link to a professional heritage was forged, providing examples of what it can mean to remain involved in the process of self—development. These relationships allowed me to tap into the kinship reminiscent of the day of the art guild. "...there was this closeness of man to man," writes Martine-Kinkead (1986), "the sense of one another's existence, and the exchange between the experienced workers and the novices: the meeting of eyes, the showing and the watching, the speaking and the listening" (p. 60). An experience of "being with" was created, which by its quality and shape strengthened the structure of the project. The active, rhythmic and consistent connection allowed me to be seen, recognized, and understood as the person I was, and the person I was becoming.

Creative experience demands a willingness to oscillate between surrender and control and diffuseness and differentiation. Inasmuch as psychotherapy is a creative venture, so too the participants involved in the interchange will experience oscillations between certainty and doubt brought about by the fluctuations of the work. Ongoing immersion in art-making sets in motion a movement away from the compulsion to hold the controllable and the known, reminding one that the most valuable things in this field cannot be learned, but must be experienced.

References

Allen, P. (1992). *Artist in residence: an alternative to "Clinification" for art therapists.* Art Therapy. Journal of the American Art Therapy Association, 9 (1), 22—29.

Allen, T. (1967). *Effectiveness of counselor trainees as a function of psychological openness.* Journal of Counseling Psychology, 14 (1), 35-40.

Arieti, S. (1976). *The magic synthesis.* NY: Basic Books

Betensky, M. (1987). *Phenomenology of therapeutic art expression and art therapy.* In Judith Rubin, ed., Approaches to Art Therapy, (pp. 149-66).

Bugental, J. (1965). *The search for authenticity; an existential-analytic approach in psychotherapy.* NY: Holt, Rinehart & Winston.
——(1987). The art of the psychotherapist. Existential Psychiatry, 6 (21), 19—34.

Carkhuff, R. & Truax, C. (1965). *Training in counseling and psychotherapy: an evaluation of an integrated didactic and experiential approach.* Journal of Consulting Psychology, 29 (4), 333—336.

Corey, G. (1977). *Theory and practice of counseling and psychotherapy.* CA: Brooks/Cole.

Dewey, J. (1977). *Art as experience.* NY: A Wideview/Perigree Book.

Dissanayake, E. (1988). *What is art for?* Seattle and London: University of Washington Press.

Douglass, B. and Moustakas, C. (1985). *Heuristic inquiry: The internal search to know.* Journal of Humanistic Psychology, 25(3), 39-55.

Ehrenzweig, A. (1967). *The hidden order of art.* Berkeley and Los Angeles: U. of California.

Erikson, J. (1988). *Wisdom and the senses.* NY and London: W. W. Norton.

Field, J. (1934). *A life of one's own*. Baltimore, MD: Penguin Books.

Fromm, E. (1959). *The creative attitude*. in Anderson, Harold H. (ed.), Creativity and its cultivation. NY: Harper and Brothers Publishers.

Ghiselin, B. (1952). *The creative process: A symposium*. Berkeley, CA: U. of California

Grudin, R. (1990). *The grace of great things: Creativity and innovation*. NY: Ticknor and Fields.

Jourard, S. (1967). *Psychotherapy as invitation*. Existential Psychiatry, 6 (21), 19-34.

Kneller, G. (1965). *The art and science of creativity*. NY: Holt, Rinehart and Winston

Kohut, H. (1959). *Introspection, Empathy, & Psychoanalysis. An Examination of the Relationship between Mode of Observation and Theory*. Journal of American Psychoanalytical Association., VII, pp. 459-483.

London, P. (1989). *No more secondhand art*. Boston and Shaftesbury: Shambhala

Luborsky, L., Singer, B. and Luborsky, L. (1975). *Comparative studies of psychotherapies: Is it true that "everyone has won and all must have prizes?"* Archives of General Psychiatry, 32, 995-1008.

Martine-Kinkead, J. (1985). *Working for a living*. In D. M. (ed.), A Way of Working, (pp. 59-65). NY: Parabola Books.

May, R. (1975). *The courage to create*. NY: W. W. Norton.

McNiff, S. (1989). *Depth psychology of art*. Springfield, IL: C. C. Thomas

Nozick, R. (1989). *The examined life*. NY: Simon and Schuster.

Nucho, A. (1987). *The psychocybernetic model of art therapy*. Springfield, IL: C. C. Thomas

Patrick, C. (1955). *What is creative thinking?* NY: Philosophical Library.

Perls, F., Hefferline, R. and Goodman, P. (1951). *Gestalt therapy: Growth and excitement in the human personality*. NY: Dell.

Robbins, A. (1973). *The art therapist's imagery as a response to a therapeutic dialogue*. Art Psychotherapy, 1, 181-184.

————(1973). *A psychoanalytic perspective towards the inter-relationship of the creative process and the functions of an art therapist*. Art Psychotherapy, 1, 7-12.

Rogers, C. (1962). *The interpersonal relationship: the core of guidance*. Harvard Educational Review, 32 (4), 416-429.

————(1976). *Toward a theory of creativity*. In Rothberg (Ed.), The Creativity Question. Durham, NC: Duke University Press.

Shainberg, D. (1983). *Teaching therapists how to be with their clients*. John Welwood (Ed.), Awakening the Heart. Boston: New Science Library.

Sloane, R., Staples, F. , Cristol, A. Yorkston, N. and Whipple, K. (1975). *Psychotherapy versus behavior therapy*. Cambridge: Harvard University Press.

Storr, A. (1980). *The art of psychotherapy*. NY: Methuen.

Strupp, H. (1958). *The psychotherapist's contribution to the treatment process*. Behavior Science, 3, 34-67.

Trungpa, Ch. (1985). *Becoming a full human being*. John Welwood (Ed.) Awakening the Heart. Boston: New Science Library.

Vaughan, T. (1987). *On not predicting the outcome: creativity as adventure*. The Journal of Creative Behavior, 21(4), 300-311.

Winnicott, D. W. (1971) *Playing and reality*. NY: Basic Books.

Zinker, J. (1977). *Creative process in gestalt therapy*. NY: Vintage Books.

Free Arts for Abused and Neglected Children,
A Testing Ground for Potential Art Therapists
by Elda Unger, M.A., A.T.R.

Elda Unger, president of the Southern California Art Therapy Association and former director of the art therapy program at Pine Grove Hospital, received the 1991 Special Award by the County of Los Angeles Task Force to Promote Self-Esteem. Through Free Arts For Abused Children, Ms. Unger, as vice-president and president for 14 years, has helped bring the arts to thousands of children in over 75 residential care facilities in Los Angeles. She has appeared before the U. S. Senate Children's Caucus on behalf of abused children.

Therapeutic art by non-therapist artists is a controversial yet growing concept developed by the Free Arts for Abused Children organization in Los Angeles and Orange counties. Many art therapists value the work done by FAAC, introducing art where it has not been used before, and introducing the concept of it being therapeutic and diagnostic as well. Others feel that the volunteers are taking jobs away from professional art therapists. But the concept seems to have caught on. Started in 1977, FAAC now has over 750 volunteer artists reaching 1500 children weekly in over 75 residential care facilities. FAAC has now expanded to Phoenix, Arizona, and has plans in the near future for the rest of the country.

The facilities for abused and neglected children in Los Angeles and Orange counties, house from six children in group homes to institutions housing as many as 125, in addition to 250 children in MacLaren Hall in El Monte. The children's ages range from newborn to 18 years.

Volunteer artists agree to commit a minimum of one hour a week with a group of children for a 20 week period. In addition. we organize Free Arts Days where a group of volunteers go into facilities two or three full days a month, usually on Sunday, from 9 am to 3 pm, working with the entire population. Depending on the size of the population of the facility, we have from 15 to 50 volunteers working with 30 to 200 children on a Free Arts Day. We work with the larger facilities and combine small group homes so that we reach about 30 of the facilities a year.

Training for the artists is ongoing, through lectures, workshops, and demonstrations by prominent professionals: art therapists, psychologists, psychiatrists, social workers. The artists are clearly made aware of their limitations and boundaries as non-professionals, and learn not to probe for problems or feelings with which they are not equipped to deal. What our volunteers do is therapeutic but they are not therapists.

Instead, the training is in useful art techniques, and attitudes of caring, genuineness, and self-knowledge. They are trained as artists, not therapists. *If problems surface, they bring it to the attention of a staff member.* They are there to share their love and creativity and do not present themselves as therapists.

FAAC was started in 1977 when several of us, who had successfully worked with children at risk, set out to reach them through the arts. We incorporated as a non-profit organization in 1978, obtaining grants to continue and enlarge our organization. As a founding member and president for many years, I recognized the need for further training for myself, and became a registered art therapist in order to properly and professionally guide FAAC.

Many art therapy interns have chosen to use our program as part of their training. Many of our volunteers have sought professional training and have become art therapists after experiencing the need for this modality and the results they achieved with these children. We have encouraged many of the facilities that we serve to budget for the hiring of professional art therapists. The staff at these facilities are impressed with the healing effects of the arts and how well the children have responded. Without exception, all of the facilities we serve plan on having an art therapist on staff when their budgets permit.

Two years ago, we received a grant from a Texas foundation to start our PACT (Parents and Children Together) program. Concerned with family preservation, we work with at-risk families who have been assigned by the courts to help them fight the cycle of abuse and be able to keep their children while receiving this help. Our creative arts volunteers work in an 8 week program showing these families how to work with each other through the arts and develop new means of communication and play, release some of their frustration and learn how to do creative and enjoyable things together.

Our PACT program has now been extended to the new children's court house in Monterey Park, Los Angeles, where child abuse cases are heard. Art volunteers do art projects with most of the 100 families waiting for their hearings. Because of this, both the children and parents are found to deal with the court room experience with more equanimity. Judges and lawyers are surprised to hear the children ask if they can come back to the court house and do more art instead of responding to the experience with the usual trepidation and trauma.

A striking 2-story enamel on copper mural of 36 self-portraits of children made with FAAC volunteers now greet all visitors upon entering the court house building.

FAAC was ahead of its time in addressing the newly defined traumatology relating to abused children, and the healing effects of art. Art is not a luxury, but a necessity for survival for a large portion of our population. Free Arts For Abused Children (FAAC) is probably the only non-profit organization that actively recruits, screens, trains and places arts volunteers in residential care facilities for abused and neglected children.

FAAC has been funded largely by our fundraising events, grants from private foundations and corporations. All of our Free Arts Days are underwritten by individuals and organizations. Donations of tickets to shows and concerts are given to the facilities by performing artists and interested supporters of FAAC.

FAAC appears to have struck a responsive chord in the arts and entertainment community, and has been liberally supported by their donations, and appearances by Hollywood celebrities at our fund-raising affairs. They have also generously donated time on radio and TV public services supporting our work. Volunteers have been recruited through our public service announcements, and through help from local universities. Public relations firms have donated their services as well. We now have a paid staff of five whose salaries are funded by monies raised from corporate grants, individual sponsors, membership dues and our fundraisers. All of these activities have made the public aware of the healing effects of the arts. As a result, the demand for our kind of services has increased and we have started our first pilot program toward national expansion in Phoenix, Arizona.

An executive board in Phoenix has been formed to organize and oversee this new program, under a charter of the parent organization, using our by-laws and articles of incorporation, and a complete organizational layout for board and committees. The executive director in Phoenix, a registered art therapist, is organizing our program there using our extensive material for screening applicants and manuals for training volunteers. She will provide training for the volunteers with the help of other mental health professionals. Her salary is being raised by the Arizona board with her assistance. She has attended Los Angeles board meetings, program development meetings, teacher training sessions, and participated in Free Arts Days and PACT Programs.

The first Free Arts For Abused Children of Arizona program took place in September, 1993. We expect that, as the demand for this program becomes more widespread, it will be repeated elsewhere. Our expansion plans call for registered art therapists to be the first paid executive directors of each new chapter, which will be organized in a similar manner to the Phoenix pilot program.

Art Projects for FAAC Volunteers

The following are some of the art projects that non-professional FAAC volunteers do with the children. These are non-invasive, non-judgmental and allow the children to express themselves freely, some of them for the first time.

• Constructions

The children are given scraps of wood (odd shapes donated by carpenters and builders), stones, dried vegetation and wooden flat bases along with pieces of metal, rock, plexiglas with glue and paint, whatever we have of interest. From this they form imaginative environments that make them feel good about themselves.

• T-Shirt Designing

The children paint with fast drying fabric paint directly on the shirts or draw a design on sand paper with crayon which we iron onto the shirts.

• Clones

Children lie down on a doubled sheet of vinyl (discarded rolls donated by wallpaper stores) or heavy butcher or wrapping paper, and their bodies are traced in whatever position they wish (football player, ballet dancer, guitar player, basketball player, etc.). After the life-size pattern is cut out and painted (both front and back), it is partially stapled, stuffed tightly with news-

414

paper, then closed, creating a dramatic "clone."

• Decorating Flower Pots

The children are given pots and fast drying acrylic paints. After they decorate the pots, they put plants in them to take to their rooms. They are shown how to care for the plants in order for them to thrive, a lesson in responsibility and pride in creation.

• Painting Colorful Art without Paint

Each child is given a sheet of white construction paper, colorful tissue paper that bleeds, a paint brush and liquid starch. Each little piece of tissue paper that they lay on the construction paper is painted on with liquid starch. They continue to realize various shapes and forms overlapping each other as they paint with the starch. This creates a beautiful abstract which can be made into a light print by blotting another sheet on top, giving them a monoprint of the original. Many use the print for a greeting card and we frame the original.

• Clay Work

The children roll clay into balls. From these balls we ask them to allow various forms and creatures to emerge. As they create, they talk about their creations while carefully smoothing all the rough spots and cracks with their fingers and water.

• Thumb and Pencil Art

The only supplies needed are paper, a soft graphite pencil and thumbs. The edges of randomly shaped scrap paper are covered with graphite. This paper is placed on 2x2 squares of paper or cardboard so that, holding the paper firmly in place, the children can smear the graphite onto the square with their thumbs. When several graphite shapes are rubbed onto the cardboard, a beautiful abstract picture appears.

• Collages

Choosing from a large supply of pre-cut words and magazine pictures, the children cut and paste onto large sheets of colored construction paper any images they like. They are encouraged to further decorate their collage with markers.

• Monoprints

Each child is given 2 small pieces of plexiglass (about 4" x 6"), scraps donated from plexiglass shops. They paint any design they choose on one of the plexiglas sheets with acrylic paint. Then they take the second piece of plexiglas and press it on top of the first until the plexiglas feels glued together. Then carefully, without sliding them, they pull them apart. The suction creates intricate patterns which can be printed as greeting cards getting at least 2 prints from each piece of plexiglas.

• Creating and Drawing a Story

They are told to draw a story which becomes a cartoon strip for some of the children and an imaginative painting for others. They enjoy telling the story they have drawn. Young children as well as adolescents participate in this process.

Conclusion

Many children our FAAC volunteers see have not experienced art in any form. We are proud to bring the experience of creativity to the children in over three quarters of the 100 child care facilities in Los Angeles County, bringing hope, joy, and in many cases, a new means of communication. We are also proud to introduce artist volunteers to the process of art therapy, which in turn, has created many new professional art therapists.

References

Keyes, M. F. (1983). *The inward journey.* San Mateo, CA: Open Court Press.

Kramer, E. (1972). *Art as therapy with children.* NY: Schocken.

Linesch, D. (1992). *Adolescent art therapy.* NY: Brunner/Mazel.

Lusebrink, V. B. (1990). *Imagery and visual expression.* NY: Plenum Press.

McNiff, S. (1986). *Educating the creative arts therapist: a profile of the profession.* IL.: C. C. Thomas.

Oaklander, V. (1978). *Windows to our children.* Highland. NY: The Center for Gestalt Development.

Sperry, V. (1968). *The art experience.* Boston: Boston Book.

Virshup, E. (1979) *Right brain people in a left brain world.* Los Angeles: Guild of Tutors Press.

Reducing Student Attrition Rate Through Art
by Evelyn Virshup, Ph.D., A.T.R. and Bernard Virshup, M.A., M.D.

Author of Right Brain People In A Left Brain World, *Evelyn Virshup teaches creativity and stress reduction at Art Center College of Design, art therapy at Cal State University, L.A., and has given art therapy workshops internationally. She has hosted and produced over 150 cable TV programs, discussing psychological issues and the use of art with mental health professionals. In 1987, her documentary,* Suicide, A Teenage Dilemma, *won an EMMY. A past president of the Southern California Art Therapy Association, she is presently Public Relations Chair of the American Art Therapy Association.*

A retired cardiologist, Bernard Virshup teaches physicians, medical students at University of Southern California and UCLA, and art students at Art Center College of Design ways of dealing with the stresses of professionalization. He is the author of numerous articles and several books on the subject including Coping in Medical School.

The process of art can be used effectively to help students cope better with the stresses of school, improve their academic and social skills, and lower their dropout rate.

A major problem educators face today is lowering the large dropout rate, students who never finish school. In colleges, the rate averages 50% attrition across the country; in many high schools, the figure is about 30%. We must add to these dismal figures the students who fail to take full advantage of our educational system, and those who turn to drugs, teen-age suicide, and other anti-social and self-destructive coping efforts.

Art therapists have an opportunity to help reverse this trend. Art Center College of Design in Pasadena had a dropout rate of about 33% when, in

1982, we began an elective course to help students learn ways of coping better with these stresses. In 1986, a new administration made such a course, of 2 1/2 hours once a week for five weeks mandatory for the entire second term class. Over the next two years, the attrition rate dropped to 8%.

Although geared at Art Center to art students, the principles are universal. We first began teaching them to medical students at the University of Southern California School of Medicine, and at a UCLA credit program for teachers in primary and secondary schools. We have presented them in many workshops to many different populations, and have concluded that they can be applied to any student or indeed, any child or adult. At Art Center, the course is taught by four different teachers, all with their own personal philosophies and styles but with a general approach on which all four agree.

The emphasis of the course is not on reducing the stress of the school, but on improving the students' coping skills.

Stress has two major definitions. One is that of external stress, a difficult situation. The other is that of internal stress, that is, the thoughts and feelings of the individual exposed to a difficult situation. Engineers refer to these as stress, which is the pressure on a material, and strain, which measures how much the material is "bent out of shape."

Developing coping skills implies that individuals can learn how to handle situations that are difficult for them, and that these are behavioral skills that can be taught. We are more concerned with helping them learn how to cope with the stress, than with reducing it. We must emphasize that this is not 'therapy', that is, it is not intended to *rehabilitate* the individual. It is educational, in that it teaches new coping attitudes and behaviors.

The 3 major strategies students learn to help cope with stress are:

- improving their feelings of identity and self worth
- helping them deal more effectively with their own internal, often excessive, criticism of themselves, and
- learning how to establish supportive relationships.

These objectives can be achieved in different ways, and, as we said, the teachers have differences in philosophy and approach, ranging in persuasion from behaviorism to supportive counseling. It is interesting that we all have found success and reinforcement for our own approaches, and it is not with any degree of competition that we wish to tell you of the success we have found with our own approach that uses art as the primary medium for promoting change and growth in our students.

We begin the first class by placing them in a circle, rather than in the usual formation in which they represent a solid phalanx of resistance, opposed to the teacher, who is then almost compelled to play out the expert teacher role. In a circle, they become more interactive, with teachers and with each other, and we all feel more comfortable with each other.

Exercise 1: Drawing Initials

In the first class "warm-up," the students each draw their names very large on a sheet of paper, and then, in and around the letters draw symbols of how they see themselves—who they are, what they do, what their interests are—that they are willing to share with the rest of the class. Everyone enjoys this, and it sets the tone for sharing, for admiring each other, for symbolization, and for safe self-revelation.

The first major issue we deal with is identity and self-worth.

Exercise 2: Short-Form Jungian Types Test

We give them all a short-form Jungian Types Test. Jung identified various tendencies in people, which he called functions. Katherine Briggs and her daughter, Isabel Myers devised a test for these functions, the *Myers-Briggs Type Inventory*, which gives a score for the Extrovert-Introvert, Sensate-Intuitive, Thinking-Feeling, and Perceptive-Judging pairs of functions. For our purposes, we give a simplified adaptation of the *Hogan and Champagne Inventory* which is short, easy to self-score, and appears reasonably reliable.

Comment: The United States is dominated by an extrovert-sensate culture. In one of their early samples of 3503 high school males in a college preparatory program, Myers and Briggs found extroverts outnumbered introverts by 61.5% to 38.5%, and sensates outnumbered intuitives by 57.9% to 42.1%. According to Keirsey and Bates, there are 3 times as many extroverts as introverts, and 3 times as many sensates as intuitives. Extrovert and sensate functions are emphasized in most schools, and are the gold standard for "normal" behavior, while the introvert and intuitive functions are either denied or overlooked.

Sensate people are described by these and other authors as depending on the information taken in through the five senses. They believe in what they can see, touch, smell, hear, taste.

Sensate people are:
- "good" steady workers and allocate time well
- patient with routine

419

- good at precise work
- seldom make errors of fact
- good students.

They like:

- standard ways of solving problems
- established ways of doing things
- skills they have already learned.

Now let us draw you a picture of the intuitive person. Intuitive people:
- See patterns and possibilities invisible to others

- Look for relationships between ideas, and the meaning behind the obvious; they put two and two together quickly

- Like solving problems and are patient with complicated situations

- Value imagination and inspiration

- Work in bursts of energy powered by enthusiasm, with slack periods in between

- Get bored with repetition

- Are impatient with the practical and with routine details

- Dislike taking time for precision

- Are dreamers and innovators, with artistic and spiritual values.

We tend to see the intuitive function as the prime and necessary characteristic of the creative individual. In his study of art students, Stephens found that 27 of 31 artists (87%) were Intuitive. We found that two thirds of over 300 Art Center students tested were introverts, and nine tenths intuitives.

Not everyone has a complimentary view of the intuitive function. In a world of practical, realistic sensates, intuitives are :

- Irrational, undisciplined, contrary, unrealistic, impractical, and inadequate daydreamers.

- Their values are unusual, their perception of life is strange, and they come to different conclusions about the world.

- They often do poorly in school, are given poor grades and are often undervalued by society.

- They are frequently a source of concern and frustration to their parents and teachers.

Scientists are not free of this bias. Some researchers have looked at this richness of imagination, intensity of experience, bursts of productive energy, and loose and novel associations, and seen only a syndrome suggesting mental illness. They call it:

- "Input dysfunction"
- "A defect in the cognitive mechanisms which filter stimuli"
- "Fundamental breakdown in inhibitory mechanisms"
- " 'Subclinical' or 'early' " expressions of potential bipolar lability;" i.e, manic-depressive disorder.

To us, however, their depression is usually situational and reversible, and not necessarily a reflection of bipolar depression.

Most Art Center students agree that before they came to Art Center they felt "different," and not "like" everyone else. And most of them, like many minorities, had drawn the wrong conclusion—that there was something wrong with being different, that there was something wrong with them.

When these students take the Types test and find that they are indeed in a minority in the country but that there are many other students at Art Center like them, and many successful people of their type, there is a palpable change in self-esteem. We give them the description of their type to read, and they compare it with others in the room. As a homework assignment, they take the test home and give it to their partner, or room-mate or parent—someone with whom they have a relationship. They write a paper (often misspelled) saying if and how the test has given them a different understanding of their relationship. (They get an automatic A on the paper for turning it in.)

One student wrote, "The surprising part is when I gave this test to my boyfriend and he turned out to be an INFJ as well. This is especially shocking when you take into consideration that only 1% of the population are quoted as testing out to be INFJ's. We have been together for 4 years now and I've always been amazed at how alike we are and what a good strong relationship we have maintained." Another wrote, ""The category ENFJ reflex (sic) my personality like a mirror. I can really relate to it. It is exactly me. I am really amazed. I asked my boyfriend to take this test and he is a ISTJ which is very opposite of what I am. The funny thing about that is we are so diverse but yet we get along so well. I think this test can really help people to understand and be more aware of themselves and others."

The students develop an esprit de corps, of patriotism toward their type, of being part of a favored minority, and also an understanding and tolerance for those of other types.

Next, we make use of the fact that art, like dreams, is a royal road to the unconscious.

We all have definite resistance to allowing the unconscious to enter consciousness. One of Freud's legacies is the unfortunate concept of the unconscious as being a dangerous and unpleasant place. After all, Freud dealt with neurotics and hysterical people, and was searching through the unconscious for painful and repressed memories.

Jung put this in perspective later by showing that for the vast majority of us the unconscious or shadow side was the road to emotional growth, not only interesting but rewarding to explore. Even more important, in our experience, what people put into their artwork they are usually willing, even eager, to talk about. We have never found anyone who got into trouble from showing his artwork, and talking about it. On the contrary, we have seen many, many people who, after talking about their artwork, were able to find solutions and paths for themselves.

We think it is important that, for students to be open and spontaneous, the teacher must:

- handle these drawings with sensitivity, caring, admiration, and respect
- reassure the students that they need not share with anyone else what they have drawn or written, and invite the student to share their thoughts and feelings about their drawings,
- and must not themselves interpret any of these drawings.

The teacher should also be aware that critiquing or grading the artwork at this stage is an almost certain way to close the channel of communication that the artwork offers, and cancels the opportunity for using the artwork for personal development. While the student might benefit in terms of artistic expertise, we believe that this type of education should follow, not precede, the student's appreciation of the opportunity that art gives for self expression and growth.

Following are some of the art exercises we use, and the implications for the students.

Exercise 3: Projection drawing

Instructions: "After creating random lines on a sheet of paper, using string dipped in ink, or feeling textures with closed eyes, look at what you have drawn from all sides until you see an image of some object or person. If no image is forthcoming, put color down intuitively until an image appears. Using colors, bring out that image. Write a short fantasy about what you have drawn; if you wish, you can start with 'Once upon a time...'

"…Does what you have drawn and written have significance for you personally?"

Comment: It is probably difficult for someone who has not actually done this exercise to realize the impact it has upon the sophisticated as well as naive artist. To suddenly really understand that art is a projection of oneself upon paper, a projection that we can look at, examine, and own for ourselves, can be an emotionally exhilarating insight, a firm basis for further personal understanding and growth. Sometimes the experience is met with denial, but this attitude generally changes when many students share their metaphoric drawings, freely.

As we said, some of Jung's ideas are very important to the artist, especially his conception of the unconscious as an interesting and friendly place. Whereas Freud's emphasis was on treatment for mental illness, Jung's emphasis was on self-exploration for the sake of growth. But also we believe, not only in individuality, but in the collective unconscious, and in the concept that great works of art are great because the artist was able to delve into himself deeply enough to come up with universal concepts, that speak truth to everyone. We believe that artists who, despite talent and competence, are unable to delve deeply into their own unconscious will not create significant work.

One metaphor for the collective unconscious is that we all have our own private deep pools, but that underneath they are all connected to the same deep water layer. The deeper we can go fishing, the more likely our catch is to have universal significance. We have adapted the following imagery from Joseph Shorr.

Exercise 4: Fishing in a deep pool (Guided imagery)

Instructions: "On wandering in a meadow on a pleasant day, you come to a *deep* pool. Throw in a line with a hook on the end. After a while, pull up the line. What is on the end of the line? Draw it. Finally, as the object you have drawn, finish the following sentences:

- I feel—–
- The adjective which best describes me is—–
- I wish—–
- I must—–
- I secretly—–
- I need—–
- I will—–
- Never refer to me as—– "

And then ask, "Does that have significance for you personally?"

423

We look at the drawing as a metaphoric image describing what we may be focusing on in our lives at the moment.

We introduce Gestalt psychology concepts when we emphasize how many parts of us there are (some of which we are more aware of than others, some of which we like more than others), and how difficult it is to acknowledge and integrate these separate parts.

Exercise 5: Two Fantasy Animals

Instructions: "Draw two separate fantasy animals on one sheet of paper. After both animals are created, write 3 adjectives about each animal that describe how they look to you. Then write a short conversation between these animals about some current concern of yours."

Comment: Almost always, these two animals represent polarities, different "parts" of the artist. Also, almost always one of these animals is critical of the other. By sharing their two animals, looking at the significance of their positions and body parts (are they facing each other, do they have mouths to communicate, ears to listen, etc.), the students begin to acknowledge their different parts, rather than needing to be like one and not the other, and they begin to accept themselves for who they are. The short dialogue then allows the student to begin integrating the two parts.

This exercise can be repeated many times, and different animals and different parts of the student can be brought out each time. Indeed, multiple animals can be created, each a different part, and the student can then have a chance to change initial self-criticism to self-acceptance.

We believe deeply in the humanistic theories of Abraham Maslow and Carl Rogers and about the importance of each individual. We quote to students what Rogers says about how difficult it is to allow oneself to understand another person. We emphasize active listening and model this, and have them practice it with us and with each other. We also emphasize the importance of non-verbal communication. One way we illustrate this is to have people draw together on the same piece of paper.

Exercise 6: Drawing Together

In pairs, students draw together without talking on the same sheet of paper. Art materials are provided, but no other explanation is given; students must choose for themselves nonverbally, individually, how they are to deal with this assignment. The students are instructed only to be aware of their feelings as they share the space.

Comment: Art mirrors the way you are in real life with people. Who went first? Who followed? Did you interact, or did you stay on your side of the paper? If the other person came onto your side, how did you feel? Change partners and try it again. Is this your nonverbal style? By learning what your style is, you are in a better position to alter it if you wish.

We have them create their own tissue paper family.

Exercise 7: Tissue Paper Family

Directions:"Using torn pieces of colored tissue paper and starch or glue, create symbols of your family, selecting a color and shape and position for each member in relation to you."

Comment: This exercise allows students to let you and others know about their family and problems as they see them. It is always informative, sometimes quite revealing, and always breaks down barriers between students. An adaptation to see their ethnological perspective is a picture or collage of how they see the world (the globe).

In addition to communication, a central humanistic issue for us is the way in which students learn to be their own source of reinforcement, as against allowing themselves to be determined by those to whom they assign power over them. In this we get a lot of help in an unlikely place, from the behaviorist, B. F. Skinner. We try to get them in touch with what they individually say are the really basic satisfactions of life for them, and how to choose for themselves the ways of achieving them that make sense to them, instead of giving away to others the power to determine what they do or how they paint.

Exercise 8: Assertiveness

We ask them to show us something they have drawn, and, using our position as teacher and authority, we express some absurd opinion, or some absurd criticism. We announce in advance what we are doing, we make it a game, we do it in very gradual steps, and we ask that they all first reflect what we say, and then say what they think. We all watch supportively as each student struggles with a vain attempt to please us, but finally expresses his own independent opinion. Little by little this sense of needing to please us extinguishes, and eventually they all reach their own sense of artistic integrity. By the end of class, they are all able to say to us, in effect, "I can see that you have strong feelings about this, but this is really is an expression of me." Establishing their own individual reinforcers is now a part of their language and their personal and artistic life.

The Process of Creativity

In addition we describe the attitudes that foster creativity such as aloneness, inactivity, gullibility, remembering and inner replaying of past traumatic conflicts, day dreaming, a strong sense of self, the ability to tolerate ambiguity and, last of all, discipline and alertness.

We also describe what the blocks to creativity may be, including an ill-defined sense of self, low self esteem, fear of criticism, passivity, conformity, comparisons/competition, having a preference for judging ideas rather than generating them and avoidance of the here-and-now.

We tell the students about the 7 different intelligences as proposed by Howard Gardner.

- Linguistic: sensitivity to the meaning and order of words; poet, translator: T. S. Eliot, Alice Walker.

- Logical-mathematical: the ability to handle chains of reasoning and to recognize patterns and order; mathematician, scientist: Einstein, Madame Curie.

- Musical: sensitivity to pitch, melody, rhythm and tone; composer, singer: Leonard Bernstein, Jesse Norman.

- Bodily-kinesthetic: the ability to use the body skillfully and handle objects adroitly; athlete, dancer, surgeon: Martha Graham, Magic Johnson.

- Spatial: the ability to perceive the world accurately and to re-create or transform aspects of that world: sculptor, architect, surveyor: Picasso, Georgia O'Keeffe.

- Interpersonal: the ability to understand people and relationships; politician, salesman, religious leader: Gandhi, Golda Meier.

- Intrapersonal: access to one's emotional life as a means to understand oneself and others; therapist, social worker: Sigmund Freud, Karen Horney.

Gardner goes beyond the theoretical by providing physiological evidence that each of the seven intelligences exists as a discrete entity.

In addition, we introduce them to the concepts of linguist Deborah Tannen regarding the different conversational styles of men and women. Dr. Tannen describes the *hierarchal, competitive language* styles that many men use in communication in contrast to *language for intimacy* attitudes of many women. These communication styles are similar to the ways Jung proposed that *Thinkers and Feelers* behave.

When we understand these many differences among ourselves, and *eliminate the concept of right and wrong ways of being,* we can comprehend and deal with the many cognitive styles and strategies which we all use. It alleviates stress in our interpersonal relationships, giving us more energy for creative problem-solving in all aspects of our lives.

Summary:

Many of the students who fail to graduate, or who turn to self-destructive or antisocial behaviors, do so because they have never learned how to cope with the stresses of life and of school. Adequate coping skills are necessary for success in school and in life, and can be taught through art exercises. Art therapists can have a central role in teaching coping skills because the student population that needs these skills most are most amenable to teaching through the arts.

We believe that many students who are poor in academic studies are of the *intuitive* type. Intuitive people have difficulty with the self-discipline and orderly thinking that are important in succeeding, or even in surviving, in school. It is our strong impression, and those of some other educators that the "problem" student who has difficulty adjusting to the school environment may often be of this type. But art comes naturally to many of these people, giving us a tool by which we can play to the strengths of these students rather than their weaknesses. Art has many dimensions, and if we use the dimension that is experiential and personal, and is for self-expression and for building good behavioral patterns, we can make an end run around resistances they have built up to school. Used in this way, teachers can help students improve self-esteem and coping behavior.

We look forward to the time when art is an integral part of education, and when a course on coping skills and improving feelings of self-worth using art is an integral part of the curriculum at art schools, colleges and high schools in general. If art educators can demonstrate by controlled studies that art-centered coping programs can reduce the student drop-out rate, art education will get the regard from administrators it deserves.

References

Arieti, S. (1976). *Creativity, the magic synthesis.* NY: Basic Books.

Briggs, K. and Myers, I. (1962). *The Myers-Briggs Type Indicator.* Palo Alto, Ca: Consulting Psychologists Press.

Burk, James E., Art Specialist, Office of Secondary Education, Los Angeles Unified School District. Unpublished communication.

Gardner, H. (1983). *Frames of mind.* NY: Basic Books.

Hogan, R. & Champagne, D. *(1980). Personal style inventory.* La Jolla, CA: University Associates.

Holden, C. *(1987). Creativity and the troubled mind.* Psychology Today: 21 (9).

Keirsey, D. and Bates, M.(1978). *Please understand me. Character and Temperament Types.* Del Mar, CA: Prometheus Nemesis.

Maslow, A. *(1968). Toward a psychology of being.* NY: Van Nostrand.

Rogers, C. (1970). *On becoming a person.* Boston: Houghton Mifflin.

Shorr, J.*(1983). Go see the movie in your head.* Santa Barbara, CA: Ross-Erikson.

Skinner, B.F. *(1953). Science and human behavior.* NY: Macmillan Co.

Stephens, W. B. (1972). *Relationship between selected personality characteristics of senior art students and their area of art study.* Unpublished doctoral dissertation, University of Florida.

Tannen, D. *(1990). You just don't understand.* NY: Morrow.

Virshup, B. (1985) *Coping in medical school.* NY: W. W. Norton.

Virshup, E. (1978). *Right brain people in a left brain world.* Los Angeles: Guild of Tutors Press.

In 1992, the city of Los Angeles erupted in violence. In an attempt to help repair the psychological damage, artists hastened to lend their services—to the disadvantaged, the children, the emotionally battered. Many of these artists had little or no therapy training. In an attempt to support their efforts, SCATA, the Southern California Art Therapy Association produced a brochure that the Los Angeles Cultural Affairs Department distributed to these artists, to give them some idea of the power of the tools they were using. A copy of this brochure is reproduced here.

 **SOUTHERN CALIFORNIA ART THERAPY ASSOCIATION**

in association with

The City of Los Angeles Cultural Affairs Department

presents

The Art of Healing Trauma
Media, Techniques, and Insights

by Evelyn Virshup, Ph. D., A.T.R., Shirley Riley, M.A., A.T.R., M.F.C.C. and Dorothy Shepherd, M.A., A.T.R., M.F.C.C.

Artists know how vital art is for self expression when words are inadequate, and that art helps communicate feelings and promotes healing. Art therapists use art therapeutically when working with clients under stress. Members of the Southern California Art Therapy Association hope that by sharing information about some psychological effects of the art process, the artist/teachers' and their student artmakers' experiences will be enhanced.

The art tools we use are a vehicle for the release of powerful emotions. The violence and trauma which are a fact of life for many Americans stimulate these emotions. As you strive to bring positive art experiences to those with whom you share your expertise, emotions associated with traumatic memories may surface and result in unexpected reactions and behavior: such is the power of art. Handled properly, this can relieve stress. Handled badly, it can create more stress.

When you work with *emotionally traumatized artmakers*, consider the following:

☐ Crayons, markers, paint and construction paper can be a magical means to help people express themselves, but you will need to decide how to balance *instruction for a quality product* with the *power and delight of personal expression.* We have learned that in budding artmakers, emotional expression is inhibited by the need to create an aesthetic product. In fact, you may influence the level of emotional expression by where you place your emphasis. If the emotion is too overwhelming, one might emphasize aesthetics. If, however, your aim is to encourage self-expression, *allow the artmaker's work to be whatever it may be.* Set aside for now your desire for an aesthetic product, and contain your need to teach them "how it should be done."

☐ *Do not critique—admire and encourage!* Your artmakers need support. *They have enough internal critics already.* Just by providing structure and opportunity, you allow the "built-in" therapeutic quality of artmaking to emerge.

☐ If the art experience is negative or stressful, encourage building on it. Suggest, "Draw what you would do if you were in charge," or "Draw your solution to the problem." Be prepared for repetition of the same theme. *It takes time to recover from trauma.*

☐ *Do not interpret.* Ask for, listen to, and accept the artmaker's story about the art product, and interpretation of the significance of the colors used. Artwork is an accurate reflection of our inner worlds. *When we interpret others' work, we frequently project our own inner worlds and confuse the artmaker.*

☐ *Create a support group* of fellow artist-volunteers to talk or make art about your experiences.

429

Different Art Media have Different Psychological Effects.

Advantages	Disadvantages
Pencils: Are familiar, allow for control, corrections, are available, give comfort and provide structure in chaotic situations. Can provide initial structure to contain "out of control" emotional expression.	Connote schoolwork, evaluation, criticism. Restrict expression. Encourage indecision, frequent erasing, changing. Lack color, inhibiting the expression of feeling.
Color pencils: Same as above. Color may help accessing feelings. Consider color pencils which can be softened by brushing with water.	Controlled. Hard to make strong statements.
Precut photo collage material: Easily controlled, instantly gratifying, requires no "talent," stimulates imagination by finding images, words and unusual juxtapositions.	Glue may replace collage as focus. If collage is not pre-cut, the artmaker may be distracted in the search for images.
Felt pens: Familiar, easily available. Color moves more freely. Can cover other media, can hide or provide structure and control amount of emotional material expressed. Can balance expressiveness with a certain amount of control.	Dry out when not cared for, and frustrate the artmaker.
Oil pastels/ Craypas: Provide a wider range of color. Move more easily, can be liberating. Have novelty, inviting exploration and expression, new possibilities for problem solving. Blend easily, can cover other colors as one can cover over a layer of feeling. Invite creativity, the user still in charge.	An unfamiliar and slightly messy medium may remind artmaker of early prohibitions agains getting dirty
Plasticene (oil-based clay): 3-D expression with fewer inhibitions regarding product perfection. Can provide opportunity to role-play with sculpted figures. Reusable, relatively clean and colorful. 3-D products can be dismantled and reconstructed at will to fill the needs of the artmaker.	Creates frustration and anger unless help is available to correct mechanical problems, such as creating armatures of tooth picks or coffee stirrers. May access strong feelings unexpectedly.
Soft pastels/Chalk: User has even more freedom with color blending. Invites spontaneous expression.	Greater freedom creates frustration because of inability to delineate forms clearly. Can foster "out of control" feelings, and reactivate more memories of early prohibitions against "getting dirty." May create strong need for assistance to turn "failure" into satisfactory experience.
Water-based paints: Can be liberating, inviting open and colorful expression, working and reworking, dramatic presentation of issues important to artmaker. Can be enhanced with more controlled media (pencils, felt-tipped pens) which provide progressive exploration of emotional content.	Can make artmaker frustrated and angry because media is difficult to control, inhibiting expression of intended content. Colors can dissolve into mud. May require close supervision. (*We suggest telling the artmaker to let the paint dry, and rework with more controlled media to create structure, thereby possibly alleviating a sense of failure.*)
Wet clay (water-based clay): Selectively offered to people when it would be advantageous to give up some control. Finished products can be fired and glazed, evoking feeling of accomplishment. Provides a highly plastic media as a positive alternative to other media. For many novices, clay evokes fewer negative messages about not having "talent."	Can easily become formless without adequate instruction. Can be extremely messy, causing severe anxiety about cleanliness and performance. Can have negative results when "out of control" feelings parallel "out of control" media.

More control ↑

Less control ↓

To increase your understanding of some psychological aspects of the art process, we suggest you note, *but do not comment on,* the following:

☐ The size of the image in relation to the size of the paper may reflect the level of self esteem. What does the artmaker say about the placement on the page?

☐ What media did the artmaker choose? The tools chosen may reflect the level of openness and freedom to express feelings. Was the person comfortable with his/her choice of tools?

☐ Rapidity of execution, inability to stay focused, and/or a low frustration level may indicate anxiety. Determine if more or less structure is needed.

☐ Lack of color may mean suppression of feelings. Does this "interpretation" concur with your observations?

☐ Excessive dependency on your expertise may reflect an unwillingness to explore or take risks. How can you nurture and at the same time encourage exploration effectively?

☐ Anxiety evoked by imagery and performance may be your clue to explore feelings verbally. Encouraging story-telling and use of metaphor may release feelings in a safe environment and alleviate anxiety.

☐ Unwillingness to share thoughts about artwork may mean the artmaker doesn't feel "safe." In addition, many people have strong internal prohibitions about revealing family "secrets" and circumstances.

As we said earlier, we strongly recommend that you refrain from interpreting the products, the symbols and the behaviors of the artmakers in process. Accept that just the "doing" will reduce some of stress they are experiencing, as will your acceptance and admiration.

We also recommend empathic listening: reflect their thoughts, accept their feelings, admire their efforts. Avoid denying feelings ("you shouldn't feel that way,")— or advice-giving. By allowing them to problem-solve themselves (with your support) you can help your student artmakers feel that *their art is seen and their voices heard.*

If you are interested in exploring for yourself the use of media from an art therapy point of view, members of SCATA are available for workshops and consultations. For further information, please write, phone or FAX:

Southern California Art Therapy Association*

Box 4455
Sunland, CA 91041-4455
Phone (213) 343-4010
FAX (818) 225-7001

*SCATA 1992 BOARD: Evelyn Virshup, *Pres.*, Elda Unger, *Pres.-Elect,* Thelma Kornreich, *Treasurer,* Dorothy Shepherd, *Corres. Sec,* Deborah Mosbrooker, *Membership,* Patti Wallace, *Nat. Delegate,* Joan Landon, *Program Chair.*